D0407459

CONFLICT OF INTEREST
IN MEDICAL RESEARCH, EDUCATION, AND PRACTICE

Bernard Lo and Marilyn J. Field, *Editors*

Committee on Conflict of Interest in
Medical Research, Education, and Practice

Board on Health Sciences Policy

INSTITUTE OF MEDICINE
OF THE NATIONAL ACADEMIES

THE NATIONAL ACADEMIES PRESS
Washington, D.C.
www.nap.edu

THE NATIONAL ACADEMIES PRESS 500 Fifth Street, N.W. Washington, DC 20001

NOTICE: The project that is the subject of this report was approved by the Governing Board of the National Research Council, whose members are drawn from the councils of the National Academy of Sciences, the National Academy of Engineering, and the Institute of Medicine. The members of the committee responsible for the report were chosen for their special competences and with regard for appropriate balance.

This study was supported by Contract No. N01-OD-4-2139, TO # 201 of the National Institutes of Health, Contract No. 63229 of the Robert Wood Johnson Foundation, The Greenwall Foundation, the ABIM Foundation, Contract No. S07-2 of the Josiah Macy Jr. Foundation, Contract No. 1007182 of the Burroughs Wellcome Fund, and also the endowment fund of the Institute of Medicine, all contracts between the National Academies. Any opinions, findings, conclusions, or recommendations expressed in this publication are those of the authors and do not necessarily reflect the view of the organizations or agencies that provided support for the project.

Library of Congress Cataloging-in-Publication Data

Conflict of interest in medical research, education, and practice / Bernard Lo and Marilyn J. Field, editors ; Committee on Conflict of Interest in Medical Research, Education, and Practice, Board on Health Sciences Policy.
p. ; cm.
Includes bibliographical references and index.
ISBN 978-0-309-13188-9 (hardcover)
1. Business and medicine. 2. Conflict of interests. I. Lo, Bernard. II. Field, Marilyn J. (Marilyn Jane) III. Institute of Medicine (U.S.). Committee on Conflict of Interest in Medical Research, Education, and Practice. IV. National Academies Press (U.S.)
[DNLM: 1. Conflict of Interest. 2. Biomedical Research—ethics. 3. Education, Medical—ethics. 4. Ethics, Clinical. W 50 C748 2009]
RA394.C665 2009
174.2—dc22
2009020634

Additional copies of this report are available from the National Academies Press, 500 Fifth Street, N.W., Lockbox 285, Washington, DC 20055; (800) 624-6242 or (202) 334-3313 (in the Washington metropolitan area); Internet, http://www.nap.edu.

For more information about the Institute of Medicine, visit the IOM home page at: **www.iom.edu.**

Printed in the United States of America

The serpent has been a symbol of long life, healing, and knowledge among almost all cultures and religions since the beginning of recorded history. The serpent adopted as a logotype by the Institute of Medicine is a relief carving from ancient Greece, now held by the Staatliche Museen in Berlin.

Suggested citation: IOM (Institute of Medicine). 2009. *Conflict of Interest in Medical Research, Education, and Practice*. Washington, DC: The National Academies Press.

"Knowing is not enough; we must apply.
Willing is not enough; we must do."
—Goethe

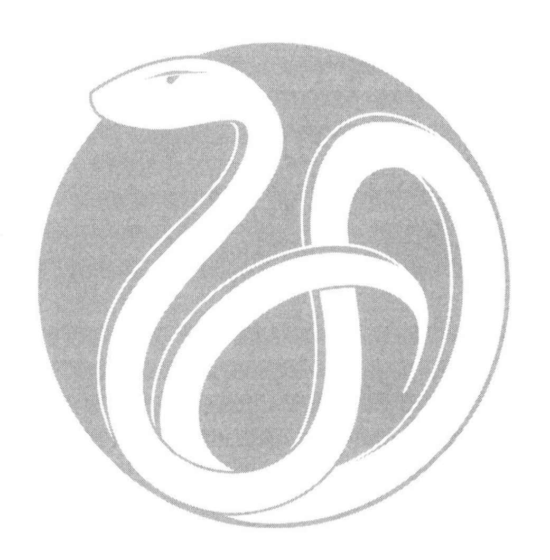

INSTITUTE OF MEDICINE
OF THE NATIONAL ACADEMIES

Advising the Nation. Improving Health.

THE NATIONAL ACADEMIES

Advisers to the Nation on Science, Engineering, and Medicine

The **National Academy of Sciences** is a private, nonprofit, self-perpetuating society of distinguished scholars engaged in scientific and engineering research, dedicated to the furtherance of science and technology and to their use for the general welfare. Upon the authority of the charter granted to it by the Congress in 1863, the Academy has a mandate that requires it to advise the federal government on scientific and technical matters. Dr. Ralph J. Cicerone is president of the National Academy of Sciences.

The **National Academy of Engineering** was established in 1964, under the charter of the National Academy of Sciences, as a parallel organization of outstanding engineers. It is autonomous in its administration and in the selection of its members, sharing with the National Academy of Sciences the responsibility for advising the federal government. The National Academy of Engineering also sponsors engineering programs aimed at meeting national needs, encourages education and research, and recognizes the superior achievements of engineers. Dr. Charles M. Vest is president of the National Academy of Engineering.

The **Institute of Medicine** was established in 1970 by the National Academy of Sciences to secure the services of eminent members of appropriate professions in the examination of policy matters pertaining to the health of the public. The Institute acts under the responsibility given to the National Academy of Sciences by its congressional charter to be an adviser to the federal government and, upon its own initiative, to identify issues of medical care, research, and education. Dr. Harvey V. Fineberg is president of the Institute of Medicine.

The **National Research Council** was organized by the National Academy of Sciences in 1916 to associate the broad community of science and technology with the Academy's purposes of furthering knowledge and advising the federal government. Functioning in accordance with general policies determined by the Academy, the Council has become the principal operating agency of both the National Academy of Sciences and the National Academy of Engineering in providing services to the government, the public, and the scientific and engineering communities. The Council is administered jointly by both Academies and the Institute of Medicine. Dr. Ralph J. Cicerone and Dr. Charles M. Vest are chair and vice chair, respectively, of the National Research Council.

www.national-academies.org

COMMITTEE ON CONFLICT OF INTEREST IN MEDICAL RESEARCH, EDUCATION, AND PRACTICE

BERNARD LO (*Chair*), Professor of Medicine and Director, Program in Medical Ethics, University of California, San Francisco

WENDY BALDWIN, Director, Poverty, Gender and Youth Program, Population Council

LISA BELLINI, Associate Dean for Graduate Medical Education and Associate Professor of Medicine, University of Pennsylvania

LISA A. BERO, Professor, Department of Clinical Pharmacy and Institute for Health Policy Studies, University of California, San Francisco

ERIC G. CAMPBELL, Associate Professor, Institute for Health Policy and Department of Medicine, Massachusetts General Hospital and Harvard Medical School

JAMES F. CHILDRESS, Hollingsworth Professor of Ethics, Department of Religious Studies and Professor of Medical Education and Director, Institute for Practical Ethics, University of Virginia

PETER B. CORR, General Partner, Celtic Therapeutics Management Company, L.L.P.

TODD DORMAN, Associate Dean and Director, Continuing Medical Education, and Professor of Anesthesiology, Johns Hopkins Medical Center

DEBORAH GRADY, Professor of Medicine and Director, Women's Health Clinical Research Center and Associate Dean for Translational Research, University of California, San Francisco

TIMOTHY S. JOST, Robert L. Willett Family Professor of Law, Washington and Lee University School of Law

ROBERT P. KELCH, Executive Vice President for Medical Affairs, University of Michigan and Chief Executive Officer, University of Michigan Health System

ROBERT M. KRUGHOFF, President, Consumer CHECKBOOK/Center for the Study of Services

GEORGE LOEWENSTEIN, Herbert A. Simon Professor of Economics and Psychology, Department of Social and Decision Sciences, Carnegie Mellon University

JOEL PERLMUTTER, Elliot Stein Family Professor of Neurology and Professor of Radiology and Physical Therapy, Washington University School of Medicine in St. Louis

NEIL R. POWE, Professor of Medicine, Epidemiology, and Health Policy and Management and Director, Welch Center for Prevention, Epidemiology, and Clinical Research, Johns Hopkins School of Medicine and Bloomberg School of Public Health

DENNIS F. THOMPSON, Alfred North Whitehead Professor of Political Philosophy, Department of Government and Professor of Public Policy, John F. Kennedy School of Government, Harvard University

DAVID A. WILLIAMS, Chief of the Division of Hematology/Oncology, Director, Clinical and Translational Research, Children's Hospital Boston and Leland Fikes Professor of Pediatrics, Harvard Medical School

Committee Consultants and Background Paper Authors

JASON D. DANA, Assistant Professor, Department of Psychology, University of Pennsylvania

MICHAEL DAVIS, Senior Fellow, Center for Study of Ethics in the Professions and Professor of Philosophy, Humanities Department, Illinois Institute of Technology

JOSEPHINE JOHNSTON, Research Associate, Hastings Center, Garrison, New York

IOM Staff

MARILYN J. FIELD, Senior Program Officer
FRANKLIN BRANCH, Research Associate
ROBIN E. PARSELL, Senior Program Assistant (from January 2008)
AFRAH ALI, Senior Program Assistant (until November 2007)
ANDREW POPE, Director, Board on Health Sciences Policy

Acknowledgments

In preparing this report, the committee and project staff benefited greatly from the assistance and expertise of many individuals and groups. Important information and insights came from four public meetings that the committee organized to collect information and perspectives from a range of academic, professional, consumer, patient, and other organizations and individuals. A number of speakers at these meetings also shared their knowledge at other times during the course of the study. Appendix A includes the agendas of the public meetings and a list of organizations that submitted written statements of views.

The committee appreciates the contributions of the authors of the background papers that appear as Appendix C (Michael Davis at Illinois Institute of Technology and Josephine Johnston at the Hastings Center) and Appendix D (Jason Dana at University of Pennsylvania). Our project officer at the National Institutes of Health, Walter Schaffer, was always helpful in getting our questions answered. We also called on Daniel Wolfson at the American Board of Internal Medicine Foundation for information. In addition, Ariel Winter of the Medicare Payment Advisory Commission helped by answering questions about the commission's work. Mary Nix at the Agency for Healthcare Research and Quality provided data from the National Guidelines Clearinghouse that we could not obtain online. An undoubtedly incomplete list of others who assisted the committee's work includes David Atkins, James Bernat, Carol Blum, David Blumenthal, Deborah Briggs, Laura Brockway-Lunardi, Robert Campbell, Roger Chou, Vivian Coates, Allan Coukel, Bette Crigger, Susan Ehringhaus, Brian Eigel,

Susan Gilbert, Marianne Hockema, Cato Laurencin, Jeffrey Leiden, Martha Liggett, Kathleen Lohr, Peter Lurie, Charlene May, Jennifer Padberg, James Severson, Mark Sommerfeld, Gabriel Sullivan, and Myrl Weinberg.

The committee and project staff also appreciate the work of copy editor Michael Hayes. Within the National Academies, we particularly acknowledge the assistance of Clyde Behney, Judy Estep, Robert Giffin, Janice Mehler, Abbey Meltzer, Amy Packman, Donna Randall, Bronwyn Schrecker, and Jackie Turner.

Reviewers

This report has been reviewed in draft form by individuals chosen for their diverse perspectives and technical expertise, in accordance with procedures approved by the National Research Council's Report Review Committee. The purpose of this independent review is to provide candid and critical comments that will assist the institution in making its published reports as sound as possible and to ensure that the report meets institutional standards for objectivity, evidence, and responsiveness to the study charge. The review comments and draft manuscript remain confidential to protect the integrity of the deliberative process. We wish to thank the following individuals for their review of this report:

Claudia R. Adkison, Emory University School of Medicine
Robert Baron, University of California, San Francisco School of Medicine
Paul Citron, Medtronic, Inc. (Retired)
F. Sessions Cole, Washington University School of Medicine
Peter Densen, University of Iowa Carver College of Medicine
Thomas J. Fogarty, Fogarty Engineering
Leo T. Furcht, University of Minnesota
Linda Golodner, National Consumers League
Henry T. Greely, Stanford University Law School
Allen S. Lichter, American Society of Clinical Oncology
Joseph Loscalzo, Brigham and Women's Hospital
Alan Nelson, American College of Physicians Foundation

Philip A. Pizzo, Stanford University School of Medicine
Richard Schilsky, University of Chicago Medical Center
Larry J. Shapiro, Washington University in St. Louis School of Medicine
Harold Sox, Annals of Internal Medicine and American College of Physicians
Jeremy Sugarman, Johns Hopkins Medical Institutions
P. Roy Vagelos, Merck & Co., Inc. (Retired)

Although the reviewers listed above have provided many constructive comments and suggestions, they were not asked to endorse the conclusions or recommendations, nor did they see the final draft of the report before its release. The review of this report was overseen by **David Challoner,** University of Florida, and **Judith L. Swain,** National University of Singapore and University of California, San Diego. Appointed by the National Research Council and the Institute of Medicine, these individuals were responsible for making certain that an independent examination of this report was carried out in accordance with the institutional procedures and that all review comments were carefully considered. Responsibility for the final content of this report rests entirely with the authoring committee and the institution.

Preface

Hardly a week goes by without a news story about conflicts of interest in medicine. While this committee met, colleagues and friends sent me many news reports and journal articles on the topic. These reports—even if one expects that initial news reports may not always have the stories quite straight—served as continual reminders that conflicts of interest create deep concerns about the integrity of medicine and medical research and raise questions about the trustworthiness of physicians, researchers, and medical institutions.

As I look back over our deliberations, several themes stand out. First, as with all Institute of Medicine (IOM) reports, the committee was charged with making recommendations that were based on evidence and convincing reasons. Although the committee members were aware of powerful anecdotes and had personal beliefs about the issues, we repeatedly asked whether the evidence supported our conclusions and recommendations. If it did not, we developed a reasoned case on the basis of the committee's experience and the judgment of the committee members about the arguments for the use of different approaches presented in the literature or in statements submitted to the committee. Second, it is a challenge to craft policy recommendations that strike the right balance between addressing egregious cases and creating burdens that stifle relationships that advance the goals of professionalism and generate knowledge to benefit society. The committee tried to consider the possibility that well-intentioned policies may have unintended adverse consequences. Third, regulation alone may have limited effectiveness in the absence of a culture of professionalism and other incentives that are aligned to promote professional behavior. The committee considered how a variety of organizations—including those that accredit health care institutions and license health care professionals, publish the findings of medical research, use practice guidelines, and pay for medical care—can buttress the conflict of interest policies implemented by institutions that carry out medical research, provide education and patient care, and develop practice guidelines.

This report cannot and did not attempt to resolve all issues related to conflicts of interest in medicine. In view of our expansive charge, we tried to address central questions rather than the many details of this complex topic. For example, we focus on conflicts that involve financial interests because they are at the heart of concerns and debates about conflicts of interest. Furthermore, because relationships with pharmaceutical, medical device, and biotechnology companies have created the greatest concern and were central in the discussions that led the IOM to pursue this study, we focused on those relationships. The committee expects that many of the recommendations and analyses in our report will also apply more generally to professional and institutional relationships with other commercial entities, such as insurers and vendors of nonmedical products.

The committee could not resolve some important issues like harmonizing the different requirements for the disclosure of financial relationships because they would require much more time and additional expertise. Instead, to standardize aspects of disclosure policies and procedures, the committee recommended a focused consensus development process that would involve multiple stakeholders on the issue.

Our committee was diverse, involving members with different professional backgrounds and areas of expertise. These different perspectives led to spirited discussions and debates. Each of us listened to points of view and information that we had not previously considered. We tried to listen to and understand other viewpoints and be open to new perspectives, even if in the end we did not agree on all issues. Appendix F describes the different views on one issue, a proposal by some committee members for broader requirements for public disclosure. In general, the committee hoped that by explaining our reasoning on difficult issues our audiences would better appreciate the multiple considerations that a sound conflict of interest policy should address.

As chair, I want to personally thank the committee members for their hard work and their willingness to engage on difficult topics. I am deeply grateful to them for the time and effort that they took from their busy schedules to devote to this project. This report is truly a collaborative effort and is much the better, I think, for the back-and-forth discussions. I also want to personally thank our IOM staff for their tremendous efforts in making this report possible. Robin Parsell skillfully handled meeting and other logistics, and Franklin Branch provided research assistance in many areas. Marilyn Field was unstinting in her background research, drafting and revising of the manuscript, and high standards for our work. And I want to thank Lindsay Parham, my research assistant at the University of California at San Francisco, for her expert help with background research.

Bernard Lo, M.D., *Chair*
Committee on Conflict of Interest in
Medical Research, Education, and Practice

Contents

Boxes, Figures, and Tables

BOXES

FIGURES

TABLES

Summary

ABSTRACT

Patients and the public benefit when physicians and researchers collaborate with pharmaceutical, medical device, and biotechnology companies to develop products that benefit individual and public health. At the same time, concerns are growing that wide-ranging financial ties to industry may unduly influence professional judgments involving the primary interests and goals of medicine. Such conflicts of interest threaten the integrity of scientific investigations, the objectivity of professional education, the quality of patient care, and the public's trust in medicine.

This Institute of Medicine report examines conflicts of interest in medical research, education, and practice and in the development of clinical practice guidelines. It reviews the available evidence on the extent of industry relationships with physicians and researchers and their consequences, and it describes current policies intended to identify, limit, or manage conflicts of interest. Although this report builds on the analyses and recommendations of other groups, it differs from other reports in its focus on conflicts of interest across the spectrum of medicine and its identification of overarching principles for assessing both conflicts of interest and conflict of interest policies. The report, which offers 16 specific recommendations, has several broad messages.

- *The central goal of conflict of interest policies in medicine is to protect the integrity of professional judgment and to preserve public trust rather than to try to remediate bias or mistrust after it occurs.*
- *The disclosure of individual and institutional financial relationships*

is a critical but limited first step in the process of identifying and responding to conflicts of interest.

- *Conflict of interest policies and procedures can be strengthened by engaging physicians, researchers, and medical institutions in developing policies and consensus standards.*
- *A range of supporting organizations—including accrediting groups and public and private health insurers—can promote the adoption and implementation of conflict of interest policies and promote a culture of accountability that sustains professional norms and public confidence in medicine.*
- *Research on conflicts of interest and conflict of interest policies can provide a stronger evidence base for policy design and implementation.*
- *If medical institutions do not act voluntarily to strengthen their conflict of interest policies and procedures, the pressure for external regulation is likely to increase.*

Physicians and researchers must exercise judgment in complex situations that are fraught with uncertainty. Colleagues, patients, students, and the public need to trust that these judgments are not compromised by physicians' or researchers' financial ties to pharmaceutical, medical device, and biotechnology companies. Ties with industry are common in medicine. Some have produced important benefits, particularly through research collaborations that improve individual and public health. At the same time, widespread relationships with industry have created significant risks that individual and institutional financial interests may unduly influence professionals' judgments about the primary interests or goals of medicine. Such conflicts of interest threaten the integrity of scientific investigations, the objectivity of medical education, and the quality of patient care. They may also jeopardize public trust in medicine.

Surveys show the breadth and diversity of relationships between industry and physicians, researchers, and educators in academic and community settings. For example,

- gifts from drug companies to physicians are ubiquitous;
- visits to physicians' offices by drug and medical device company representatives and the provision of drug samples are widespread;
- many faculty members receive research support from industry, and industry funds the majority of biomedical research in the United States;
- many faculty members and community physicians provide scientific, marketing, and other consulting services to companies; and some serve on company boards of directors or on industry speakers bureaus; and
- commercial sources provide about half of the total funding for accredited continuing medical education programs.

Although certain of these financial relationships may be constructive, recent news reports, legal settlements, research studies, and institutional announcements have documented a variety of disturbing situations that could undermine public confidence in medicine. These situations include

- physicians and researchers failing to disclose substantial payments from drug companies, as required by universities, government agencies, or medical journals;
- settlements with the U.S. Department of Justice by medical device and pharmaceutical companies to avoid prosecution for alleged illegal payments or gifts to physicians;
- companies and academic investigators not publishing negative results from industry-sponsored clinical trials or delaying publication for over a year after the completion of a trial;
- academic researchers putting their names on manuscripts, even though they first became involved after the data were collected and analyzed and after the first drafts were written by individuals paid by industry; and
- professional societies and other groups that develop clinical practice guidelines choosing not to disclose their industry funding and not to reveal the conflicts of interest of the experts who draft the guidelines.

Although the causes of these situations are various and their extent is unclear, they highlight the tension that may exist between financial relationships with industry and the primary missions of medical research, education, and practice. In addition to these examples, research on industry gifts and other financial relationships has generated troublesome findings. For example, systematic reviews of the evidence sponsored by a pharmaceutical company are more likely than other reviews to present conclusions favorable to the company, even when the actual findings of the analysis are not favorable. In addition, articles based on company-sponsored clinical trials are more likely to draw conclusions favorable to the company's product than articles trials not sponsored by industry. Although these findings do not necessarily show that the research is biased and other explanations can be offered (e.g., companies do not fund trials unless they see a reasonable likelihood of success), they do raise legitimate questions about possible undue influence.

To cite another example, the availability of drug samples may be associated with the prescription of new brand name drugs when they are not recommended by evidence-based practice guidelines or when appropriate but less expensive drugs or generic equivalents are available for the same indication. Although one argument for the use of drug samples is that they help low-income patients, research suggests that these individuals are not the primary recipients of such samples. Also, although small gifts to physicians may seem to be inconsequential, some research suggests that small gifts can contribute to unconscious bias in decision making and advice giving. It also seems unlikely that companies would give such gifts to physicians if they did not believe that they would benefit the company in some way.

In addition to information that raises concern about the scope and consequences of industry financial ties in medicine, surveys and other studies have reported inconsistencies in the adoption and implementation of conflict of interest policies by medical institutions. Relationships and practices that are forbidden by one institution may be allowed and even encouraged by others. Reports also have described shortcomings in the oversight of conflicts of interest in research by federal agencies and medical institutions.

Unfortunately, the empirical evidence relevant to financial relationships and conflicts of interest is limited. On many topics related to conflicts of interest, no systematic studies are available. For other topics, data are suggestive rather than definitive. The studies that have been conducted have primarily been observational rather than interventional, in large part because the issues cannot be investigated using randomized controlled trials of the effects of different kinds of relationships or different approaches to identifying and managing conflicts of interest. A number of academic medical centers, professional associations, and other institutions have taken steps to strengthen their conflict of interest policies, but few data that can be used to assess the consequences—positive or negative—of these changes are available. Some prominent physicians and researchers have argued that concerns about conflicts of interest are far out of proportion to the evidence that they exist or are harmful, and some contend that measures designed to address conflicts of interest have interfered with beneficial collaborations with industry. Critics of conflict of interest policies have also charged that the great majority of individuals who have not acted in an unethical manner may be subjected to onerous regulations and tacit conclusions that they are culpable of misconduct until proven otherwise.

Responding to the situations and concerns outlined above, the Institute of Medicine appointed a committee to investigate and develop a consensus report on conflicts of interest in medical research, education, and practice and in the development of clinical practice guidelines. Consistent with its charge, the committee

- examined conflicts of interest in medical research, education, and practice and in the development of clinical practice guidelines and
- developed analyses and recommendations to inform the design and implementation of policies that identify and manage conflicts of interest in these contexts without damaging constructive collaborations with industry.

Because the evidence on many issues is limited, the committee had to rely on its experience and judgment in evaluating the analyses and arguments presented in the literature and in statements submitted to the committee. During its work, the committee kept in mind the core goals of medical research, education, and practice and practice guideline development, which include serving the best interests of patients and society through the generation of valid scientific knowledge, the independent evaluation of evidence and the application of critical thinking, and the creation and use of evidence-based recommendations for patient care.

Reflecting concerns that were raised during the planning of the project and the central issues in debates and policies on conflicts of interest in medicine, the committee focused on financial relationships involving pharmaceutical, medical device, and biotechnology companies. Although it did not investigate in depth the conflicts of interest associated with different physician payment arrangements or with physician referral of patients to facilities in which they have an ownership interest, the committee recognized the seriousness of those types of conflicts and the difficulties that policy makers have encountered in trying to eliminate or manage them. It also recognized other sources of conflicts of interest, for example, desires for professional advancement and recognition.

After examining a wide array of evidence, analyses, and perspectives on conflicts of interest, the committee reached several overarching conclusions. They are as follows:

- The goals of conflict of interest policies in medicine are primarily to protect the integrity of professional judgment and to preserve public trust rather than to try to remediate bias or mistrust after they occur.
- The disclosure of individual and institutional financial relationships is a critical but limited first step in the process of identifying and responding to conflicts of interest.
- Conflict of interest policies and procedures can be strengthened by engaging physicians, researchers, and medical institutions in developing conflict of interest policies and consensus standards.
- A range of supporting organizations—public and private—can promote the adoption and implementation of conflict of interest policies and help create a culture of accountability that sustains professional norms and public confidence in professional judgments.
- Research on conflicts of interest and conflict of interest policies can provide a stronger evidence base for policy design and implementation.
- If medical institutions do not act voluntarily to strengthen their conflict of interest policies and procedures, the pressure for external regulation is likely to increase.

PRINCIPLES FOR IDENTIFYING AND ASSESSING CONFLICTS OF INTERESTS

Chapter 2 presents the principles and conceptual framework for identifying and assessing conflicts of interest. Conflicts of interest are defined as *circumstances that create a risk that professional judgments or actions regarding a primary interest will be unduly influenced by a secondary interest.* Primary interests include promoting and protecting the integrity of research, the quality of medical education, and the welfare of patients. Secondary interests include not only financial interests—the focus of this report—but also other interests, such as the pursuit of professional advancement and recognition and the desire to do favors for friends, family, students, or colleagues. Conflict of interest policies typically focus on financial gain because it is relatively more objective, fungible, and quantifiable. Financial gain can therefore be more effectively and fairly regulated than other secondary interests.

The severity of a conflict of interest depends on (1) the likelihood that professional decisions made under the relevant circumstances would be unduly influenced by a secondary interest and (2) the seriousness of the harm or wrong that could result from such an influence. The likelihood of undue influence is affected by the value of the secondary interest, its duration and depth, and the extent of discretion that the individual has in making important decisions.

Conflict of interest policies generally emphasize prevention and management rather than punishment. They do not assume that any particular professional will necessarily let financial gain influence his or her judgment. Likewise, a judgment that someone has a conflict of interest does not imply that the person is unethical. Such judgments assume only that some situations are generally recognized to pose an unacceptable risk that decisions may be unduly influenced by considerations that should be irrelevant. Chapter 2 presents criteria, described in the list that follows, that can be used to evaluate conflict of interest policies.

- Proportionality. Is the policy effective, efficient, and directed at the most important and most common conflicts? Conflict of interest policies and procedures may create harms or burdens as well as benefits. Do the policies and their implementation unnecessarily interfere with the conduct of legitimate research, teaching, and clinical practice?
- Transparency. Is the policy comprehensible and accessible to the individuals and institutions that it may affect? Such transparency is essential to determine if conflict of interest policies are reasonable and are being implemented fairly. Transparency can also help institutions learn

from each other about more and less successful ways of handling particular situations.

- Accountability. Does the conflict of interest policy indicate who is responsible for monitoring, enforcing, and revising it? Leaders of accountable institutions explain institutional policies and monitor and accept responsibility for the consequences, both beneficial and harmful.
- Fairness. Does the policy apply equally to all relevant groups within an institution and in different institutions? In an academic medical center, the relevant groups would include faculty, medical staff, students, residents, fellows, members of institutional committees (e.g., institutional review boards, formulary committees, panels developing practice guidelines, and device purchasing committees), and senior institutional officials.

POLICIES ON CONFLICTS OF INTEREST: OVERVIEW AND EVIDENCE

Concerns about conflicts of interest in medicine have a long history, and responses to these conflicts have evolved as relationships with industry have grown more frequent and more complex and as different responses to such relationships have been tried and found in need of modification. Government regulations and voluntary codes of conduct often follow the discovery of instances of questionable or inappropriate relationships and conduct. Government scrutiny of financial relationships and conflicts of interest may also stimulate private, voluntary efforts by academic and other institutions to deal with problems and avoid regulation.

The conflict of interest policies of academic medical centers, professional societies, medical journals, and other institutions vary on many dimensions. It is not clear that all medical institutions have conflict of interest policies. Those that do have such policies vary in what they ask physicians and researchers to disclose about their financial relationships with industry. Such variations may create additional administrative burdens for physicians and researchers who act in multiple roles and make multiple disclosures of their financial relationships with industry to different institutions for various purposes related to medical research, education, and clinical care and clinical practice guideline development.

Institutions also vary in what relationships they prohibit because they view them as creating unacceptable risks of undue influence on primary interests, and they also differ in how they manage conflicts of interest that are not prohibited. The National Institutes of Health (NIH) has identified variations and deficiencies in how research institutions implement the 1995 U.S. Public Health Service (PHS) regulations on conflict of interest, and it has advised institutions on steps that they can take to strengthen their policies. Similarly, the Association of American Medical Colleges (AAMC) and the Association of American Universities (AAU) have developed recommendations and guidance on conflict of interest policies governing research with human participants, but surveys indicate that research institutions have not fully implemented these recommendations.

Although the disclosure of financial interests or conflicts of interest is a necessary part of conflict of interest policies, it is not sufficient in itself to safeguard the integrity of professional judgment or to maintain public trust. For example, when a relationship or conflict of interest is disclosed to individual patients, students, or research participants, they often lack the knowledge and perspective to assess the relationship and may have no satisfactory options if they have concerns about it. Conflicts that are disclosed but not eliminated or managed can continue to pose risks to judgment and undermine public trust.

The recommendations in Chapter 3 establish the fundamental elements of an effective policy response to conflicts of interest in medical research, education, and practice. Recommendation 3.1 calls on all institutions engaged in these activities to establish conflict of interest policies and create conflict of interest committees to evaluate and manage conflicts. Recommendation 3.2 focuses on the essential policy step of requiring physicians, researchers, and senior officials to disclose to their institutions their financial relationships with industry. Unless institutions are informed of these relationships, they cannot identify conflicts of interest or determine whether additional steps—such as the elimination or management of the conflict—are needed to reduce the risk of bias or a loss of public trust. Recommendations 3.1 and 3.2 are similar to the recommendations made in other reports on conflict of interest; but they extend to all institutions that carry out medical research, medical education, clinical care, and practice guideline development.

The disclosure of financial relationships can be effective only if it provides sufficient information for others to use in assessing a relationship and judging the severity of a conflict. At the same time, disclosure can be burdensome, particularly for physicians who must make multiple disclosures for different activities. Recommendation 3.3 calls for the standardization of disclosures with the goals of providing institutions with the specific information that they need to assess relationships while reducing the reporting burdens on physicians and researchers. Such standardization is best pursued through a consensus development process that involves a broad array of concerned parties (e.g., academic medical centers, professional societies, public interest groups, and NIH and other public agencies). On the basis of the agreements resulting from this process, the next step would be for software developers to produce computer programs that allow an individual to fill out a standard questionnaire and then format the information for different institutions and purposes. This should reduce the burden on individuals and increase the consistency of the information disclosed.

Even with further policy development and standardization, institutions will still face questions about the completeness and accuracy of the information disclosed to them. Recommendation 3.4 calls for the U.S. Congress to create a national program that requires pharmaceutical, medical device, and biotechnology companies and their foundations to publicly report payments to physicians, researchers, health care institutions, professional societies, patient advocacy and disease-specific groups, providers of continuing medical education, and foundations created by any of these entities. Although many details will need to be worked out, the information should be readily available on a secure, searchable public website that allows the identification and aggregation of all payments that an individual or institution receives from all companies. Such a program of company reporting will enhance accountability by allowing universities, journals, and others to verify the disclosures that have been made to them. It may also discourage the formation of questionable relationships that individuals or companies would prefer not be widely known.

CONFLICTS OF INTEREST IN BIOMEDICAL RESEARCH

Research partnerships among industry, academia, and government are essential to the discovery and development of new medications and medical devices that improve the prevention, diagnosis, and treatment of health problems. Chapter 4 reports on evidence that relationships between academic researchers and industry are widespread and are associated with benefits, for example, greater research productivity. At the same time, evidence suggests that these relationships have risks, including decreased openness in the sharing of data and findings and the withholding of negative results. These kinds of risks justify additional requirements and incentives, as recommended in this report, for institutions to adopt and implement policies to identify and eliminate or manage conflicts of interest.

Consistent with the recommendations of AAMC and AAU, Recommendation 4.1 calls for a general rule that researchers may not conduct research involving human participants if they have a financial interest in the outcome of the research, for example, if they hold a patent on an intervention being tested in a clinical trial. Exceptions should be allowed only if an individual's participation is judged to be essential for the safe and appropriate conduct of the research. An example might be the inventor of a complex new implanted medical device who has unique expertise and technical skills that are essential for the safe implantation of the device during pilot or early-phase studies. If a conflict of interest committee approves the involvement of such a researcher, it should take advantage of the full range of options for managing the conflict, including placing restrictions on the researcher's role in the study.

Although Recommendation 4.1 does not cover nonclinical research, financial relationships in this arena may also create risks of undue influence that institutions should assess and manage as appropriate to protect the integrity of the science. Additional studies on financial relationships in nonclinical research, their risks and consequences, and the ways in which institutions identify and respond to these relationships would help establish an evidence base that could be used to guide judgments about policies in this area.

CONFLICTS OF INTEREST IN UNDERGRADUATE, GRADUATE, AND CONTINUING MEDICAL EDUCATION

Chapter 5 presents strong evidence that relationships with industry are pervasive in undergraduate, graduate, and continuing medical education. Most medical students and residents are exposed to lunches, gifts, and other interactions with pharmaceutical company representatives on a frequent basis. Faculty members have extensive relationships with these individuals as well.

In analyzing relationships with industry in the context of medical education, the focus should be on the learning environment, the development of core competencies, and consistency between the formal curriculum and the informal or hidden curriculum. The key goals of medical education include helping learners at all levels develop the ability to think critically and appraise the evidence for clinical decision making. In controlled situations, some interactions with representatives of medical device companies may foster the goals of appropriate training, patient safety, and device evaluation. Otherwise, the committee found no bases for concluding that educational goals are promoted by other relationships involving gifts, most visits by pharmaceutical company representatives, service as a marketing consultant, participation in an industry speakers bureau, or acceptance of credit for a ghostwritten article. Indeed, the evidence suggests that some of these relationships are associated with undue influence and thus undermine the goals of medical education. Overall, the risks of these relationships outweigh any possible benefits.

Recommendation 5.1 therefore calls on academic medical centers to prohibit faculty, students, residents, and fellows from accepting gifts (including meals), making presentations that are controlled by industry, and claiming authorship for ghostwritten publications. This restriction is not intended to exclude the acceptance of scientific materials from industry scientists under appropriate material transfer agreements or the payment of reasonable honoraria to speakers who present their own material. Recommendation 5.1 also calls for restrictions on the acceptance of drug samples and visits by drug and medical device sales representatives.

For academic medical centers and community physicians, drug samples present difficult issues. Caring for indigent patients who cannot afford needed drugs is frustrating for physicians who are trying to act in their patients' best interests. Many physicians believe that drug samples allow some patients access to drugs that they could otherwise not obtain. Nonetheless, research suggests that most samples are not in fact given to patients who lack financial access to needed medications and that physicians who have access to samples may change their prescribing habits, for example, by not prescribing the drugs that they would prefer their patients to use or by prescribing drugs in ways that are not consistent with evidence-based recommendations. The committee concluded that the lack of access to affordable medications is serious and disturbing but that drug samples are not a satisfactory answer to this societal problem. Academic medical centers should, at a minimum, oversee and restrict their use.

Because faculty, students, residents, and fellows may not understand the risks posed by conflicts of interest and the rationale for conflict of interest policies, Recommendation 5.2 calls on academic medical centers and teaching hospitals, as part of their educational mission, to provide education on the avoidance of conflicts of interest and the management of relationships with pharmaceutical and medical device industry representatives. Organizations that accredit medical schools and residency programs should develop standards to reinforce this recommendation.

Questions about conflicts of interest have been particularly visible in continuing medical education. Most physicians are required to participate in accredited continuing medical education as a condition for relicensure, specialty certification, or granting of hospital medical staff privileges. Many commercial and academic providers of accredited continuing medical education receive half or more of their funding from industry, which raises concerns about industry influence over the selection of educational topics, the content of presentations, and the overall scope of educational offerings (e.g., whether they provide sufficient coverage of such issues as prevention and physician-patient communication).

Although individual continuing medical education providers and the accrediting organization for continuing medical education have taken steps to limit industry influence, the dependence of many programs on industry funding raises doubts about how successful these steps can be. Recommendation 5.3 calls for a broad-based consensus development process to propose a new system of funding accredited continuing medical education that is free of industry influence, enhances public trust in the integrity of the system, and provides high-quality education. Some members of the committee supported a total end to industry funding, but others were concerned about the potential for unintended harm from such a ban. The committee recognized that changes in the current system likely would substantially reduce industry funding for accredited continuing medical education. Even if education providers trim their expenses, the costs of accredited continuing medical education would likely increase for many physicians, which could be an economic burden for some physicians, for example, those in rural areas.

CONFLICTS OF INTEREST AND MEDICAL PRACTICE

As is the case in medical research and education, evidence shows that relationships with industry are widespread among physicians in practice. Physician acceptance of gifts and meals from industry representatives is commonplace, as are visits with company sales representatives. Company marketing strategies are sophisticated. As part of these strategies, physicians may be used as marketing agents, physicians' prescribing habits may be tracked through commercial databases, and companies may sponsor so-called seeding trials that are primarily designed to market products to participating physicians. Published studies of these strategies are limited but suggest the risk of undue industry influence on physician prescribing behavior with little or no benefit to patient care. Many physicians may view drug representatives as useful, but reliance on individuals whose charge is to increase sales is not a satisfactory solution to practitioners' need for valid, reliable, and up-to-date medical information.

Several recent policy changes may affect the relationships between industry and physicians in practice. Several drug and device companies are voluntarily making public information on their payments to physicians by physician name and the purpose and the amount of the payment; other companies have been required to do so as part of legal agreements with federal prosecutors. The Pharmaceutical Research and Manufacturers of America also recently revised its code on interactions with health care professionals to prohibit the use of certain marketing tools and gifts (including well-paid speaking engagements) as inducements or rewards for prescribing or recommending a course of treatment. Compliance is voluntary, but the organization says that it will ask member companies to declare whether they have adopted its provisions and will then post the information on its website. The Advanced Medical Technology Association has included similar provisions in its revised code for medical device companies. In addition, some professional societies have recently revised their conflict of interest policies to restrict or manage certain relationships with industry and to make their policies public.

Taking into account the weight of the evidence and the recommendations and actions of other groups or institutions, the committee recommended the elimination of some problematic relationships between practicing physicians and industry. In broad terms, Recommendation 6.1 calls on physicians in clinical practice not to accept gifts, including meals, from companies; to enter only into bona fide consultation arrangements with written contracts; to avoid presenting or publishing material whose content is controlled by industry or is ghostwritten; to set restrictions on meetings with company sales representatives; and to use drug samples only for patients who lack financial access to medications. This recommendation is generally parallel to Recommendation 5.1 (for faculty, students, residents, and fellows). Independent assessment of the evidence and the practice of evidence-based medicine are core competencies for physicians in clinical practice as well as academic practice; relationships with industry should not undermine those competencies.

Because recommendations directed to physicians are more likely to be adopted if other incentives are aligned with those recommendations, Recommendation 6.1 also calls on professional societies and institutions that provide health care (and that employ physicians or grant them staff privileges) to take actions to support physician acceptance of changes in their relationships with companies. Recommendation 6.2 calls for further revisions to industry practices to be consistent with those outlined in Recommendation 6.1. It is a separate recommendation to emphasize that relationships between physicians and industry are bilateral and that the expectations for givers and receivers in financial relationships should be parallel.

CONFLICTS OF INTEREST AND DEVELOPMENT OF CLINICAL PRACTICE GUIDELINES

Financial relationships with companies affected by clinical practice guidelines are common both for groups convening expert panels to develop guidelines and for the individuals serving on those panels. Groups often do not make public their conflict of interest policies, their sources of funding for guideline development, or the financial relationships of the panel members. This lack of transparency makes it difficult for the readers and users of guidelines to assess the potential for undue influence and bias.

The committee found examples of alleged undue industry influence on the development of clinical practice guidelines but little systematic research. The risks that result from the acceptance of industry funding and the inclusion of individuals with industry ties on guideline development panels include possible bias in the recommendations made in guidelines and possible harm to patients because guidelines may influence physician practice behavior, quality improvement measures, reimbursement incentives, and insurance coverage decisions.

Recommendation 7.1 calls on groups that develop guidelines not to accept direct funding for guideline development from industry and generally to exclude individuals with conflicts of interest from guideline development panels. Because it may be impossible in some situations to obtain the needed expertise from individuals who have no conflicts, the recommendation also includes measures to limit the likelihood of undue influence if panels include members with conflicts of interest. These measures include requiring that chairs of guideline development panels have no conflicts of interest, limiting members with conflicts of interest to a small minority of the panel membership, and precluding such members from voting on topics in which they have a financial interest. The committee also calls for groups that develop guidelines to involve the public in attempts to identify experts without conflicts of interest, to make such efforts public, and to disclose publicly any conflicts of interest of those selected for membership on panels.

Recommendation 7.2 calls for organizations that have an interest in the use of evidence-based clinical practice guidelines to establish incentives to encourage the developers of guidelines to adopt the committee's recommendations. For example, the National Guideline Clearinghouse could require that the guidelines that it posts include information about the sources of funding for a guideline, the sponsor's conflict of interest policy, and the financial interests of the expert panel members. Similarly, public and private health plans and accreditation and certification bodies could avoid the use of clinical practice guidelines that lack information that allows users to identify conflicts of interest and assess the risks that they pose.

INSTITUTIONAL CONFLICTS OF INTEREST

Institutional conflicts of interest arise when an institution's own financial interests or the interests of its senior officials pose risks to the integrity of the institution's primary interests and missions. Institutional conflicts typically appear when research conducted within an institution could affect the value of equity that the institution holds in a company or the value of a patent that the institution licenses to a company. Institutional conflicts of interest have not received as much attention as individual conflicts of interest, but their consequences can also be damaging. If they are not properly identified and managed, institutional conflicts can undermine the work and reputation of an entire institution, including employees or members who are themselves strictly avoiding individual conflicts of interest.

Recommendation 8.1 calls for the boards of trustees of institutions to establish a conflict of interest committee to make judgments about institutional relationships with industry, including the relationships of senior officials. In their fiduciary role, members of the board oversee the long-term interests of the institution. They stand at a greater distance from the day-to-day pressures of decision making, which should help them assess more judiciously the potential risks posed by a particular financial interest to the institution's core missions. This committee of the board of trustees could be supported by staff committees on institutional conflict of interest. Recommendation 8.2 calls for NIH to develop regulations requiring institutions covered by the 1995 PHS regulations to adopt institutional conflict of interest policies.

THE ROLE OF SUPPORTING ORGANIZATIONS

In carrying out medical research and education, providing patient care, and developing practice guidelines, physicians, researchers, and the institutions in which they work are part of complex intersecting systems. These systems can amplify or mitigate the pressures that individuals and institutions may experience to expose their primary professional obligations or social missions to undue influence from secondary interests, such as financial gain. Within these systems, a variety of organizations—public and private—can influence the policies and practices of institutions and support the norms of professional integrity. For example, accreditation and certification organizations set standards for medical schools, residency and fellowship programs, and individual physicians. State agencies license and relicense individual physicians, and specialty boards certify and recertify them. Journals publish medical research. The National Guideline Clearinghouse posts clinical practice guidelines. Public and private health insurers use a variety of financial and other incentives to influence the practices of institutions and individual clinicians. The U.S. Department of Justice and the Office of the Inspector General of the U.S. Department of Health and Human Services enforce laws limiting or prohibiting certain conflicts of interest, and NIH is responsible for overseeing compliance with PHS policies covering its grantees.

In addition to discussing incentives for policy adoption and implementation, the final chapter of the report discusses the roles of collaboration and consensus building in building conflict of interest policies that win acceptance and avoid needless burdens. Although the emphasis should be on preventing problems, policies should also be backed by enforcement and appropriate sanctions as well as assessment of their effectiveness.

Recommendation 9.1 proposes that groups such as accrediting organizations, public and private health insurers, and associations of medical journal editors develop incentives to make institutions more accountable for preventing, identifying, and managing conflicts of interest. The accompanying discussion gives examples of such incentives. The final recommendation, Recommendation 9.2, calls for more research to assess the positive and negative consequences of conflict of interest policies and provide a stronger evidence base for improving conflict of interest policies and their application.

Society has traditionally granted the medical profession considerable autonomy to regulate itself. Society may be willing to continue do so in the case of conflicts of interest; but concern is growing in the U.S. Congress, state legislatures, federal agencies, and elsewhere that stronger measures are needed. Physicians and researchers can play a vital role in designing responsible and reasonable conflict of interest policies and procedures that reduce the risks of bias and the loss of trust while avoiding undue burdens or even harms. They and the institutions that carry out medical research, education, clinical care, and practice guideline development must recognize public concerns about conflicts of interest and take effective measures soon to maintain public trust.

OVERVIEW AND LIST OF RECOMMENDATIONS

TABLE S-1 Report Recommendations in Overview

Recommendation Number and Topic	Primary Actors
General policy	
3.1 Adopt and implement conflict of interest policies	Institutions that carry out medical research and education, clinical care, and clinical practice guideline development
3.2 Strengthen disclosure policies	Institutions that carry out medical research and education, clinical care, and clinical practice guideline development
3.3 Standardize disclosure content and formats	Institutions that carry out medical research and education, clinical care, and clinical practice guideline development and other interested organizations (e.g., accrediting bodies, health insurers, consumer groups, and government agencies)
3.4 Create a national program for the reporting of company payments	U.S. Congress; pharmaceutical, medical device, and biotechnology companies
Medical research	
4.1 Restrict participation of researchers with conflicts of interest in research with human participants	Academic medical centers and other research institutions; medical researchers

TABLE S-1 Continued

Recommendation Number and Topic	Primary Actors
Medical education	
5.1 Reform relationships with industry in medical education	Academic medical centers and teaching hospitals; faculty, students, residents, and fellows
5.2 Provide education on conflict of interest	Academic medical centers and teaching hospitals; professional societies
5.3 Reform financing system for continuing medical education	Organizations that created the accrediting program for continuing medical education and other organizations interested in high-quality, objective education
Medical practice	
6.1 Reform financial relationships with industry for community physicians	Community physicians; professional societies; hospitals and other health care providers
6.2 Reform industry interactions with physicians	Pharmaceutical, medical device, and biotechnology companies
Clinical practice guidelines	
7.1 Restrict industry funding and conflicts in clinical practice guideline development	Institutions that develop clinical practice guidelines
7.2 Create incentives for reducing conflicts in clinical practice guideline development	Accrediting and certification bodies, formulary committees, health insurers, public agencies, and other organizations with an interest in objective, evidence-based clinical practice guidelines
Institutional conflict of interest policies	
8.1 Create board-level responsibility for institutional conflicts of interest	Institutions that carry out medical research and education, clinical care, and clinical practice guideline development
8.2 Revise PHS regulations to require policies on institutional conflicts of interest	NIH
Supporting organizations	
9.1 Provide additional incentives for institutions to adopt and implement policies	Oversight bodies and other groups that have a strong interest in or reliance on medical research, education, clinical care, and practice guideline development
9.2 Develop research agenda on conflict of interest	NIH, Agency for Healthcare Research and Quality, and other agencies of the U.S. Department of Health and Human Services

RECOMMENDATION 3.1 Institutions that carry out medical research, medical education, clinical care, or practice guideline development should adopt, implement, and make public conflict of interest policies for individuals that are consistent with the other recommendations in this report. To manage identified conflicts of interest and monitor the implementation of management recommendations, institutions should create a conflict of interest committee. That committee should use a full range of management tools, as appropriate, including elimination of the conflicting financial interest, prohibition or restriction of involvement of the individual with a conflict of interest in the activity related to the conflict, and providing additional disclosures of the conflict of interest.

RECOMMENDATION 3.2 As part of their conflict of interest policies, institutions should require individuals covered by their policies, including senior institutional officials, to disclose financial relationships with pharmaceutical, medical device, and biotechnology companies to the institution on an annual basis and when an individual's situation changes significantly. The policies should

- request disclosures that are sufficiently specific and comprehensive (with no minimum dollar threshold) to allow others to assess the severity of the conflicts;
- avoid unnecessary administrative burdens on individuals making disclosures; and
- require further disclosure, as appropriate, for example, to the conflict of interest committee, the institutional review board, and the contracts and grants office.

RECOMMENDATION 3.3 National organizations that represent academic medical centers, other health care providers, and physicians and researchers should convene a broad-based consensus development process to establish a standard content, a standard format, and standard procedures for the disclosure of financial relationships with industry.

RECOMMENDATION 3.4 The U.S. Congress should create a national program that requires pharmaceutical, medical device, and biotechnology companies and their foundations to publicly report payments to physicians and other prescribers, biomedical researchers, health care institutions, professional societies, patient advocacy and disease-specific groups, providers of continuing medical education, and foundations created by any of these entities. Until the Congress acts, companies should voluntarily adopt such reporting.

RECOMMENDATION 4.1 Academic medical centers and other research institutions should establish a policy that individuals generally may not conduct research with human participants if they have a significant financial interest in an existing or potential product or a company that could be affected by the outcome of the research. Exceptions to the policy should be made public and should be permitted only if the conflict of interest committee (a) determines that an individual's participation is essential for the conduct of the research and (b) establishes an effective mechanism for managing the conflict and protecting the integrity of the research.

RECOMMENDATION 5.1 For all faculty, students, residents, and fellows and for all associated training sites, academic medical centers and teaching hospitals should adopt and implement policies that prohibit

- the acceptance of items of material value from pharmaceutical, medical device, and biotechnology companies, except in specified situations;
- educational presentations or scientific publications that are controlled by industry or that contain substantial portions written by someone who is not identified as an author or who is not properly acknowledged;
- consulting arrangements that are not based on written contracts for expert services to be paid for at fair market value;
- access by drug and medical device sales representatives, except by faculty invitation, in accordance with institutional policies, in certain specified situations for training, patient safety, or the evaluation of medical devices; and
- the use of drug samples, except in specified situations for patients who lack financial access to medications.

Until their institutions adopt these recommendations, faculty and trainees at academic medical centers and teaching hospitals should voluntarily adopt them as standards for their own conduct.

RECOMMENDATION 5.2 Academic medical centers and teaching hospitals should educate faculty, medical students, and residents on how to avoid or manage conflicts of interest and relationships with pharmaceutical and medical device industry representatives. Accrediting organizations should develop standards that require formal education on these topics.

RECOMMENDATION 5.3 A new system of funding accredited continuing medical education should be developed that is free of industry influence, enhances public trust in the integrity of the system, and provides high-quality education. A consensus development process that includes representatives of the member organizations that created the accrediting body for continuing medical education, members of the public, and representatives of organizations such as certification boards that rely on continuing medical education should be convened to propose within 24 months of the publication of this report a funding system that will meet these goals.

RECOMMENDATION 6.1 Physicians, wherever their site of clinical practice, should

- not accept of items of material value from pharmaceutical, medical device, and biotechnology companies except when a transaction involves payment at fair market value for a legitimate service;
- not make educational presentations or publish scientific articles that are controlled by industry or contain substantial portions written by someone who is not identified as an author or who is not properly acknowledged;
- not enter into consulting arrangements unless they are based on written contracts for expert services to be paid for at fair market value;
- not meet with pharmaceutical and medical device sales representatives except by documented appointment and at the physician's express invitation; and
- not accept drug samples except in certain situations for patients who lack financial access to medications.

Professional societies should amend their policies and codes of professional conduct to support these recommendations. Health care providers should establish policies for their employees and medical staff that are consistent with these recommendations.

RECOMMENDATION 6.2 Pharmaceutical, medical device, and biotechnology companies and their company foundations should have policies and practices against providing physicians with gifts, meals, drug samples (except for use by patients who lack financial access to medications), or other similar items of material value and against asking physicians to be authors of ghostwritten materials. Consulting arrangements should be for necessary services, documented in written contracts, and paid for at fair market value. Companies should not involve physicians and patients in marketing projects that are presented as clinical research.

RECOMMENDATION 7.1 Groups that develop clinical practice guidelines should generally exclude as panel members individuals with conflicts of interest and should not accept direct funding for clinical practice guideline development from medical product companies or company foundations. Groups should publicly disclose with each guideline their conflict of interest policies and procedures and the sources and amounts of indirect or direct funding received for development of the guideline. In the exceptional situation in which avoidance of panel members with conflicts of interest is impossible because of the critical need for their expertise, then groups should

- publicly document that they made a good-faith effort to find experts without conflicts of interest by issuing a public call for members and other recruitment measures;
- appoint a chair without a conflict of interest;
- limit members with conflicting interests to a distinct minority of the panel;
- exclude individuals who have a fiduciary or promotional relationship with a company that makes a product that may be affected by the guidelines;
- exclude panel members with conflicts from deliberating, drafting, or voting on specific recommendations; and
- publicly disclose the relevant conflicts of interest of panel members.

RECOMMENDATION 7.2 Accrediting and certification bodies, health insurers, public agencies, and other similar organizations should encourage institutions that develop clinical practice guidelines to adopt conflict of interest policies consistent with the recommendations in this report. Three desirable steps are for

- journals to require that all clinical practice guidelines accepted for publication describe (or provide an Internet link to) the developer's conflict of interest policies, the sources and amounts of funding for the guideline, and the relevant financial interests of guideline panel members, if any;
- the National Guideline Clearinghouse to require that all clinical practice guidelines accepted for posting describe (or provide an Internet link to) the developer's conflict of interest policies, the sources and amounts of funding for development of the guideline, and the relevant financial interests of guideline panel members, if any; and
- accrediting and certification organizations, public and private health plans, and similar groups to avoid using clinical practice guidelines for performance measures, coverage decisions, and similar purposes if the guideline developers do not follow the practices recommended in this report.

RECOMMENDATION 8.1 The boards of trustees or the equivalent governing bodies of institutions engaged in medical research, medical education, patient care, or practice guideline development should establish their own standing committees on institutional conflicts of interest. These standing committees should

- have no members who themselves have conflicts of interest relevant to the activities of the institution;
- include at least one member who is not a member of the board or an employee or officer of the institution and who has some relevant expertise;
- create, as needed, administrative arrangements for the day-to-day oversight and management of institutional conflicts of interest, including those involving senior officials; and
- submit an annual report to the full board, which should be made public but in which the necessary modifications have been made to protect confidential information.

RECOMMENDATION 8.2 The National Institutes of Health should develop rules governing institutional conflicts of interest for research institutions covered by current U.S. Public Health Service regulations. The rules should require the reporting of identified institutional conflicts of interest and the steps that have been taken to eliminate or manage such conflicts.

RECOMMENDATION 9.1 Accreditation and certification bodies, private health insurers, government agencies, and similar organizations should develop incentives to promote the adoption and effective implementation of conflict of interest policies by institutions engaged in medical research, medical education, clinical care, or practice guideline development. In developing the incentives, these organizations should involve the individuals and the institutions that would be affected.

RECOMMENDATION 9.2 To strengthen the evidence base for the design and application of conflict of interest policies, the U.S. Department of Health and Human Services should coordinate the development and funding of a research agenda to study the impact of conflicts of interest on the quality of medical research, education, and practice and on practice guideline development and to examine the positive and negative effects of conflict of interest policies on these outcomes.

1

Introduction

Patients and the public benefit from constructive collaboration between academic medicine and pharmaceutical, medical device, and biotechnology companies. At the same time, medical leaders, public officials, public interest groups, and others have raised concerns about the risks associated with the extensive financial ties that link industry with the individuals and institutions that carry out medical research, medical education, patient care, and practice guideline development. The risks are that individual and institutional financial interests may unduly influence professional judgments involving these primary institutional missions. Such conflicts of interest threaten the integrity of scientific investigations, the objectivity of medical education, the quality of patient care, and the public's trust in medicine.

The benefits of collaboration with industry are most evident in biomedical research. New medications and medical devices have significantly improved outcomes for people with a range of serious and common diseases, including—among many others—coronary artery disease, congestive heart failure, hypercholesterolemia, several types of cancers, and peptic ulcer disease. Such successful products result from a long, complex, and often unpredictable process of translating basic science discoveries into new preventive, diagnostic, or therapeutic products and services. The basic discoveries often come from the laboratories of university and government scientists; but their development into actual products available to clinicians and patients usually depends on the technical, production, and financial resources of pharmaceutical, medical device, or biotechnology companies. It is estimated that it takes an average of 15 years and more than $800 million to discover and develop a new drug, and only about 10 percent of the drugs that enter clinical testing are actually approved for marketing (DiMasi et al., 2003, 2004; FDA, 2004a). Chapter 4 and Appendix E further examine the nature and value of university-industry collaboration in medical research.

With the benefits of research collaboration and the expansion of financial relationships in other areas have also come conflicts of interest and evidence of bias. For example, in clinical research, unfavorable results in some major industry-sponsored trials have been withheld from publication, thus distorting the totality of the findings included in the scientific literature. These trials involved drugs commonly prescribed for arthritis, depression, and elevated cholesterol levels, among other medications (Wright et al., 2001; Gibson, 2004; Whittington et al., 2004; Kastelein et al., 2008). Not publishing negative results undermines evidence-based medicine and puts millions of patients at risk for using ineffective or unsafe drugs. One striking case involves the withholding of negative findings from pediatric clinical trials of the effects of selective serotonin reuptake inhibitors on depression (Healy, 2006; Turner et al., 2008). Findings were withheld so frequently that although one meta-analysis of the published literature (ACN, 2004) concluded that these drugs were safe and effective, another meta-analysis (Whittington et al., 2004) that took into account unpublished as well as published data concluded the opposite: that the risks outweigh the benefits for all but one drug in this class of antidepressants. A recent analysis found that more than half of the trials used to support Food and Drug Administration approval for the marketing of a drug or medical device had not been published within 5 years after approval (Lee et al., 2008). In addition, litigation has revealed documents that link bias in publications to financial relationships with pharmaceutical manufacturers (Steinman et al., 2006; Psaty and Kronmal, 2008; Ross et al., 2008). As discussed in Chapter 4, the statistical associations involving industry sponsorship do not prove causality, but they do raise serious concerns about undue industry influence and have prompted a range of responses, including the creation of publication protections in university-industry research contracts and the issuance of regulations and other requirements that the results of clinical trials be reported in clinical trial registries.

In medical education, it is particularly troublesome when a faculty member is a promotional speaker for a pharmaceutical, medical device, or biotechnology company or agrees to be listed as an author for a ghostwritten publication. This is because faculty members are expected to present unbiased information and objective assessments of the scientific literature and to help medical students, residents, and fellows develop life-long habits of exercising independent judgment and critically evaluating scientific evidence. They are also expected to serve as role models of professionalism. These expectations may be undermined by some financial relationships between faculty and industry and by failures to disclose such relationships.

In clinical care, patients need to trust that their physicians' recommendations are not distorted by commercial interests. Such trust may contribute to the healing process and to patients' sense of well-being. Some financial relationships between physicians and industry raise concerns about the risk of bias in clinical decisions. For example, companies have paid some physicians large but generally undisclosed amounts to give talks to other physicians, whose prescribing practices were then tracked by company sales representatives (Elliott, 2006; Carlat, 2007). Drug samples and other gifts to physicians by company sales representatives are major marketing tools that evidence suggests influence prescribing choices (see Chapter 5). Furthermore, during the last decade, several federal prosecutions alleging that companies made illegal payments to physicians to induce them to use the companies' drugs or medical devices have led to settlements in which the companies agreed to modify various marketing practices and, in some cases, to post publicly their payments to physicians (see Chapter 6). The prevalence of illegal payments is not known.

Another area of concern is clinical practice guidelines. Clinical practice guidelines influence patient care, quality and performance standards, and reimbursement for health care professionals and institutions. If a risk exists that guidelines are biased or may be viewed as biased in favor of the products of the companies that sponsored the guideline development process or companies that have financial relationships with experts involved in the process, then patients may be harmed and users' trust in the guidelines may be undermined. Evaluating the potential for such bias is often difficult, however, because many entities that develop practice guidelines do not have clear conflict of interest policies for this activity, do not disclose their funding sources, and do not reveal the relevant financial relationships or conflicts of interest for the experts responsible for developing a set of guidelines. A review of clinical practice guidelines that do include information on financial relationships of the participants suggests that conflicts of interest are common (for examples, see Chapter 7 and guidelines posted on the website for the National Guideline Clearinghouse).

Conflicting interests are, to some degree, both ubiquitous and difficult to avoid. For example, regardless of how they are paid for their services (e.g., on a fee-for-service or a capitated basis), physicians will face some incentives that may at times conflict with their professional responsibility to provide care that best serves their patients' interests. Medical school faculty may face conflicts in the time and energy that they devote to each element of their academic responsibilities—research, teaching, and clinical care.

Many conflicts are unavoidable features of multifaceted professional roles and obligations. Others are optional, for example, the creation of a consulting or a speaking agreement with a pharmaceutical, medical device, or biotechnology company. These kinds of financial relationships with industry are the focus of this report.

As explained further in Chapter 2, this report specifically defines a conflict of interest as existing when an individual or institution has a secondary interest (e.g., an ownership interest in a start-up biotechnology company) that creates a risk of undue influence on decisions or actions affecting a primary interest (e.g., the conduct of objective and trustworthy medical research). This definition frames a conflict of interest in terms of the risk of such undue influence and not the actual occurrence of bias.

Some argue that concerns about conflicts of interest are overstated and that policy responses have been excessive, inconsistent, and unduly burdensome on physicians and researchers (see, e.g., Stossel [2005, 2007], Duvall [2006], Borgert [2007], and Bailey [2008]). According to that viewpoint, problems related to conflicts of interests are rare. Thus, the vast majority of scientists, educators, and clinicians should not be subject to onerous conflict of interest rules and regulations because of a few miscreants. The argument continues that burdensome rules and regulations stifle valuable collaborations between industry and academia. Moreover, allegations of conflict of interest inappropriately call into question the motives and integrity of individual scientists and clinicians, because a financial relationship related to one's research, teaching, or clinical practice does not prove the actual presence of bias in decisions or judgments. Consequently, it would be better to focus on detecting and minimizing bias rather than on disclosing, limiting, or managing financial relationships with industry. Furthermore, some of the intended beneficiaries of conflict of interest policies—for example, research participants—do not seem to be concerned about the financial interests of the investigators (see, e.g., Hampson et al. [2006] and Weinfurt et al. [2006a] and the further discussions in Chapters 3 and 4). Another criticism is that the focus on conflicts of interest related to financial ties with industry distracts attention from other threats to objectivity and public trust, such as career ambitions, a desire for recognition, intellectual bias, personal ties, and physician payment methods.

As discussed in Chapter 2, many objections to conflict of interest policies are based on misunderstandings of their purpose and nature. If they are correctly explained, the policies should not be seen as impugning anyone's motives. They are, in fact, a way of avoiding intrusive investigations into people's motives. They also protect against bias or distrust when other methods (e.g., assessments of actual bias after the fact) are not feasible or sufficient. Although other secondary interests may inappropriately influence professional decisions and additional safeguards are necessary to protect against bias from such interests, financial interests are more readily identified and regulated.

Opposition to conflict of interest policies often focuses on what might be lost with further restrictions on ties to industry. For example, eliminating industry support for accredited continuing medical education might result in increases in the fees that physicians must pay for such education, a reduction in the number of accredited courses, and a drop in income for institutions that provide continuing medical education. To cite another example, if universities insist on contract terms that restrict a company's ability to withhold or censor research findings, then companies might move more research contracts elsewhere (e.g., to contract research organizations or overseas research centers that do not have such restrictions). Similarly, some faculty members may leave a university if that university restricts faculty members' financial ties with industry. Such losses (costs) tend to be immediate, easily identifiable, and tangible.

In contrast, the costs of conflicts of interest and the benefits of mitigating or eliminating them tend to be less tangible, less immediate, and more diffuse. Eliminating direct industry funding of continuing medical education, for example, could increase evidence-based physician prescribing practices, which over time could reduce wasteful health care spending and improve the quality of patient care, but demonstrating such causal relationships could be difficult or impossible. Another benefit of dealing with conflicts of interest that is even harder to define and document but that is significant could be the maintenance of public trust in medical professionals and institutions. Indeed, the maintenance of trust is a major objective of conflict of interest policies across a broad range of professions, in addition to medicine (see Appendix C).

Research suggests that people are generally not good at making trade-offs between costs and benefits that are immediate and tangible and those that are less immediate and less tangible (for a review, see Rick and Loewenstein [2008]). People tend to put a disproportionate emphasis on costs and benefits that are immediate and tangible. For example, the impact of a single, free drug company-sponsored lunch on a physician's prescribing practices or on public trust may be small to insignificant, but the cumulative consequences of many lunches to many physicians may be great. The human tendency to overweight the immediate and tangible compared with the delayed and intangible thus complicates efforts to understand and respond to conflicts of interest.

OVERVIEW AND THEMES OF REPORT

This Institute of Medicine (IOM) report examines the extent of financial relationships with industry and conflicts of interest in medical research, education, and practice and in the development of clinical practice guidelines. It reviews policies that have been adopted or proposed to avoid or manage these conflicts and recommends steps that can be taken to improve the design, implementation, and evaluation of these policies. The report builds on the analyses and recommendations of other groups. It is different, however, in its focus on conflict of interest across the spectrum of medicine and in its identification of overarching issues and strategies that can be used to limit the negative effects of conflicts of interest while preserving the benefits of collaboration with industry, particularly in moving discoveries from basic science into improved patient care. The report has several broad messages.

1. *The goal of conflict of interest policies in medicine is to protect the integrity of professional judgment and to preserve public trust rather than to try to remediate problems with bias or mistrust after they occur.*

In all aspects of medicine, judgments must inevitably be made, and reasonable people will disagree over some judgments. Both science and medicine depend on public trust that judgments are made in good faith and are not unduly influenced by the financial interests of professionals or the institutions with which they are affiliated. Well-formulated and well-explained conflict of interest policies can help identify individual and institutional relationships that could reasonably be questioned and allow judgments to be made prospectively about whether particular relationships should be eliminated, permitted, or managed.

It is prudent to require physicians and medical researchers to avoid or manage situations that offer a significant possibility of bias rather than to wait to investigate allegations of bias or misconduct until after they occur. Investigations performed to uncover bias after the fact can be difficult, time-consuming, and heavily burdensome for all involved. Furthermore, when bias occurs in clinical research, medical education, or practice guideline development, it can harm research participants or patients, waste scarce resources, and damage individual and institutional reputations, including the reputations of those whose relationships with industry are appropriately structured and disclosed and serve the public good. If trust is eroded by continuing revelations of withheld negative research findings, promotional relationships disguised as consulting services, and similarly troublesome situations, it may be hard to restore.

2. *Disclosure of individual and institutional financial relationships is a critical but limited first step in the process of identifying and responding to conflicts of interest.*

Institutions that carry out medical research, medical education, patient care, and practice guideline development depend on individuals' disclosure of their financial relationships with industry. Without such disclosure, institutions will lack the information they need to identify and assess conflicts of interest and determine what additional steps—such as eliminating or managing the conflicting interest—may be necessary. Disclosure by institutions is likewise important because institutions may also have financial relationships that create conflicts of interest. The disclosures need to be sufficiently specific and comprehensive to allow an initial assessment of the risk of undue influence. At the same time, the harmonization of disclosure requirements and procedures can reduce administrative burdens for researchers and physicians who must make multiple disclosures to different institutions for different purposes.

Disclosure does not resolve or eliminate conflicts of interest. Institutions must also evaluate and act upon the disclosed information. Actions might include the elimination of a relationship, further disclosure (e.g., to research participants, patients, or the public), or other types of management (e.g., restricting the participation of a researcher with a conflict of interest in the enrollment of study participants or analysis of study data).

3. Conflict of interest guidelines and policies can be strengthened by engaging physicians, researchers, and medical institutions in developing policies and consensus standards.

For conflict of interest policies to be truly effective, buy-in from physicians and researchers will be important, so that they regard conflict of interest policies as a means to help them fulfill their professional responsibilities and not as externally imposed nuisances. Furthermore, if those who are subject to conflict of interest policies participate in policy development, they may suggest how the policies can be framed to avoid unintended adverse consequences and undue administrative burdens. In several areas in which substantial policy variation or disagreement exists and greater agreement is needed, the report proposes the creation of consensus development panels with a broad range of participants, including consumer representatives. Two areas that are ripe for consensus building involve the standardization of information that physicians and researchers are required to disclose (Chapter 3) and the development of a new system of financing continuing medical education (Chapter 5).

4. A range of organizations—public and private—can promote the adoption and implementation of conflict of interest policies and help create a culture of accountability that sustains professional norms and promotes public confidence in professional judgments.

Institutions that carry out medical research, medical education, clinical care, and practice guideline development have the primary responsibility for addressing conflicts of interests in these activities. These institutions do not, however, act in isolation. Rather, they interact with many other organizations—including academic and trade membership associations, accreditation and certification bodies, patient advocacy groups, health plans, and federal and state agencies—that have a stake in reducing the severity of individual and institutional conflicts of interest. As discussed in Chapter 9, these organizations can create incentives to encourage institutions to adopt and implement policies that are consistent with the recommendations of this committee and other organizations, such as the Association of American Medical Colleges, the Association of American Universities, and the International Committee of Medical Journal Editors. Such incentives would encourage and reinforce professional responsibility and promote public trust.

5. *Research on conflicts of interest and conflict of interest policies can provide a stronger evidence base for policy design and implementation.*

The current evidence base for conflict of interest policies is not strong. A program of research on conflicts of interest and conflict of interest policies could provide policy makers with a better evidence base and a basis for understanding the nature and consequences of conflicts of interest in different situations. It could likewise guide policy makers as they revise policies and procedures to make them more effective and less burdensome.

6. *If medical institutions do not act voluntarily to strengthen their conflict of interest policies and procedures, the pressure for external regulation is likely to increase.*

The continuing publicity about conflicts of interest in medicine and the failure of individuals and institutions to adhere to conflict of interest policies has prompted calls for government regulation. Indeed, this report recommends some areas for government action, but it also emphasizes that risks as well as the potential benefits of regulation should be considered.

Origins of the Study

This study grew out of discussions within the IOM about the threats to objectivity and public trust in biomedical research and medicine created by conflicts of interest related to certain types of financial relationships between industry and researchers based in universities and federal agencies. Consideration of the topic was further stimulated by inquiries from groups outside the IOM about whether the IOM would examine conflicts of interest and industry ties as they might affect the publication of research and the development of clinical practice guidelines. In response, the IOM proposed a broad-ranging study that would examine conflicts of interest across medical research, medical education, clinical practice, and practice guideline development.

The IOM appointed a 17-member committee to oversee the study and develop the study report. (See Appendix A for more information about study-related activities.) Consistent with its charge, the committee

- examined financial relationships with industry and conflicts of interest in medical research, education, practice, and practice guideline development and
- developed analyses and recommendations to inform the design and implementation of policies for the identification and management of

conflicts of interest in these contexts without damaging constructive collaborations with industry.

To address this broad charge, the committee consciously adopted a crosscutting perspective and tried to view medicine as a complex system with many interacting components and interested parties. It drafted its report for a diverse audience of academic, scientific, professional, medical institution, industry, consumer, news media, and government leaders. Their understanding of the hazards of conflicts of interest and the elements of effective, balanced policies aimed at preventing conflicts of interest from occurring is essential.

During the course of its work, the committee searched for and assessed empirical evidence relevant to its charge, and it read and heard a wide range of views. The analyses and recommendations in this report reflect the committee's conscientious effort to understand and take these views into account. The committee also examined how conflicts of interest are handled in other professions (see Appendix C).

Focus and Concepts

Given the breadth of its charge, the committee focused on conflicts of interest involving *physicians, biomedical researchers, and senior institutional officials*. These individuals have been at the center of most controversies about conflicts of interest and most proposals for policy change. Many of the conclusions and recommendations presented in this report will, however, be generally relevant to nursing, pharmacy, dentistry, and other health professions and to other health researchers. In some cases, institutional policies may extend beyond researchers, professionals, and senior officials. For example, professional society policies governing members of a panel developing clinical practice guidelines will cover all members, including consumers, patients, and the representatives of health insurers.

This report generally uses the term *institutions* to refer to academic medical centers; professional societies; patient or consumer groups; and other entities that carry out medical research, provide medical education and clinical care, or develop clinical practice guidelines.[1] The report also distinguishes (particularly in Chapter 9) supporting *organizations*, such as accrediting agencies and state licensure boards, that may create incentives

[1] For the purposes of this report, the committee distinguished companies that produce commercial medical products from other mostly noncommercial medical institutions (and their personnel) that these companies seek to influence. (Some providers of continuing medical education are for-profit concerns.) The committee recognized that commercial companies conduct or sponsor research and may undertake activities with educational value.

for institutions to adopt and implement effective and credible conflict of interest policies or codes of conduct and for individuals to follow these policies or codes. Some entities, such as medical journals, cross these definitional boundaries and are covered by recommendations related to both institutions and organizations.

Reflecting the discussions that led to this study and the emphasis of much research, press coverage, and public and professional debate, this report emphasizes *financial interests and relationships* involving *pharmaceutical, medical device, and biotechnology companies* that make—or that are developing—medical products used in patient care. (For convenience, the report sometimes refers to these companies as "industry" or "medical product companies," although some start-up biotechnology and other companies may not yet have products approved for marketing.) Other interests, such as the desire for public recognition, may also threaten objectivity and public trust, but financial interests are the central focus of conflict of interest debates and policies.

Notwithstanding the prominence of medical product companies in discussions of conflicts of interest in medicine, the committee recognized that significant conflicts of interest in medical research, education, and practice can be created by financial relationships involving many other kinds of companies. These include health insurers; prescription drug and other benefit management companies; law firms; investment companies; and suppliers of food, office supplies, and other nonmedical goods and services. Much of the discussion in this report about the adoption of policies and the disclosure of information should be relevant to financial relationships involving these other commercial entities.

The committee also understood that serious conflicts of interest may arise from the way in which physicians are paid for their clinical services and from physician ownership interests in hospitals, diagnostic centers, and facilities. The IOM did not plan this study to investigate these issues, but they are briefly discussed in Chapter 6.

Although the analyses presented in this report build on a series of reports on responsible research and integrity in science issued by the IOM and the National Research Council, those earlier reports did not examine conflict of interest in depth. Nonetheless, they provide useful perspectives. In particular, the reports *Integrity in Scientific Research* (IOM/NRC, 2002) and *Responsible Research* (IOM, 2003) underscore the importance of creating organizational and social environments that support and encourage responsible and ethical behavior by individuals and institutions. This report also builds on recommendations made in other reports that called for the undertaking of more and better comparative effectiveness studies and other steps needed to build and communicate the evidence base for clinical practice (see, e.g., previous IOM studies [1991, 2007]). One recommendation of this report (Recommendation 9.2) is that the evidence base for conflict of interest policies needs to be strengthened to help policy makers identify effective policies and avoid unwanted consequences.

HISTORICAL AND POLICY CONTEXT

Concerns about conflicts of interest have a long history; and the responses to these conflicts have evolved as relationships with industry in medical research, education, and practice have grown more frequent and more complex. They have also evolved as different responses to such relationships have been tried and found to be in need of modification.

The following brief review indicates, first, that both government regulations and voluntary codes of conduct often follow the discovery of instances of questionable or inappropriate relationships and conduct. This is similar to the pattern in other areas, such as the oversight of research involving human participants.[2] Second, government scrutiny of conflicts of interest may stimulate private, voluntary efforts by academic and other institutions to deal with problems and avoid regulation. Third, when these efforts are found to be wanting and government acts, legislators and administrators may still delegate to regulated institutions many of the details of policy development, implementation, and monitoring.

Expanding Relationships Between Industry and Medicine

Relationships between physicians, medical researchers, and medical schools and companies that produce medical products have a long history, as have efforts to encourage such relationships. For example, in the early 1920s, Eli Lilly worked with researchers at the University of Toronto to manufacture insulin in quantities adequate for research and then clinical use; the university also granted royalty-free patents to other companies to expand the drug's availability worldwide (Thayer, 2005). In 1925, the National Research Council (which the National Academy of Sciences established at the request of President Woodrow Wilson to organize scientific research) created a short-lived National Research Fund that raised money from private companies to support research in academic institutions (Swann, 1988).

The mixing of product marketing and medical information for physicians likewise has a lengthy history (see, e.g., Podolsky and Greene [2008]).

---

[2] In general, this report follows the practice of recent IOM reports in referring to research participants rather than research subjects (IOM, 2001, 2003, 2004; NBAC, 2001). This report uses the latter terminology when quoting and sometimes when referring to reports that employ that terminology.

More than a century ago, a review in the *Chicago Medical Recorder* of *Merck's Manual of the Materia Medica* (now the *Merck Manual of Diagnosis and Therapy*) observed: "[a]lthough this little book is gotten out by a manufacturing firm and with some view towards its advertising value, it nonetheless is of such merit that it is deserving of mention in this column" (quoted by Lane and Berkow [1999, p. 112]). Then, as now, recognition of the value of industry contributions can coexist with unease about commercial motivations and potential bias.

Professional societies and the medical products industry also have long-standing relationships, for example, industry advertising in journals sponsored by medical societies. As early as the late 1940s and early 1950s, the American Medical Association (AMA) began to market information from its new physician database to pharmaceutical companies and to commission studies of the effectiveness of different marketing techniques, the results of which were sent to pharmaceutical and device companies—along with pamphlets promoting advertising in the *Journal of the American Medical Association* (Greene, 2007). This AMA business has generated some controversy and is discussed further in Chapter 6 (see also Steinbrook [2006]).

Biomedical research saw a marked expansion of government funding after World War II. By 1965, spending by the National Institutes of Health (NIH) and other federal agencies accounted for almost two-thirds of the total funding for biomedical research, whereas it was about 7 percent in 1940 (Ginzberg and Dutka, 1989). Then, in the late 1970s, the balance began to shift toward commercial funding. By the turn of the 21st century, the share of health research and development funding accounted for by industry reached 55 to 60 percent (see Chapter 4). New relationships and collaborations between universities and industry during the late 1970s and 1980s were stimulated by a combination of economic conditions, pressures on the federal budget, scientific discoveries, needs for expertise outside universities, and other factors, including legislative incentives for universities to develop discoveries commercially. A Congressional Research Service report noted that another factor in universities' pursuit of industry funding was a "desire to lessen the regulations associated with the expenditure of Federal dollars" (Johnson, 1982, p. 2).

Industry has also become a major source of funding for medical education, particularly continuing medical education. Between 1998 and 2007, the share of continuing medical education provider income accounted for by commercial sources, excluding advertising and exhibits, grew from 34 to 48 percent, with higher rates for some providers, such as for-profit education and communication companies and medical schools (ACCME, 2008a). Through their support for professional society journals and meetings, pharmaceutical and medical device companies are also important sources of income for professional societies, often accounting for 30 to 50 percent or more of the total income of professional societies (see Chapter 8).

Growing Concerns About Relationships with Industry

As they have evolved, relationships between industry and medicine have brought many benefits, primarily in biomedical research. They have also raised concerns that such relationships can—if they are not properly managed—threaten the objectivity of medical research, education, and practice and undermine public trust in critical American institutions.

Table 1-1 lists some notable events in the emergence of relationships with industry and conflict of interest as a concern in medicine. They include congressional hearings in the 1980s that posed questions about whether conflicts of interest were reducing openness in universities and biasing the advice given to policy makers. A Congressional Research Service report on the commercialization of academic biotechnology research observed that "the credibility of university scientists associated with industry has fallen into question" (Johnson, 1982, p. 5). An article in *Science* from the same period titled The Academic-Industrial Complex (Culliton, 1982) summarized the ethical concerns that these relationships presented to university administrators and faculty:

> How can universities preserve open communication and independence in the direction of basic research while also meeting obligations to industry? Is it acceptable for one corporation to dominate research in an entire department? Are there adverse consequences in terms of collaboration among faculty in various departments if one group must worry about protecting corporate rights to licenses? Will patent and licensing provisions delay scientific publication? Should corporate sponsorship be subject to peer review? Under what conditions may a faculty member have an equity position in industry? Do such ties compromise loyalty to university teaching and research? Will graduate students be compromised or poorly served? Will extensive corporate ties erode public confidence in university faculty as disinterested seekers of truth? (Culliton, 1982, p. 961)

Concerns about conflict of interest beyond the research context were also growing during the 1970s and 1980s. Some concerns related to questions about commercial bias in scientific publications. Others focused on physician referral of patients to specialty centers in which they had a financial interest and on the prevalence of company-provided gifts, lavish entertainment, marketing activities that were disguised as scientific information, and other relationships in both community and academic medical settings.

TABLE 1-1 Timeline of Selected Events Relevant to the Evolution of Conflict of Interest Principles, Policies, and Practices

Year	Event
1959	Senator Estes Kefauver initiates hearings on pricing practices in the pharmaceutical industry that expand to cover marketing practices
1962	President John F. Kennedy issues a memorandum, Preventing Conflict of Interest on the Part of Advisers and Consultants to the Government (27 FR 1341)
1964	American Association of University Professors and American Council on Education (ACE) issue a statement on conflicts of interest in government-sponsored research
1971	The National Academy of Sciences (NAS) approves a letter (On Potential Sources of Bias) to ask members of its study committees to describe financial and other factors that in their judgment "others may deem prejudicial"
1972	The U.S. Congress passes the first antikickback statute (P.L. 92-603)
1978	The U.S. Congress enacts the Ethics in Government Act (P.L. 95-521) to promote confidence in the integrity of government officials and prevent conflict of interest
1980	Patent and Trademark Amendments of 1980 (P.L. 96-517) (Bayh-Dole Act) and Stevenson-Wydler Technology Innovation Act (P.L. 96-480) encourage the commercial development of federally developed or funded technologies
1981	Economic Recovery Tax Act of 1981 (P.L. 97-34) provides a 25 percent tax credit for 65 percent of private investments in universities for basic research
1982	U.S. House of Representatives holds hearings on university-industry cooperation in biotechnology
	The presidents of five leading universities meet with scientists and industry leaders to discuss conflict of interest and university-industry ties (Pajaro Dunes Conference)
1983	California Fair Political Practices Commission orders an investigation of the University of California's enforcement of rules on disclosure of corporate support of faculty research after finding that more than 50 faculty members had financial interests in companies that were funding their research
1984	Association of American Universities (AAU) conducts a survey of university policies on conflict of interest in privately funded research
	Editorial in the *New England Journal of Medicine* announces policy on conflict of interest
1985	AAU issues the report *University Policies on Conflict of Interest and Delay of Publication*
1986	ACE issues the report *Higher Education and Research Entrepreneurship: Conflicts Among Interests*
1987	U.S. Public Health Services (PHS) issues Grants Policy Statement, which states that grant recipients should have written guidelines on conflict of interest
	Accreditation Council for Continuing Medical Education (ACCME) adopts Guidelines for Commercial Support (revised and issued as standards in 1992)
1988	U.S. House of Representatives holds hearing on scientific misconduct and hears concerns about conflicts of interest. Additional hearings follow (one is titled Is Science for Sale?)

TABLE 1-1 Continued

Year	Event
	International Committee of Medical Journal Editors (ICMJE) develops a statement of requirements for authors that includes a provision for authors to voluntarily disclose relevant financial interests and expands the scope of the policy in 1993 and 1998
1989	The U.S. Congress passes a law (Omnibus Budget Reconciliation Act of 1989) barring self-referral arrangements for clinical laboratory services under Medicare; legislation passed in 1993 and 2004 expands and refines the restrictions
	Ethics Reform Act of 1989 (P.L. 101-94) allows federal advisory committee members (special government employees) to participate, despite a conflict of interest, if an agency determines that the need for the individual to participate outweighs the conflict
	The National Institutes of Health (NIH) issues and then withdraws draft guidelines on policies on conflict of interest for recipients of PHS research grants
1990	A U.S. House Committee on Government Operations report (*Are Scientific Misconduct and Conflicts of Interest Hazardous to Our Health?*) recommends the development of PHS regulations that "clearly restrict financial ties for researchers who conduct evaluations of a product or treatment in which they have a vested interest"
	Association of American Medical Colleges publishes *Guidelines for Dealing with Faculty Conflicts of Commitment and Conflicts of Interest in Research*
	American Medical Association (AMA) adopts statement on inappropriate gifts to physicians from industry
	American College of Physicians issues a position paper on physicians and the pharmaceutical industry
1992	NAS report *Responsible Science* (1992) concludes, "The issues associated with conflict of interest in the academic research environment are sufficiently problematic that they deserve thorough study and analysis by major academic and scientific organizations" (p. 78)
1993	ICMJE approves statement on conflict of interest in peer review and publication
	Minnesota law limits drug company gifts to physicians and requires company disclosure of payments to physicians (excluding drug samples and educational materials)
1994	The National Science Foundation (NSF) issues Investigator Financial Disclosure Policy "to help ensure the appropriate management of actual or potential conflicts" (effective 1995)
1995	PHS (60 FR 35815, 42 CFR 50) publishes regulations on the responsibility of grant applicants for promoting objectivity in research
1998	The Food and Drug Administration publishes regulations requiring disclosure by clinical investigators of certain financial relationships (63 FR 5233)
1999	The death of Jesse Gelsinger in a gene transfer experiment provokes controversy after it is revealed that the principal investigator and his university had ownership interests in the company making the interventional product

See Table 1-2 for reports issued after 1999

Continued

TABLE 1-1 Continued

Year	Event
2001	ICMJE publishes new, more stringent policies on conflict of interest
	Vermont requires pharmaceutical companies to disclose payments to doctors and certain health care organizations related to marketing activities
	To promote adherence to its ethical guidelines, AMA, with funding from industry, initiates the campaign "What you should know about gifts to physicians from industry"
2003	HHS issues Compliance Program Guidance for Pharmaceutical Manufacturers, which observes that gifts "potentially implicate the anti-kickback statute if any one purpose of the arrangement is to generate business for the pharmaceutical company"
2004	The U.S. Congress questions NIH about the apparent failure of dozens of employees to disclose relationships with industry
	NIH issues stringent new policies for employees and later moderates them
	HHS issues final guidance to institutional review boards on financial relationships in clinical trials
	ACCME issues revised Standards for Commercial Support
2007	The U.S. Department of Justice announces deferred prosecution or nonprosecution agreements that allow five orthopedic device companies to avoid criminal prosecution for providing financial inducements for surgeons to use their products
2008	The Pharmaceutical Research and Manufacturers of America releases revised *Code on Interactions with Healthcare Professionals* and recommends an end to some gift-giving practices
	The Advanced Medical Technology Association issues revised *Code of Ethics*
	HHS issues regulations requiring physician-owned hospitals and physician owners of hospitals to disclose physician ownership interest to patients
	Massachusetts limits gifts and payments to physicians from pharmaceutical and device companies and requires companies to publicly disclose certain payments
2009	Federal legislation proposed to require disclosure of company payments to physicians and others and reporting of physician ownership interests in health care facilities

SOURCES: This timeline draws on a variety of materials, including the websites of the organizations cited above. Other resources include Johnson (1982), Budiansky (1983), OTA (1984), Steneck (1984), IOM (1991), Maatz (1992), Frankel (1996), Lemmens and Singer (1998), McCanse (2001), Krimsky (2003), Rapp (2003), Huth and Case (2004), Kassirer (2004), NIH (2004), Brody (2007), Parascandola (2007), Ross et al. (2007), Emanuel and Thompson (2008), ORI (2008), Lopes (2009), MedPAC, (2009), and Carpenter (in press).

Evolving Public and Private Responses to Concerns About Conflict of Interest

In the early 1960s, in recognition of the importance of outside advice on complex scientific and policy questions from objective experts, the federal government (through a presidential memo) established policies to limit conflicts of interest among special government employees serving as advisory committee members and consultants. In the academic community, the American Association of University Professors (AAUP) and the American Council on Education (ACE) issued a joint statement, On Preventing Conflicts of Interest in Government-Sponsored Research at Universities (AAUP/ACE, 1965). The statement spoke of the importance of university-industry relationships but stressed the need to protect the integrity of educational institutions in the face of ties between these institutions and both government and industry. It called for universities to advise government research agencies about the steps they were taking to avoid problems. According to McNeil and Roberts (1991), this statement forestalled government regulation and led to the adoption of policies by most major research universities of "very general guidelines" on conflict of interest that relied on faculty-initiated disclosure (p. 149). By 1967, a number of universities, including Yale, Harvard, Stanford, Michigan, Chicago, Minnesota, and California, had adopted conflict of interest policies that had been approved by the Federal Office of Science and Technology (Wellman, 1967).

A few years after AAUP and ACE issued their statement and after some incidents that raised concerns about bias and conflict of interest, the National Academy of Sciences approved a letter, On Potential Sources of Bias, which it issued in 1971. The letter asked members of the organization's scientific study committees to describe financial and other factors that in their judgment "others may deem prejudicial" (quoted in Parascandola [2007]). According to Parascandola, "[s]cientists universally opposed the policy, however, for a range of reasons—while some argued that all experienced and knowledgeable experts were inherently conflicted, others were offended at the suggestion that any expert could be biased" (p. 3774).

Such negatives responses to conflict of interest policies continue. Nonetheless, the adoption of policies has expanded as the scope and complexity of relationships with industry have increased and instances of questionable or illegal behavior have accumulated—with the attendant negative publicity.

In 1984, the Association of American Universities declined to propose conflict of interest policies for its members, but it did undertake a survey of university policies (OTA, 1984; McNeil and Roberts, 1991). It found that 19 of the 46 responding institutions relied on faculty members to determine whether they had a possible conflict of interest and then to initiate disclosure; 26 institutions had a university-initiated, annual disclosure process (reported in Maatz [1992]). In addition, 21 schools had policies on faculty equity or managerial ties to industry that required disclosure and approval.

In what appears to be the first policy of its sort, the editor of the *New*

England Journal of Medicine announced in 1984 that the journal would ask authors to disclose their relationships with companies that could be affected by their published findings (Relman, 1984). By 1990, the Association of American Medical Colleges had issued for its members guidelines on dealing with conflicts of interest, and AMA had provided guidance to physicians on accepting gifts from industry.

Congressional concerns about financial relationships between physicians or researchers and commercial entities have led to legislation on several occasions and also to threats of legislation. As early as 1972, the U.S. Congress prohibited companies from offering and physicians and others from accepting overt or covert payments or other rewards in return for the referral of patients or ordering of services paid for by Medicare or Medicaid. Beginning in 1989, the Congress also enacted a series of restrictions (known as the "Stark laws," after their sponsor) on self-referral arrangements, which occur when physicians refer patients to specialty hospitals, imaging centers, or other facilities in which they have a financial interest. Also, in 1989, congressional hearings and other pressures prompted NIH to issue draft guidelines on conflict of interest for its grantees. The agency then withdrew these guidelines after criticism that they were too restrictive and would "devastate productive relationships between university researchers and industry, deny scientists outlets for their discoveries at the bench and interfere with the technology transfer" (Mazzaschi, 1990, p. 137). The U.S. Public Health Service eventually issued regulations in 1995 (see Appendix B).

In recent years, members of Congress have raised questions about industry support for continuing medical education, industry payments to physicians, and faculty member disclosure of such payments. As discussed in later chapters, members of Congress have proposed legislation that addresses some of these questions. Some proposals would require companies to report consulting and other payments to physicians, and other proposals promote alternatives to pharmaceutical company sales representatives as sources of information for physicians about medications.[3] A few states have adopted policies requiring companies to disclose certain payments to physicians, and some states have created alternative education programs for physicians and other prescribers of medications.

In the 1990s, social science research techniques and findings began to influence understandings of the relationships between physicians and

[3] Examples of legislation that was proposed but not enacted by the 110th Congress (2007-2008) include S. 2029 (Physician Payments Sunshine Act of 2007), S. 3343 (Medicare Imaging Disclosure Sunshine Act of 2008), and H.R. 6752 (Independent Drug Education and Outreach Act of 2008). The first proposal has been revised and reintroduced in the 111th Congress (Grassley, 2009).

industry. For example, in an analysis of marketing literature and interactions between physicians and industry representatives, Roughead and colleagues (1998) noted that "[r]eciprocity is one of the norms by which society abides. . . . The provision of gifts by sales personnel encourages an automatic response of indebtedness on the part of the receiver who will then look for ways to make repayment" (p. 307). Other research has documented the importance of unconscious bias (see Appendix D).

Since 2000, a number of private and public groups have issued reports on conflict of interest in aspects of medical research, education, or practice. Table 1-2 lists some of the more prominent reports, several of which are discussed in later chapters of this report. Most reports have focused on research. Most have recognized the value of legitimate and properly designed research, educational, and technical relationships; but several have recommended some restrictions on other types of relationships and the more effective implementation of policies. In addition, the Pharmaceutical Research and Manufacturers of America (PhRMA) revised its voluntary *Code on Interactions with Healthcare Professionals* (effective January 2009) to more strongly discourage noninformational gifts, such as providing tickets to sporting events and token consulting arrangements (PhRMA, 2008). The Advanced Medical Technology Association has also revised its *Code of Ethics* for medical device manufacturers (effective July 2009) to include generally similar provisions (AdvaMed, 2008). (Other countries also have industry codes on relationships between the pharmaceutical industry and physicians [Jost, 2009].)

The recommendations in the reports listed in Table 1-2 are often similar (but not entirely consistent) in calling for more accountability and openness and more effective implementation. The policies of particular institutions vary, and some individuals may be subject to multiple policies that apply to their different roles and activities. To the extent that the adoption and implementation of policy recommendations have been evaluated, the results are mixed, as discussed in Chapter 3.

Evolution of Other Strategies to Limit Bias in Medical Research, Education, and Practice

At the same time that policy makers, universities, professional groups, and others were responding to concerns about conflict of interest, methodologists, statisticians, and scientists were working to develop and refine methods for designing and conducting research and analyzing data in ways that limit bias—whatever the source—during all stages of scientific investigation, from protocol design through the reporting of the results (see Chapter 4). In addition, academic medical centers have instituted education on evidence-based medicine to instruct future physicians on how to evaluate

TABLE 1-2 Selected Reports on Conflict of Interest Released Since 2000

Date	Organization	Title of Report or Paper
2001	Association of American Medical Colleges	*Protecting Subjects, Preserving Trust, Promoting Progress: Policy and Guidelines for the Oversight of Individual Financial Interests in Human Subjects Research*
2001	Association of American Universities	*Report on Individual and Institutional Financial Conflict of Interest*
2001	General Accounting Office	*Biomedical Research: HHS Direction Needed to Address Financial Conflicts of Interest*
2001	National Bioethics Advisory Commission	*Ethical and Policy Issues in Research Involving Human Participants*, Volume 1 (see the subsection on conflict of interest in Chapter 3)
2001	National Human Research Protections Advisory Committee	*Recommendations on HHS's Draft Interim Guidance on Financial Relationships in Clinical Research*
2002	Association of American Medical Colleges	*Protecting Subjects, Preserving Trust, Promoting Progress II: Principles and Recommendations for Oversight of an Institution's Financial Interests in Human Subjects Research*
2002	Council on Government Relations	*Recognizing and Managing Personal Conflicts of Interest*
2003	Council on Government Relations	*Approaches to Developing an Institutional Conflict of Interest Policy*
2004	American Association of University Professors	*Statement on Corporate Funding of Academic Research*
2004	National Institutes of Health	*Report of the National Institutes of Health Blue Ribbon Panel on Conflict of Interest Policies*
2007	Committee on Finance, U.S. Senate	*Use of Educational Grants by Pharmaceutical Manufacturers*
2007	Federation of American Societies for Experimental Biology	*Call to Action: Managing Financial Relationships Between Academia and Industry in Biomedical Research*
2007	National Institutes of Health	*Targeted Site Reviews on Financial Conflict of Interest: Observations*
2008	American Council on Education	*Working Paper on Conflict of Interest*
2008	Association of American Medical Colleges	*Industry Funding of Medical Education*
2008	Association of American Medical Colleges/ Association of American Universities	*Protecting Patients, Preserving Integrity, Advancing Health: Accelerating the Implementation of COI Policies in Human Subjects Research*

NOTE: These reports do not include organizational codes of conduct or institutional policies. Full citations for these reports are included in the References at the end of the main text of the report.

critically the evidence presented in (or absent from) journal articles, practice guidelines, and other sources of clinical information and advice (see, e.g., Bennett et al. [1987] and EBM Working Group [1992]). Others have worked to shift methods for the development of clinical practice guidelines away from unsystematic expert opinion and consensus processes toward formal, objective procedures for identifying and reviewing the relevant evidence and linking the strength and quality of the evidence to recommendations (see Chapter 7). These techniques and strategies work together with conflict of interest policies to reduce the risk of bias and maintain public trust in medical research, education, and practice.

ORGANIZATION OF REPORT

Chapter 2 sets forth a normative and conceptual framework for the report, including definitions and the criteria used to assess the potential benefits and harms created by financial relationships. Chapter 3 presents an overview of conflict of interest policies and what is known about their impact.

Chapters 4 through 7 are devoted to examinations of industry relationships and conflicts of interest in the domains of medical research, medical education, clinical practice, and practice guideline development, respectively. Chapter 8 discusses the importance of policies on conflicts that arise at the level of the institution. Finally, Chapter 9 discusses the role that accrediting and other supporting organizations can play in promoting the adoption and implementation of conflict of interest policies by the institutions that are on the front lines of medical education, research, and practice. Several appendixes provide additional background about the report or topics mentioned in the report.

2

Principles for Identifying and Assessing Conflicts of Interest

Relationships between physicians and biomedical researchers on the one hand and pharmaceutical, medical device, and biotechnology companies on the other hand are widespread and have produced important benefits, particularly in the development of new tests and treatments. At the same time, these relationships have also created significant risks that the financial goals of industry may conflict with the professional goals of medicine. The goals of for-profit medical companies are to produce products that improve health and, at the same time, to ensure a financial return to shareholders. The primary goals of medicine include improving health by providing beneficial care to patients, conducting valid research, and offering excellent medical education. In pursuing those goals, individual professionals, health care institutions, and research organizations have obligations to put patient interests first, carry out unbiased research, critically appraise information, and serve as role models of professional behavior for students. The problem of conflict of interest arises because in some circumstances in modern medicine these goals and obligations are at risk of being compromised by the undue pursuit of financial gain or other secondary interests.

Medicine today faces many difficult challenges, including, among others, high costs of treatment and associated pressures to cut costs, lack of availability of health insurance, and persistent medical errors. In comparison, the problem of conflict of interest may seem less significant. However, none of the other challenges can be adequately met if conflicts of interest are not well managed. For example, patients and the public need to be able to trust that the high costs of health care and health insurance arise from the provision of services that are beneficial, necessary, appropriately priced, and not inappropriately driven by the financial interests of physicians, other health care providers, or medical product companies. Failure to deal with the problem of conflict of interest can undermine efforts to address the other serious challenges that medical professionals and researchers face today.

This chapter develops a conceptual framework for identifying and assessing conflicts of interests.[1] In addition to defining the concept of conflict of interest and clarifying some common misunderstandings about its applications, the chapter presents principles to guide the formulation and implementation of conflict of interest policies. The principles take the form of (1) statements of the purposes of conflict of interest policies, (2) criteria for assessing the content of these policies, and (3) criteria for evaluating the implementation of policies. The principles do not directly yield decisions in particular cases or even rules that could be directly enforced, nor do they determine in advance the relative importance of all the values involved in making decisions. In applying them to particular policies and individual cases, there is no substitute for judicious practical judgment sensitive to the institutional context. However, the principles provide an essential framework for formulating and implementing any conflict of interest policy. They focus attention on the most important factors that should be considered when professionals and institutions make decisions and policies regarding conflicts of interest, select the agents who should be responsible for implementing and enforcing those policies, and choose the methods that they will use to regulate conflicts of interest.

WHAT IS A CONFLICT OF INTEREST?

Although conflict of interest policies are now widespread in many areas of medicine, the meaning and purposes of these policies are not always clearly understood. The term "conflict of interest" is used in many different and often inconsistent ways. Nonetheless, institutional and public policies on conflicts of interest need to define what the policies cover and what they do not cover.

The definition that the committee adopted is consistent with the core meaning of the concept as it is used in many institutional policies. It is, however, formulated to clarify key elements that are sometimes obscured in discussions of those policies.

---

[1] The discussion in this chapter draws on work by Thompson (1993) and Emanuel and Thompson (2008). The committee also consulted other definitions and frameworks, including those of Davis (1998), AAMC (2001), Davis and Stark (2001), NIH (2004), Moore et al. (2005), Lurie (2007), Sage (2007), AAMC-AAU (2008), and Beauchamp and Childress (2009).

A conflict of interest is a set of circumstances that creates a risk that professional judgment or actions regarding a primary interest will be unduly influenced by a secondary interest.

To avoid common misunderstandings of the concept that can lead to misplaced and ultimately ineffective or counterproductive policies, the committee stresses the importance of each of the three main elements of a conflict of interest: the primary interest, the secondary interest, and the conflict itself.

The primary interest that conflict of interest policies seek to protect varies according to the purpose of a professional activity. Primary interests include promoting and protecting the integrity of research, the welfare of patients, and the quality of medical education. Physicians and medical researchers accept the primacy of these interests when they act in their professional roles. Physicians and researchers exercise judgment and discretion in their work. Patients, the public, research participants, medical students, residents, and fellows need to trust physicians and researchers to act and make judgments in ways that are consistent with these primary interests. These primary interests are sometimes stated as ends or goals (e.g., promoting patient welfare), as obligations (e.g., the physician's obligation to promote patient welfare), or as rights (e.g., the patient's right to have the doctor promote his or her welfare). The committee uses the term primary "interests" to encompass all of these values, however they are stated. Whatever the primary interests are, the point of regulating conflicts of interest is to try to ensure that secondary interests do not subvert physicians' and researchers' decisions and actions regarding those primary interests and do not undermine trust in their clinical or scientific judgment. Furthermore, medical institutions—including medical schools, research institutes, professional societies, scientific journals, patient advocacy organizations, or government health agencies—should also keep these primary interests paramount, as discussed further in Chapter 8.

To be sure, identification of the exact primary interest in specific situations may sometimes be challenging, and primary interests sometimes conflict with each other. For example, in public health emergencies or under conditions of dire resource scarcity, physicians may have fundamental obligations to the population as a whole that may compete with their obligations to individual patients. In clinical research, the welfare of the participants in a study and the study's successful completion may be in conflict. Nonetheless, it is almost always clear that a primary interest should take precedence over a secondary interest.

The second main element of a conflict of interest is the secondary interest. Secondary interests may include not only financial gain but also the desire for professional advancement, recognition for personal achievement, and favors to friends and family or to students and colleagues. Conflict of interest policies typically and reasonably focus on financial gain and financial relationships. The reason is not that financial gains are necessarily more corrupting than the other interests but that they are relatively more objective, fungible, and quantifiable. A financial interest therefore tends to be more effectively and fairly regulated than other secondary interests. Furthermore, for-profit companies exert influence primarily through their financial relationships with physicians and researchers. They cannot bestow professional rewards such as prestigious scientific prizes that may also lead to conflicts of interest.

Most secondary interests, including financial interests, are—within limits—legitimate and even desirable goals. The secondary interests are objectionable only when they have greater weight than the primary interest in professional decision making. For example, for a researcher or a teacher, financial interests should be subordinate to presenting scientific evidence in an unbiased manner in publications and presentations.

A financial interest does not have to be great for the influence to be undue. Indeed, social science research suggests that gifts of small value may influence decisions (see Appendix D). It also suggests that influence may operate without an individual being conscious of it. When a secondary interest has inappropriate weight in a decision and distorts the pursuit of a primary interest, it is exerting undue influence.

The third key element of the definition is the conflict itself. It is not an occurrence in which primary interests are necessarily compromised but, rather, a set of circumstances or relationships that create or increase the risk that the primary interests will be neglected as a result of the pursuit of secondary interests. A conflict of interest exists whether or not a particular individual or institution is actually influenced by the secondary interest. The claim that a conflict of interest exists is based on common experience and social science research. Both experience and research indicate that under certain conditions there is a risk that professional judgment may be influenced more by secondary interests than by primary interests.

Some of these elements of a conflict of interest refer to degrees or quantities (e.g., more or less influence), but they are not directly quantifiable. What counts as undue is a matter of judgment and depends on the context. It is not a numerical probability but a judgment in a particular situation about whether a risk is undue or inappropriate. The standards for making such a judgment should be transparent and clearly specified in actual policies rather than in vague statements that professionals should avoid "undue influence." Subsequent chapters examine what situations or relationships may be considered inappropriate in research, patient care, medical education, and practice guideline development. Appendix C offers perspectives on conflicts of interest in other professions.

Conflicts of interest should be distinguished from other closely related conflicts. Not all conflicts in medicine are conflicts between a primary and a secondary interest. A conflict of obligation arises when an individual or institution has duties that require different actions but only one of these actions can be taken in the given circumstance. Dilemmas in medical ethics often take this form, that is, the need to make hard choices between two values, neither one of which is clearly superior to the other. A common example is maintaining the confidentiality of a patient with a contagious disease, which may conflict with preventing that patient from harming someone else. There is no conflict of interest in this example because both interests have plausible claims to be considered primary. Conflicts of obligation are essentially conflicts among different primary interests. Both obligations or interests are legitimate, often equally so, and it cannot be said in advance which one should take priority.

Conflicts of commitment are closer to conflicts of interest. They often involve a conflict between what institutions view as employees' primary responsibilities to the institution and the employees' outside commitments, such as voluntary community service, participation in a political campaign, or teaching or conducting research for another institution. Like conflicts between primary interests, conflicts of commitment involve two perfectly respectable activities (indeed, in some cases, identical activities, except that they are conducted at different institutions). Also, like conflicts of interest, the institution can legitimately claim in advance that one activity takes priority over the other if they come into conflict in any way. The concern is not usually about the risk of undue influence over specific decisions (e.g., the prescribing of a particular medication or the reporting of research findings). Rather, the concern is about time and effort, for example, whether individuals are devoting sufficient attention to their responsibilities within their own primary institution. Conflicts of interest and conflicts of commitment are sometimes covered in the same institutional policy; but the circumstances, risks, and evaluative frameworks are sufficiently different that they warrant separate consideration. Nevertheless, it makes sense for the policies to be covered in the same documents and information resources and to be administered by the same officials and committees.

WHAT ARE THE PURPOSES OF CONFLICT OF INTEREST POLICIES?

Institutions, professional organizations, and governments establish policies to address the problem of conflict of interest on behalf of the public. Conflict of interest policies are attempts to ensure that professional decisions are made on the basis of primary interests and not secondary interests. (See the discussion of the policies of other professions in Appendix C.)

As discussed further in Chapter 9, such policies work best when they are preventive and corrective rather than punitive. To the extent that they are effective, they serve two overarching purposes: maintaining the integrity of professional judgment and sustaining public confidence in that judgment. That professionals should promote these purposes constitutes the fundamental principle underlying any respectable conflict of interest policy.

First, the most obvious way in which the integrity of professional judgment can be compromised is through bias. Other practices can also undermine that integrity when they violate standards of professional conduct, such as the failure to publish research findings in a timely manner, the failure to treat students and postdoctoral fellows fairly, and a lack of openness with patients. Conflict of interest policies seek to minimize the influence of secondary interests in all these practices. They most significantly guard against the risk that financial interests will have excessive weight in decisions about the conduct of research, teaching, the provision of patient care, and the development of practice guidelines.

Such policies do not assume that any particular professional will necessarily let financial gain influence his or her judgment, nor do they imply that the individual researcher or physician is an unethical person. They assume only that under some conditions a risk exists that the decisions may be unduly influenced by considerations that should be irrelevant. Nonetheless, physicians and researchers are sometimes offended by assertions that they have conflicts of interest, believing that such assertions impugn their ethical integrity.

To avoid what they believe to be the negative connotations of "conflict of interest," some institutions use such phrases as "relationships with industry" or "financial relationships" to describe not only relationships that may be evaluated for the presence of potential conflicts but also relationships that are judged to be conflicts of interest. This less direct language has the effect of obscuring the serious risks that conflicts pose. Such language is not necessary if it is recognized that the determination that an individual or institution has a conflict of interest is a judgment about the situation and not about the professional who happens to be in that situation.

The second purpose of conflict of interest policies—to help sustain public confidence in professional judgment—is less appreciated but no less important. Here the goal is to minimize conditions that would cause reasonable individuals to suspect that professional judgment has been improperly influenced by secondary interests, whether or not it has. The public includes not only patients and research subjects but also editorial writers and journalists, officials at nonprofit foundations, public officials, and other opinion leaders. When or if the public and public officials distrust physicians, researchers, or educators, they are likely to seek greater government regulation, withhold funding, and take other steps that could jeopardize future programs of patient care, research, or education.

When a physician, researcher, or educator acts in ways that lead to distrust, the consequences may affect colleagues, patients, students, and the institution or profession as a whole. Similarly, institutional practices can be the source of distrust, and the effects of such distrust may be even more widespread and damaging than distrust of an individual. Physicians retain a high standing with the public compared with the standing of many other professional groups; but physicians should be vigilant, because once public confidence is undermined, it may be difficult to restore.

As discussed in Appendix C, other professions—law, accounting, engineering, and architecture—have also recognized the importance of conflict of interest policies and ethical codes to promote objectivity in decision making and sustain public confidence. In some recent cases, most notably, accounting, failure to adhere to these codes has led to increased government regulation.

WHY NOT EXAMINE THE MOTIVES OF THE DECISION MAKER OR THE VALIDITY OF THE DECISION?

Individuals accused of having a conflict of interest often say that they would never let financial interests influence their decisions. This objection to conflict of interest policies misses the point. Because (as noted above) the conflict is a set of circumstances or conditions involving a risk rather than a specific individual decision, the existence of a conflict of interest does not imply that any individual is improperly motivated. Nevertheless, an individual professional might still object that it is not fair to generalize in this way. He or she may want to say: "Look at my actual decisions and consider my distinguished reputation." However, conflict of interest policies are by their nature designed to avoid the need to investigate individual cases in this way. For at least two reasons, such policies do not focus on the motives in a particular case.

First, reliably ascertaining or inferring motives in this context is usually impossible for those assessing whether a relationship constitutes a conflict of interest. Generally, medical research, patient care, and education involve multiple considerations and many small judgments and decisions that are impractical to review; and even if they were reviewed, they would likely not yield a clear picture of the underlying motivation. Thus, readers of journal articles, medical students, patients, and conflict of interest committees are not in a good position to judge whether secondary interests motivated a decision. The motives behind institutional decisions are usually even more opaque.

Second, any thorough effort to determine motivation in a particular case would be improperly intrusive and highly time-consuming. Fair hearings could not be held and reliable conclusions could not be reached without risking violation of the rights of privacy of the many individuals who might be involved and without distracting many people from other important work.

Sometimes another, closely related objection to a claim that an individual has a conflict of interest is raised. This objection accepts that motives should not be considered but denies the relevance of the conditions under which decisions are made: "Judge my decision—the results of the research, the content of the lecture, the prescription of the drug—and not my financial interests." Here again the problem is that many people affected by professional decisions are not in a position to judge the validity of those decisions. In addition, those who are competent to judge may not be able to do so until after the damage has occurred. Furthermore, the argument for judging outcomes ignores one of the two main purposes of conflict of interest policies: the maintenance of public confidence. Even valid decisions and research may not be widely accepted as such if they occur under conditions in which secondary interests are prominent. Moreover, many decisions in research and clinical care are close calls. Plausible reasons can be cited for each of several alternative choices. The decisive factor in whether a judgment or an action is accepted as valid may turn on whether a researcher or a clinician can be trusted to be acting for the sake of scientific truth and the best interests of patients.

Because it is both intrusive and usually impracticable to investigate motives and because the competent and timely appraisal of decisions is often difficult, it may be tempting to conclude that patients, the public, and researchers simply need to trust physicians. Trust is important, but generalized trust and reliance that medical professionals act in accord with primary professional interests may be difficult to maintain in the face of evidence that this trust is sometimes abused. Furthermore, creating trust in medical professionals who conduct research or develop practice guidelines is hard because they have little or no contact with many of the people who are affected by their decisions and who have only limited knowledge with which to evaluate the decisions. Trust is necessary and desirable, but it must be based on reasonable expectations. Those who rely on professionals must have good reason to trust their decisions. In short, they need assurance that the professionals are trustworthy. Policies designed to reduce conflicts of interest and mitigate their impact provide an important foundation for public confidence in medical professionals and institutions.

SHOULD POLICIES ALSO REQUIRE THAT PROFESSIONALS AVOID THE "APPEARANCE OF CONFLICT OF INTEREST"?

Some conflict of interest policies refer to actual or perceived conflicts of interest and state that professionals should avoid "even the appearance of a conflict of interest." That requirement may lead to confusion. All conflicts of interest involve perceptions or appearances because they are specified from the perspective of people who do not have sufficient information with which to assess the actual motives of a decision maker and the effects of those motives on the decisions themselves.

Policies that contrast actual and perceived conflicts of interest give rise to two problems. First, the contrast suggests that there is no conflict (only an appearance of a conflict) unless the decision maker actually favors secondary interests over primary interests. The implication, then, is that conflict of interest policies should treat a perceived conflict as less serious than an actual conflict. However, when a professional's judgment is actually distorted by the acceptance of a gift or the prospect of influencing a stock in which the professional has an interest, the violation is no longer principally a conflict of interest but becomes a different kind of offense, one that may involve malpractice, scientific misconduct, or kickbacks. Those violations call for the use of procedures quite different from those on which conflict of interest policies should concentrate.

Second, the creation of a category of perceived conflicts, as distinct from actual conflicts, opens the door to overly broad and excessively subjective rules. If perceived conflicts are treated as different from the other (so-called actual) conflicts that the policy regulates, conduct that is perfectly proper can be unfairly called into question. With a loose notion of the perception or the appearance of a conflict of interest, circumstances that are suspicious only to uninformed people or predisposed reporters can be the basis of indiscriminate charges of conflicts of interest. Charges of conflicts of interest should be limited to circumstances specified by policies that are objectively grounded in past experience and reasonably interpreted on the basis of relevant and accessible information.

HOW CAN CONFLICTS OF INTEREST BE ASSESSED?

Conflicts are not binary; that is, they are not simply either present or absent. They can be more or less severe. The severity of a conflict depends on (1) the likelihood that professional decisions made under the relevant circumstances would be unduly influenced by a secondary interest and (2) the seriousness of the harm or wrong that could result from such influence. As discussed later in this chapter, the criterion of proportionality in conflict of interest policies provides that the expected benefits of a relationship may

TABLE 2-1 Criteria for Assessing the Severity of Conflicts of Interest

Likelihood of undue influence
- What is the value of the secondary interest?
- What is the scope of the relationship?
- What is the extent of discretion?

Seriousness of possible harm
- What is the value of the primary interest?
- What is the scope of the consequences?
- What is the extent of accountability?

be considered, and conflicts of interest may be allowed to continue if those benefits outweigh the risks and safeguards that are instituted.

Table 2-1 lists the questions that need to be asked when the severity of a conflict of interest is assessed in particular cases. These questions express criteria or principles that identify the most important factors to be considered in formulating policies and making decisions about conflicts of interest. Assessments of the likelihood of undue influence and the seriousness of the consequences usually reflect general judgments about situations—on the basis of experience—rather than evaluations of the character of the individual in question. The individual's behavior in similar situations in the past might, however, be taken into account. The next two sections discuss the criteria in more depth.

Assessing the Likelihood of Undue Influence

In assessing the likelihood of undue influence, it is reasonable to assume that the greater that the value of the secondary interest is (e.g., the greater that the size of the financial gain is), the more probable is its influence. Thus, equity or other ownership interests in a small biotechnology company have great potential for an increase in value on the basis of the results of a clinical trial (as well as the potential for no value). Large fees for serving on a company advisory board are more valuable than occasional small honoraria for talks. Although absolute value is important, the secondary interest should generally be measured in relation to the typical income for the relevant class of professionals or in relation to the value of a research project, institutional budget, or medical practice.

However, the monetary value of a secondary interest is not the only appropriate measure of its potential impact. The economic value of pens, inexpensive meals, and other nominal gifts or relationships is low; but as explained in Appendix D, small gifts may help to create and sustain relationships, for example, between a physician and a pharmaceutical company and its representatives. The influence of such gifts and relationships may be subtle and the individual receiving such gifts may not even be conscious of their influence. It may therefore be necessary to manage or prohibit conflicts of interest even when the value of the secondary interest, as measured only by monetary value, is low and the likelihood of harm or wrong in a single instance is low.

Other aspects of relationships besides their dollar value may also increase their general value and therefore the risk of a conflict of interest. For example, payments that augment the income of an individual professional may create more concern than those that exclusively support the academic activities of a whole institution. A consulting arrangement that increases a researcher's income will tend to create more concern than one in which payments are made to the institution, department, or research group as a whole and disbursed under institutional oversight. Similarly, a research contract that is reviewed by a university for consistency with policies on data access, sponsor review, and publication rights will generally create less risk of a conflict of interest than a consulting arrangement that does not receive such review or that is reported only in very general terms (e.g., as involving payments over $20,000 when the actual amount is $200,000).

A second factor affecting the likelihood of undue influence is the scope of a relationship, which refers to its duration and depth. Longer and closer associations increase the scope and therefore the risk. Examples of such associations include a multiyear consulting agreement, a continuing leadership position as a member of a company board, or the weekly or monthly provision of free lunches at a physician's office. Likewise, long-term funding of a university or commercial continuing medical education program has more potential for influence than a one-time grant. Similarly, serving on a company's scientific advisory board, which more intimately ties the professional to the company over time, is more likely to affect the professional's judgment than accepting a fee for speaking about a company-sponsored research project.

The extent of discretion, that is, how much latitude a professional enjoys in making important decisions, is also pertinent. Even though some of their judgments are subject to various kinds of review, the principal investigator in a clinical trial exercises considerable discretion over innumerable, wide-ranging, and often hidden decisions, for example, decisions regarding the eligibility of patients to enter the clinical trial, determinations of clinical end points, ascribing of adverse events to the study intervention, the type of statistical analyses to be used, and the reporting of the results. This discretion is often limited by an independent oversight body, for example, a data and safety monitoring board, an independent panel that adjudicates adverse events, a medical monitor of adverse events, or an external auditor for data collection at individual research sites. Such oversight is usually required for any clinical trials whose results will be presented to the Food and Drug Administration for regulatory approval of a drug or medical device. In assessing such limits on discretion, it is also important to consider the independence of the judgment of the members of any oversight body. Furthermore, the more closely that the research and data analysis methods follow standard methods, the less room there is for improper influence. Similarly, the more conventional the subject matter of educational presentations, the less scope there is for bias that is not easily detected.

Authority and discretion often vary by role. Principal investigators can influence multiple dimensions of a research project, whereas laboratory technicians or research assistants have less scope for influence in most situations. Deans and chancellors, through their power to control appointments, promotions, salaries, and space, wield great power, although they are typically several steps removed from conducting research projects or teaching courses. At the other extreme, most administrative staff members have little power to influence a university's research or teaching mission.

Assessing the Seriousness of Possible Harm

The starting point in assessing the seriousness of possible harm from a conflict of interest is to identify or specify the value of the primary interest. This report concentrates on the primary goals of medicine, particularly patient care, research, and medical education. Assessing the severity of a conflict requires an examination of the specific primary goal or goals at risk in a particular situation.

A second consideration is the scope of the consequences. The greater that the scope is, the more serious is the potential for harm. Conflicts of interest that may affect multiple patient care decisions have a large scope. For example, practice guidelines that set standards of care and criteria for insurance coverage may affect millions of patients. The results of a clinical trial for a common condition can affect how thousands of physicians prescribe a specific medication. Results from a pivotal trial of a novel type of therapy that may dramatically alter patient care are likely to have a larger scope than other trials that will influence care only at the margins. Thus, conflicts of interest in clinical trials deserve special attention because of the potentially large scope of their effects.

A conflict of interest may also have negative effects on an individual's colleagues or institution. Such effects need to be taken into account even if they do not occur frequently. A pharmaceutical or medical device company's sponsorship of a research project could raise questions about the work of other researchers in the institution and weaken their ability to raise funds from other sources. A professor's close connections with a company not only could raise doubts about the objectivity of his class materials and presentations, but these connections could also have negative effects on the careers of his teaching assistants and the collegial culture of the institution. In view of such possible consequences, the fact that an individual has a right to engage in an activity should not be allowed to obscure the equally important fact that his or her actions may affect the rights of colleagues and students. The claim of an individual right by a professional does not preclude the possibility that this right may be regulated.

Finally, the seriousness of the possible harm depends in part on the extent of accountability. In general, a conflict of interest is more serious when the level of accountability of the physician, researcher, or educator to his or her peers, institution, licensing board, or similar entity is less extensive. If accountability for decisions is bolstered by an independent review of those decisions by colleagues or other authorities, there is generally less potential for harm and less cause for concern. However, the reviewers must be and must be viewed as being effective and independent and must have no conflicts of interest of their own. Accountability is also greater to the extent that sanctions for serious violations of policies are significant and imposed in a timely fashion, and it is further enhanced if the results of the disciplinary proceedings are regularly disclosed.

In summary, an overall assessment of whether a financial relationship constitutes a conflict of interest and, if so, how severe it is and how it should be managed depends on several considerations: the importance of the financial or other relationship for furthering primary medical values, the likelihood and seriousness of possible harm to those primary values, and the availability of measures that can reduce the likelihood or severity of harm. Chapter 3 discusses such measures and also the procedures applied by universities and other institutions to identify, limit, and manage conflicts of interest.

HOW CAN CONFLICT OF INTEREST POLICIES BE EVALUATED?

The discussion above focused on several questions and factors that should be considered in assessing the severity of a conflict of interest in financial relationships. They are intended to provide guidance for the formulation of the content of policies for controlling conflict of interest, for example, the specification of the information needed from individuals that will be sufficient to evaluate financial relationships, assess the severity of conflicts of interest, and guide responses to identified conflicts. Additional criteria are needed to evaluate the implementation or actual operation of the policies (Table 2-2). Even if policies are well formulated, they must also be well administered.

TABLE 2-2 Criteria for Evaluating Conflict of Interest Policies

Criterion	Description
Proportionality	Is the policy most efficiently directed at the most important conflicts?
Transparency	Is the policy comprehensible and accessible to the individuals and institutions that may be affected by the policy?
Accountability	Does the policy indicate who is responsible for enforcing and revising it?
Fairness	Does the policy apply equally to all relevant groups within an institution and in different institutions?

Proportionality

First, the criterion of proportionality calls for policies to be efficient and effective in addressing serious conflicts of interest in a preventive or a corrective way. Complicated rules and elaborate procedures can become merely bureaucratic obstacles unless they are implemented and regularly reviewed with the goals of the policy in mind. Do the policies actually address the most important and common conflicts? Are the policies practical; that is, can they actually be effectively implemented at an acceptable cost? Are the policies administered in a way that appropriately considers the likelihood of bias, the seriousness of the harm, and the potential benefits of the conflicting secondary interest (as noted above)? Do the policies and their application unnecessarily interfere with the conduct of legitimate research, teaching, and clinical practice? Do the anticipated benefits of the policies outweigh their various costs, such as administrative burdens, and any negative consequences? The effectiveness of a specific policy can be judged only after that policy has been in use for a period of time. Insofar as experience and evaluations have raised questions about the effectiveness of similar policies already adopted, however, these questions can guide the design and implementation of new policies. Finally, whether policies can achieve their overall aims will also depend on their congruence with other criteria, such as fairness and transparency, that contribute to effectiveness and that are also important for their own sake.

The criterion of proportionality should also be applied in individual situations when an assessment is made of whether a financial relationship constitutes a conflict of interest and, if there is a conflict, how it should be handled. For example, when a researcher's financial relationship with a company is evaluated, its expected benefits as well as its risks should be considered. As discussed in Chapters 1 and 4, industry support for well-designed and scientifically meritorious research tends to advance a primary goal of generating valid scientific knowledge. This may sometimes mean that an institution should allow an individual with a conflict of interest to participate in an activity because the expected benefits exceed the risks and because the risks have been lowered to an acceptable level. For example, an academic medical center may allow a scientist who holds the patent on a promising discovery to participate in developing a product and designing an early-stage clinical trial to evaluate an intervention because his or her involvement may be necessary to ensure that the product is safely and correctly administered. (These kinds of situations, which should be exceptional, are discussed further in Chapters 4 and 7.)

Transparency

Just as disclosure is usually necessary—even if it is insufficient—in dealing with conflicts of interest, so too is transparency necessary in administering conflict of interest policies. Transparent policies are readily available in clear and simple language, together with explanations and essential information about their application. They are also available not only to those who are subject to them (e.g., researchers, authors of journal articles, or members of practice guidelines panels) but also to other stakeholders, including the public. Transparency is essential to determine whether conflict of interest policies are reasonable and if they are being implemented fairly.

Conflict of interest policies may require the public disclosure of financial and some other relationships under certain circumstances, as described in Chapter 3. These disclosure policies reflect the institutions' ethical and sometimes legal responsibility to disseminate relevant information to appropriate parties. In addition, the values of transparency are also served when institutions explain their judgments in certain cases, for example, when they allow an investigator with a financial stake in the outcome of a study with human participants to conduct that research (see Chapter 4).

Rights of privacy and protection of confidentiality place some limits on how much information an institution discloses and to whom. For example, physicians have a countervailing privacy interest when it is proposed that their financial relationships (and perhaps those of their family members) be disclosed to the public, as noted in the discussion in Appendix F of public disclosure of personal information reported to academic medical centers and other institutions. Disclosures beyond the institution can be limited to the minimum amount of identifiable personal information that is needed to carry out policy goals. For some purposes, reporting aggregate or deidentified information to the public is sufficient.

Transparency can also help improve conflict of interest policies across institutions. Information about the way that one institution has handled a particular case or type of case can enable other institutions to learn about more and less effective practices and adjust their own policies and behaviors accordingly.

Accountability

Accountable individuals and institutions explain and take responsibility for their conduct and decisions. Thus, just as a physician explains the rationale for clinical decisions to patients and researchers explain the rationale for research and research procedures, so too will leaders of accountable institutions explain their policies and their application to the individuals who are directly affected and respond to questions and suggestions.

Taking responsibility for the consequences of individual or institutional actions and decisions may involve offering apologies or compensation to those harmed by these actions and acknowledging the appropriateness of penalties when a representative of the institution has acted improperly or illegally. To demonstrate that it is accountable, an institution not only will develop explicit conflict of interest policies and procedures for implementing its policies but also will devise ways to communicate how they are applied in practice. Institutional leaders will be prepared to explain how judgments about conflicts of interest are reasonably consistent across similar cases and why, for example, they determined that it was sufficient to require only the disclosure of a relationship in one case but appropriate to manage or prohibit the relationship in another case. Finally, institutional leaders will be ready to respond to questions about their own interests and impartiality. As discussed in Chapter 8, leaders should establish procedures for dealing with the conflicts that their own institutions may have.

Public engagement is often important for accountability. For example, accountability is generally enhanced if public representatives serve on institutional panels that review individual relationships that may present conflicts of interest. To cite a somewhat parallel situation, federal regulations require institutional review boards to include at least one member not affiliated with the institution. Also, as part of a commitment to openness and accountability, organizations may invite public comment on their conflict of interest policies and may take seriously suggestions for revisions. Public participation can enhance the credibility and trustworthiness of decisions about individual cases as well as more general policies.

A final aspect of accountability is a commitment to improving conflict of interest policies and their implementation. Setting benchmarks for performance and tracking outcomes can stimulate quality improvement activities, as has been demonstrated with other activities in health care organizations.

Fairness

The formal principle of fairness requires similar treatment for those in relevantly similar situations and different treatment for those in relevantly different situations. This principle has at least two implications for the application of conflict of interest policies.

First, these policies should apply to all employees or members of an institution who make significant decisions for the institution or who have substantial influence over these decisions. In academic medical centers, these decisions may involve medical education, medical research, or clinical care. Thus, residents, fellows, faculty, members of institutional committees (e.g., institutional review boards, formulary committees, and device purchasing committees), and senior institutional officials are all subject to conflict of interest policies and procedures. Although medical students do not usually have an influence over decisions that are made, they too should be expected to follow conflict of interest rules, which are among the important professional norms they are learning as they prepare for their future careers. At the same time, to be fair, conflict of interest policies and procedures may reasonably differ for people in different roles. For a medical student or resident, the policy issue might be accepting mugs, pens, and lunches from companies. For a senior leader in the institution, the issue might be serving on the board of directors of a company manufacturing medical products and receiving personal compensation for this position. In some cases, the policy response might be to prohibit a practice overall, whereas in other instances management of the conflict could be an option, depending on the specifics of the situation, as assessed by the standards listed in Table 2-1.

Second, fairness requires that individuals in different institutions who are in situations that are similar in all ethically relevant ways be treated similarly. Otherwise, the ethical basis for policies may be called into question and conflict of interest policies and decisions may be regarded as arbitrary. Although conflict of interest regulations for U.S. Public Health Service grantees and policies recommended by the Association of American Medical Colleges allow institutions discretion in setting and implementing policies to take account of local circumstances, it is important to justify such variation in ways that are understandable by and plausible to affected individuals, oversight agencies, and the public.

CONCLUSION

The purposes of conflict of interest policies are expressed in the principles that hold that professionals should act to protect the primary interests of medical practice, education, and research and to maintain public confidence in the integrity of those activities. The problem of conflict of interest is more complex than is often appreciated. As a result, both critics and defenders of conflict of interest policies sometimes misunderstand or misapply them.

A conflict of interest is not an actual occurrence of bias or a corrupt decision but, rather, a set of circumstances that past experience and other evidence have shown poses a risk that primary interests may be compromised by secondary interests. The existence of a conflict of interest does not imply that any individual is improperly motivated. To avoid these and similar mistakes and to provide guidance for formulating and applying such policies, a framework for analyzing conflicts of interest is desirable.

This chapter has presented principles for assessing conflicts of interest and evaluating policies designed to deal with such conflicts. Conflicts should be assessed by considering various factors that determine their likelihood and seriousness. Likelihood depends on the value of the secondary interest, the scope of the relationship between the professionals and the commercial interests, and the extent of discretion that the professionals have. Seriousness depends on the value of the primary interest, the scope of the consequences that affect it, and the extent of accountability of the professionals. Conflict of interest policies should be evaluated by considering their effectiveness, transparency, accountability, and fairness.

A better understanding of the nature of conflicts of interest and the clearer and fairer formulation of rules can support greater confidence in the medical profession and thereby enable physicians, educators, and investigators to concentrate on their primary missions of treating patients, teaching students, and conducting research. With robust conflict of interest policies in place, they can continue to carry out their respective activities not in wary confrontation but in beneficial cooperation with the representatives of industry.

3

Policies on Conflict of Interest: Overview and Evidence

Current conflict of interest policies and practices have evolved over more than four decades of increasing relationships with industry in medical education, research, and practice. The increase has been accompanied by intensifying discussions about how the risks and the expected benefits of these relationships should be evaluated and balanced. Since 1995, the U.S. Public Health Service (PHS) has required most research grantees to establish policies and procedures to ensure that the design, conduct, or reporting of research funded by PHS grants not be "biased by any conflicting financial interest of an Investigator" (42 CFR 50.601). The regulations, which are included in Appendix B, allow grantees considerable discretion in formulating policies and procedures. To provide more specific and comprehensive guidance to academic institutions on conflict of interest policies, the Association of American Medical Colleges (AAMC, 2001, 2002, 2008c), the Association of American Universities (AAU, 2001), AAMC and AAU jointly (AAMC-AAU, 2008), and the Council on Government Relations (COGR, 2002) have issued several reports with recommendations. The Federation of American Societies for Experimental Biology (FASEB) created a conflict of interest tool kit that offers extensive online resources and guidance for academic institutions, researchers, academic and professional societies, journal editors, and industry (FASEB, 2008). In 2008, the trade associations representing major pharmaceutical and medical device companies revised their codes on company interactions with health care professionals (AdvaMed, 2008; PhRMA, 2008). In addition, a number of academic medical centers, professional societies, medical journals, and other institutions have revised their policies in recent years.

Criticisms of current policies and their application come from different directions. Some object that policies requiring the disclosure of financial interests can be carried too far, encouraging "readers to make *ad hominem* judgements" (Rothman, 2001, p. 1275) or shifting "attention away from the merits of the work and toward the biography of its author" (Jansen and Sulmasy, 2003, p. 40). Another critic describes disclosure policies as a kind of "new scientific McCarthyism" that assumes that researchers with industry ties are "tainted and untrustworthy" (Whelan, 2008, p. A19). One researcher has criticized "conflict of interest vigilantes" who "search for evidence that doctors have failed to disclose corporate connections in publications or in presentations" (Stossel, 2007, p. 59). He has also argued that continuing medical education disclosure policies mainly serve to protect bureaucrats rather than students, are based on ideology rather than evidence, and "are deeply disrespectful of physicians and researchers" (Stossel, 2008, p. 476). (See Chapter 1 for additional criticisms.)

Others, however, argue that conflict of interest policies—when they exist—are often weak, inconsistent, and inadequately administered and enforced. For example, the American Medical Student Association (AMSA) assessed the conflict of interest policies of medical schools and concluded that the policies of the majority of the schools that responded either lacked important elements or were unlikely to influence behavior (AMSA, 2008b).[1] Whether or not one agrees with how AMSA rated the policies, the actual texts of the policies (available at or through the AMSA website) reveal considerable variability, which is consistent with the findings of this report. Members of the U.S. Congress have strongly criticized physicians and researchers who have failed to report substantial financial relationships with industry, as they were required to do, and have proposed that pharmaceutical and medical device companies be required to report publicly their payments to physicians (see, e.g., Grassley [2008b, 2009]). Also in response to concerns about the nature of financial ties between physicians and industry and the lack of disclosure of such ties, Massachusetts enacted legislation in 2008 that requires companies to report payments to physicians, researchers, and medical societies and further provides for a marketing code of conduct

[1] In AMSA's assessment, 9 medical schools received a rating of A and 19 received a rating of B for their policies; 44 schools received a rating of F (18 for the contents of the policies that they submitted, 9 for their refusal to submit policies, and 17 for their lack of a response after repeated requests). Another 46 schools had policies under revision. (The numbers of schools are based on the ratings listed as of February 13, 2009, at http://www.amsascorecard.org/.) The project's methodology, included the rating system, is available at http://amsascorecard.org/methodology and states that "[e]ach policy was graded by two independent assessors, blinded to the institution of origin. Any differences in scoring between the two assessors were resolved by a consensus process. The assessors received formal training in the use of the scoring system, independently evaluating and coming to a consensus on five training policies before beginning to evaluate the medical school policies."

that will prohibit or limit certain of these payments (Wallack, 2008; Lopes, 2009).

This chapter outlines the basic elements of conflict of interest policies, reviews empirical data about the characteristics and consequences of those policies, and concludes with recommendations. Much of the research and descriptive information located by the committee examined the policies of academic institutions and medical journals; but the recommendations apply broadly to all institutions engaged in medical research, medical education, clinical care, or practice guideline development. The specific elements of the policies may vary according to the size, complexity, and other characteristics of different types of institutions (e.g., academic medical centers, professional societies, patient advocacy groups, and nursing homes).

The focus in this chapter is on policies affecting individuals, primarily physicians and biomedical researchers (as explained in Chapter 1). Chapter 8 examines and makes recommendations about policies that govern institutional conflict of interest, which is defined to include the interests of senior institutional officials.

OVERVIEW OF CONFLICT OF INTEREST POLICIES

Most conflict of interest policies include the basic elements of the disclosure of financial relationships, the prohibition of certain relationships, and the management of conflicts of interest that have been identified. All of these elements are sometimes described under the general rubric of managing conflicts of interest.[2] Other common elements of conflict of interest policies include definitions, specification of who is subject to the policies, enforcement provisions, and identification of which officials or units within an organization are responsible for administering and monitoring conflict of interest policies and procedures. Depending on the circumstances and the type of institution, the person responsible for reviewing initial disclosures may be a department chair, the chair of a professional society committee developing practice guidelines, the editor or deputy editor of a journal, or the chair of a continuing medical education program. When an initial review identifies a possible conflict of interest, the case may be referred to a conflict of interest committee or a more senior official for further evaluation and response.

Building on Chapter 2, Box 3-1 outlines a conceptual model of the

[2] PHS rules refer to procedures to "identify and manage, reduce, or eliminate conflicting interests." Federal government policies for its employees are sometimes described in terms of the "'three-D' method of conflict of interest regulation, that is: disclosure, disqualification and divestiture" (Maskell, 2007, p. 3). Disqualification includes recusal from participation in a specific decision.

BOX 3-1
Model of Steps Used to Identify and Respond to a Conflict of Interest

Step 1 Obtain the disclosure of information about financial and other relationships that could constitute a conflict of interest.

No relationships reported: stop. Relationships disclosed: go to Step 2.

Step 2 Evaluate the disclosures—in light of the individual's responsibilities or specific activities (e.g., research, teaching, and patient care)—to determine whether a conflict of interest exists. If necessary, collect additional information to assess the likelihood of undue influence and the seriousness of possible harms.

No conflict exists: stop. Conflict exists: go to Step 3.

Step 3 Determine whether the relationship is one prohibited under institutional or other policies or whether the risks of the relationship are so serious that the individual should either eliminate it or forgo participation in the activity put at risk by the relationship.

Conflict elimination necessary: go to Step 5.
Elimination not necessary: go to Step 4.

Step 4 If management is appropriate, devise and implement a plan to manage the conflict. Go to Step 5.

Step 5 Monitor conflict elimination or management plan and assess adherence.

Plan followed. Plan not followed: go to Step 6.

Step 6 Determine the nature of the noncompliance and the appropriate response (e.g., education, penalty, or revision of the plan) and implement the response.

steps that institutions with a comprehensive conflict of interest policy and implementation strategy might follow when determining whether an individual has a conflict of interest and, if so, how to respond. It shows the elimination of an identified conflict of interest as an early step, although the committee's experience suggests that the elimination of a conflicting relationship is often considered a last option.

A given individual may be covered by several conflict of interest policies. For example, a medical school faculty member may have to understand and follow the policies not only of the medical school but also those of several other institutions. Depending on his or her activities, these other policies might include those of a medical journal, a provider of continuing medical education, a professional society, or a federal advisory committee. If a faculty member is engaged in research to support an application for marketing approval of a medical product by the Food and Drug Administration (FDA), the researcher can expect the study's sponsor to ask for the disclosure of his or her financial interests related to the company and the investigational product so that the sponsor can submit the required information to the FDA (FDA, 2001). (A recent report by the Office of the Inspector General [OIG] of the U.S. Department of Health and Human Services criticized the administration of these policies and indicated that they were deficient in several respects [OIG, 2009].) Private organizations that fund research, such as the Howard Hughes Medical Institute, also may have conflict of interest policies, which they may oversee directly rather than following the practice of the National Institutes of Health (NIH) of delegating most administrative responsibility to the research institution (Cech and Leonard, 2001). In addition, the faculty of public institutions will likely be covered by state conflict of interest policies.[3]

The committee found few reviews or studies documenting and comparing the conflict of interest policies of institutions engaged in medical research, medical education, or clinical care. It found even less information about the implementation and effects of these policies. Most studies examine the policies of academic institutions, medical and scientific journals, or government agencies. Journal articles or news stories sometime report on individual professional societies and patient or consumer groups.

In addition, through its literature review, public meetings, and other information-collecting activities, the committee identified various examples of institutional policies.[4] Although these examples are not necessarily representative, they helped the committee better understand the nature of policy variability and, in some cases, the rationale for policy differences. Institutions differ considerably in the conflict of interest policy information that they make public on their websites; and even if they are available, online information is not necessarily comprehensive, clear, or current. Since the committee began work, a number of medical schools, professional societies, and other groups have announced changes in their conflict of interest

[3] The state of Washington recently changed its policies on the use of certain university resources for outside work for faculty and some other university employees to "encourage the ethical transfer of technology for the economic benefit" of the state (University of Washington, 2008).

[4] During the study, the committee benefited from initiatives by AMSA and the Institute on Medicine as a Profession to make medical center policies available online. These databases have been useful, although they are not complete, and many schools have indicated that they are updating their policies.

policies and practices. Thus, even relatively recent overviews of conflict of interest policies may be somewhat out of date.

DISCLOSURE: AN ESSENTIAL BUT INSUFFICIENT ELEMENT OF POLICY

Disclosure—that is, revealing to others information that may otherwise be private or confidential—is a frequent response to concerns about conflicts of interest in various sectors of society. Disclosure by physicians and researchers to their academic or other institution is essential because institutional officials cannot evaluate and respond to individuals' relationships with industry if they are not aware of them. Consistent with the conceptual framework outlined in Chapter 2, disclosures should provide sufficient information about the nature, scope, duration, and monetary value of relationships to allow institutions to assess the risk that secondary interests might unduly influence judgments about research, clinical care, education, or other primary interests.

The committee distinguished disclosure to the physician's or researcher's institution from disclosure beyond the institution, for example, to patients, research participants, or the public.[5] One rationale for disclosure—especially public disclosure—is the deterrence of questionable or inappropriate relationships. As Supreme Court Justice Louis Brandeis (1914) famously expressed it, "sunshine is said to be the best of disinfectants." In a similar vein, the code of ethics of the American College of Physicians suggests that physicians considering the acceptance of gifts or other relationships with companies should ask themselves what their patients, the public, or their colleagues would think about the arrangement (Snyder and Leffler, 2005; see also Chapter 6). The *Nature* publishing group urges authors to avoid "any undeclared competing financial interests that could embarrass you were they to become publicly known after your work was published" (NPG, 2008).

Disclosure should have beneficial consequences if it leads physicians to avoid gifts, the use of industry-controlled presentations, and other relationships that create a risk of compromising their decisions and their professional independence. It could also have harmful consequences if physicians or researchers react by avoiding relationships that promote im-

[5] Some analyses refer to the provision of information to institutional officials as "reporting" and reserve the term "disclosure" for the revelation of information to members of the public (e.g., journal readers or patients) (see, e.g., AAMC [2001]). In contrast, some policies refer to reporting of information to external groups. This report follows the common usage (including in federal policies and guidance) and applies the term "disclosure" to the provision of information to internal parties as well as to external parties.

portant societal goals and that are accompanied by adequate measures to protect objective judgment.

What Is Known About Disclosure Policies, Practices, and Consequences

This section first reviews information about the characteristics of disclosure policies and practices. It then turns to evidence about the effectiveness of disclosure.

Presence and Scope of Disclosure Requirements

Medical schools The most recent comprehensive study of medical school conflict of interest policies reports on a 2003 AAMC survey of member schools (response rate of 82 percent) that was designed to characterize their policies and assess the extent to which they were consistent with the association's 2001 recommendations on conflict of interest in clinical research (Ehringhaus and Korn, 2004).[6] It found considerable variation. Almost all (95 percent) of the respondents reported that their policies covered all research involving human participants regardless of the funding source.[7] Sixty-eight percent of the schools used the PHS threshold ($10,000)[8] for individuals to disclose certain financial interests to the institution, whereas 27 percent reported a lower threshold. For elements not required by the PHS regulations, more than 60 percent of the respondents requested disclosure to the institution of equity in nonpublicly traded companies, regardless of the percent share (61 percent) or the estimated valuation (64 percent). The majority requested the disclosure of royalty income either above a certain threshold (38 percent) or regardless of the amount (33 percent).

In addition to requiring disclosure to the institution, policies may also require that financial relationships or conflicts of interest be disclosed to individuals who might be affected by the relationship. These might include research colleagues, research participants, journal readers, students, or

[6] The committee also reviewed several earlier studies for additional context and understanding of policy evolution (see, e.g., Cho et al. [2000], Lo et al. [2000], and McCrary et al. [2000]).

[7] In 2004, the Government Accountability Office reported that 79 percent of universities responding to their survey said that they had a single conflict of interest policy that covered all research. This is consistent with the recommendation of the AAU Task Force on Research Accountability that "all research projects at an institution, whether federally funded, funded by a non-federal entity, or funded by the institution itself, should be managed by the same conflict of interest process and treated the same" (AAU, 2001, p. 5).

[8] The PHS regulations state that individuals do not need to report "salary, royalties or other payments that *when aggregated for the Investigator and the Investigator's spouse and dependent children* over the next twelve months, are not expected to exceed $10,000" (NIH, 2008a, question C6, emphasis added). A similar rule applies to the disclosure of equity interests.

TABLE 3-1 Percentage of Medical Schools Requiring Further Disclosures for Researchers with a Significant Financial Interest in Their Research

Further Disclosure Required	Percentage of Medical Schools
To research participant in informed consent forms	74
To sponsors or funders of the research	65
To editors of journals to which papers or reports of research are submitted	64
In oral presentations of research results	60
In multicenter trials, to investigators, sponsors, and other institutional review boards participating in the trial	42
Other	23

SOURCE: Adapted from Ehringhaus and Korn, 2004.

patients. Again, the AAMC survey showed variation in medical school policies (Table 3-1).

A study by Weinfurt and colleagues (2006b) also reported on variations in disclosure policies. Forty-eight percent of medical schools had policies that mentioned the disclosure of researchers' financial conflicts of interest to research participants. The policies varied in what information was to be disclosed.

Medical and scientific journals The International Committee of Medical Journal Editors (ICMJE) has proposed Uniform Requirements for Manuscripts Submitted to Biomedical Journals that include explanations and provisions about conflicts of interest (ICMJE, 2008). The ICMJE website lists several hundred journals that follow these requirements, but the group does not verify the extent to which a journal does so. The World Association of Medical Journal Editors (WAME) has also made recommendations on conflict of interest policies (WAME, 2008).

Even journals that adopt conflict of interest policies may not apply them equally to industry-funded journal supplements that present papers from a conference or collections of papers on a particular topic. These supplements are generally not peer reviewed and have been criticized for including articles of lower quality (Bero et al., 1992; Rochon et al., 1994). The National Library of Medicine will not cite and index articles from certain types of sponsored supplements unless they include specific disclosures about "any financial relationship the guest editors and authors have with the sponsoring organization and any interests that organization represents, as well as with any for-profit product discussed or implied in the supplement and/or individual articles" (NLM, 2007, unpaged).

Journals may also vary their policies for review articles and editorials or may not apply their policies to review articles and editorials, which arguably offer more room for bias than original research articles. For example, a 2004 editorial in the *Journal of the American College of Cardiology* stated that the editors generally decline publication of review articles disclosing industry input out of concern for external influence and subtle bias (DeMaria, 2004). Editors of another journal initially declared that they would not accept review articles written by authors with conflicts of interest and then decided that it would accept such articles if the conflicts were not significant (e.g., they involved payments that were less than $10,000) (Drazen and Curfman, 2002).

Two recent analyses found considerable variability in the conflict of interest policies of medical and scientific journals. Cooper and colleagues (2006b) found that 93 percent of biomedical journals reported that they had conflict of interest policies applicable to authors, 46 percent reported that they had policies applicable to reviewers, and 40 percent reported that they had policies applicable to editors. Fifty-seven percent reported that they published disclosures for all articles. Earlier studies reported that the percentage of biomedical journals with disclosure policies was lower (see, e.g., McCrary et al. [2000] and Krimsky and Rothenberg [2001]). Ancker and Flanagin (2007) were able to locate online conflict of interest policies for only 33 percent of 84 "high-impact, peer-reviewed" journals in 12 scientific disciplines, but a subsequent survey found that 80 percent of the 49 responding journals reported that they had policies in place.

Journals vary in whether they give specific guidance to authors regarding what financial relationships or conflicts of interest must be disclosed. Ancker and Flanagin (2007) found that 68 percent of journals provided examples of conflicts of interest and 46 percent defined the term. The committee's review of a convenience sample of journal policies revealed differences in the specificities of the policies. One journal advises simply, "[a]uthors are required to disclose any sponsorship or funding arrangements relating to their research and all authors should disclose any possible conflicts of interest" (AJN, 2008). In contrast, the *New England Journal of Medicine* states that disclosures are to include "all of the authors' relationships with companies that make products studied or discussed in the article, companies that make related products, and other pertinent entities with an interest in the topic" (NEJM, 2008). Some journals ask authors about several specific types of relationships and also ask them to indicate explicitly if they have no relationships. One journal's manuscript agreement form asks authors to certify that their manuscript has not been sponsored by a commercial entity and that if their manuscript includes no acknowledgments, it means that nonauthors have made no substantial contribution to it (AFMI, 2008).

Professional societies and patient advocacy groups The committee found no published reviews of the disclosure policies of professional societies. It examined a convenience sample of professional society documents and websites and found considerable variation in the content and accessibility of those policies. (Unlike professional society codes of ethics or codes of conduct, disclosure policies do not apply to members generally but are limited to individuals holding positions of responsibility, for example, officers or members of policy-making committees.) Some societies had disclosure forms with a simple, open-ended question about relevant relationships, whereas other forms included specific categories of relationships and required that respondents either report such a relationship or check a box stating that they had none. The policies of some professional societies that develop clinical practice guidelines are discussed further in Chapter 7.

The committee did not attempt to conduct a systematic review of the policies of patient advocacy and disease-specific groups. It found little information on such policies in its initial search of organizational websites and other resources. To the extent that these groups engage in activities such as the development of clinical practice guidelines or the provision of accredited continuing medical education, many of the recommendations in Chapter 7, in this chapter, and elsewhere in this report will apply.

Disclosure by Companies of Payments to Physicians

District of Columbia, Maine, Massachusetts, Minnesota, Vermont, and West Virginia require pharmaceutical manufacturers to report their financial relationships with physicians; and a number of other states are considering such requirements (Wallack, 2008; Lopes, 2009; MedPAC, 2009). Minnesota and Massachusetts make the information public. Vermont requires the state's attorney general to make an annual public report based on the information that the pharmaceutical manufacturers have disclosed. Two states also require the reporting of payments by pharmaceutical manufacturers to hospitals and nursing homes. One state requires medical device companies as well as pharmaceutical companies to report payments to physicians. In general, state policies are relatively new, and their implementation and effectiveness have not been formally assessed.

Some pharmaceutical and device companies have voluntarily acted to disclose publicly certain of their payments to physicians (see Chapter 6). The specific details of company plans vary and appear to be evolving as the discussion of public reporting of payments continues. Several companies have been required to make such public disclosures as a condition of settlements with the U.S. Department of Justice (Demske, 2008; see Chapter 6 for additional discussion). In 2007, bills were introduced in the U.S. Congress to establish a requirement for companies to report publicly their payments to physicians (S. 2029 and H.R. 5605, 110th Congress). As discussed in the final section of this chapter, the Medicare Payment Advisory Commission (MedPAC), which advises the Congress on a range of Medicare policy issues, has recommended a more comprehensive policy for company reporting of payments (MedPAC, 2009).

Time Frame for Disclosure

For employees and others who are involved with an institution for an extended period, disclosure policies generally require an initial disclosure and then periodic (e.g., yearly) disclosures as well as interim disclosures when new relationships arise or when specific events occur (e.g., the submission of a new grant proposal or an application to license intellectual property). For researchers, policies may require the disclosure of financial ties before a study begins (e.g., to university administrators and institutional review board members), during a study, (e.g., to the research team, students, or research subjects), and after the study is completed (e.g., to journal editors when papers are submitted for publication in peer-reviewed journals).

The conflict of interest policies that the committee reviewed varied considerably in the time periods for which disclosure is required. Typically, policies require the disclosure of relationships that are current or that occurred during the previous year. Some policies ask about relationships that are pending, in negotiation, or expected in the next 12 months. The PHS regulations for grantees do not specify a reporting period, except that in determining whether financial relationships exceed the $10,000 threshold for reporting, researchers must consider individual and family financial relationships projected for the next 12 months.

Some organizations require disclosure for periods longer than the previous year (e.g., the American Thoracic Society requires disclosure for the previous 3 years [ATS, 2008] and the *Journal of the American Medical Association* requires disclosure for the previous 5 years [Flanagin et al., 2006]). The requirements may vary by type of relationship. For example, the policy of the American Society of Clinical Oncology specifies disclosure within 2 years for certain relationships (e.g., honoraria and consulting arrangements) but not for others (e.g., research funding) (ASCO, 2007).

Administrative Burden of Disclosure Policies

Disclosure to multiple organizations with various policies can clearly be burdensome for individuals who have received multiple grants, write many papers, serve on various committees and advisory panels, and make many continuing medical education presentations. The committee found little empirical information on the administrative burden of disclosure or other elements of conflict of interest policies for either individuals or institutions.

A 2007 faculty burden survey undertaken for the Federal Demonstration Partnership reported that respondents assigned conflict of interest monitoring an average burden rating of about 1.8 (with a rating of 1 being no burden and 5 indicating a great deal of burden), whereas grants progress reporting received a rating of 3.4 (with a rating of 3 being some burden) (Decker et al., 2007).[9] Some other government-led initiatives to streamline regulatory policies and practices mention conflict of interest policies and practices but generally do not identify them as a critical issue or problem.[10]

The committee found examples of efforts to make it easier for individuals to comply with disclosure policies. For example, to assist their employees in determining whether they have a relationship with a "substantially affected organization" (as described in NIH intramural conflict of interest policies), NIH has developed a searchable list of such organizations (http://ethics.od.nih.gov/topics/sao/sao-list.aspx). Similarly, to help committee members identify and report pertinent relationships, some federal advisory committees and at least one professional society (the American Society of Clinical Oncology) have developed lists of for-profit companies that make products that might be affected by committee decisions on a particular issue (ASCO, 2008).

[9] The response rate for the survey, which was directed to faculty at major research institutions, was less than 40 percent. The Federal Demonstration Partnership, which involves 10 federal agencies and approximately 100 institutional recipients of federal funds, is a cooperative initiative whose goal is to reduce the administrative burdens associated with research grants and contracts (http://thefdp.org/). An earlier partnership survey found that conflict of interest monitoring was cited among the tasks for which respondents received the least institutional assistance (Wimsatt et al., 2005).

[10] For example, the Research Business Models subcommittee, which is under the Committee on Science of the National Science and Technology Council, has, among other priorities, the development of "specific guidance or regulations concerning institutional financial conflicts of interest, and to resolve differences in conflict of interest interpretations and terms and conditions of Federal grant awards" (http://rbm.nih.gov/priorities/sa3.htm). At NIH, the Clinical and Translational Science Awards (CTSA) program has established a research ethics oversight committee, which has in turn created a work group on conflict of interest policies to survey CTSA sites and gather information on policies. The NIH initiative to "reengineer the clinical research enterprise" does not feature conflict of interest policies as part of its assessment of clinical research policies (http://nihroadmap.nih.gov/clinicalresearch/overview-policy.asp). Nonetheless, the presentation to the IOM committee by NIH Director Elias Zerhouni stated that improving conflict of interest administration for grantees was important to NIH (Zerhouni, 2007).

Accuracy and Completeness of Disclosures

Although most organizations are reluctant to publicize violations of their policies, instances of incomplete and inaccurate disclosure periodically make news. For example, in 2008, investigations by U.S. Senate Finance Committee staff led to a front-page story in the *New York Times* on the failure of three Harvard faculty members to disclose in full—even after they were asked to file amended disclosure forms—the substantial payments that they had received from pharmaceutical companies over the period from 2000 to 2007 (Harris and Carey, 2008; see also Grassley, 2008b). (The Senate committee staff obtained the data through separate inquiries to companies and medical schools and then compared the responses.) In some cases, it appeared that the disclosures that had been omitted involved companies whose products the researchers were investigating. The present Institute of Medicine (IOM) committee understands that one of the questions about these cases is whether the institution's disclosure policy actually requested all the information specified in the PHS regulations, but further details of investigations into the matter had not been released as this report was being completed.

Although the IOM committee did not examine the issue, it notes that journalists often fail to report the sources of funding for research that they publicize (see, e.g., Cook et al. [2007]). In addition, journalists themselves may report stories involving pharmaceutical, medical device, or biotechnology companies with which they have conflicts of interest, for example, the acceptance of company-sponsored travel or prizes for reporting or the reliance on opinion leaders suggested and paid by companies (see, e.g., Schwartz et al. [2008]).

Newspapers have also publicized examples of failures by NIH intramural scientists to disclose relationships with industry as required by agency rules and examples of scientists who have maintained relationships that would likely not have been approved under the rules. For example, journalists reported the apparent failure of dozens of NIH scientists to disclose relationships with industry, although only 20 or so actual cases were confirmed in a subsequent investigation performed by NIH (see, e.g., Weiss [2005]). Another story reported on a researcher who was found by an internal investigation to have "actively" chosen in "at least 38 separate instances . . . not to adhere to policies because it was inconvenient or time-consuming; he knew it was likely his participation [with the pharmaceutical companies] would have been disapproved" (Willman, 2006). A report from the OIG of the U.S. Department of Health and Human Services criticized the agency for not obtaining adequate documentation for the outside financial relationships that it explicitly approved (OIG, 2005).

Although cases of nondisclosure may receive considerable publicity, the frequency and extent of deliberate or unintentional underreporting is unknown, and alternative methods for improving the accuracy of disclosure have not been tested.[11] Weinfurt and colleagues (2008c) reported incomplete and inconsistent disclosure in articles on coronary stents published in 2006. They found that 75 authors disclosed at least one relationship with a pharmaceutical company or other organization, but for only 2 of those authors was that relationship disclosed in all of the authors' articles. Weinfurt and colleagues did not, however, take into account whether some journals either did not require certain relationships to be disclosed or chose not to publish the disclosures with an article. If a national system of public disclosure of payments by pharmaceutical, medical device, and biotechnology companies is enacted, institutions could verify the disclosures that they receive.

Monitoring and Enforcement

The committee found no peer-reviewed studies on the monitoring or enforcement of disclosure requirements specifically or conflict of interest policies generally. One study of journal policies reported that of the 28 journals that had a disclosure policy for authors, 13 had policies that were silent on procedures for responding to an author's failure to make a disclosure (Ancker and Flanagin, 2007). As a means of informing readers and also of promoting adherence to their policies, journals from time to time report on cases in which authors did not disclose pertinent relationships with industry (see, e.g., Petersen [2003], Armstrong [2006], Chabner [2008], DeAngelis and Fontanarosa [2008], and Ross et al. [2008]). They sometimes require these authors to write a letter to the editor acknowledging the error (see, e.g., Kurth et al. [2006], Matteson and Bongartz [2006], and Henschke and Yankelevitz [2008]).

A few journals have more stringent penalties. For example, after problems with authors' failures to disclose, the journal *Environmental Health Perspectives* adopted a policy that (1) imposes a 3-year ban on the publication of articles by authors who have "willfully failed to disclose a competing financial interest" and (2) provides for the publication of a retraction if the editors conclude that they would have rejected the article initially had they known of the undisclosed relationships (EHP, 2009). In general, however, journals decline "to become the COI [conflict of interest] investigative

---

[11] Although the committee did not locate assessments of different disclosure forms, two studies have assessed procedures for obtaining information about the contributions of the listed authors to a submitted manuscript (e.g., analysis of data and drafting of the manuscript) (Marusič et al., 2006; Ivanis et al., 2008). One found that open-ended forms yielded significantly less information than forms with explicit response categories (Marusič et al., 2006). Those studies were also replicated using different disclosure formats.

squad" and "count on . . . authors to be forthright with us" (Goldsmith, 2006, p. 2148). In addition to exposing offenders to negative publicity, journal reports about failures to make the necessary disclosures may have other consequences for authors. In one case, the Mayo Clinic required investigators found to have made incomplete disclosures to a journal to undergo an internal investigation and to participate in remedial activities (Matteson and Bongartz, 2006).

AAMC has recommended that academic medical centers specify the possible sanctions for noncompliance with policies governing conflicts of interest in research involving human subjects and then regularly assess compliance (e.g., through internal audit mechanisms and other self-evaluation strategies) (AAMC, 2001). A 2003 AAMC survey, which did not review actual policies but which relied on responses to survey questions, found that 80 percent of respondents reported that their policies had sanctions for violations (Ehringhaus and Korn, 2004).

The AMSA assessment cited earlier suggests variability in the oversight and enforcement of conflict of interest policies. On the basis of a review of medical school policies, the report categorized institutions as either having or not having provisions for oversight and enforcement (AMSA, 2008b).[12] Of the 58 schools that initially responded to the survey and supplied written policies for review, 55 percent were characterized as having oversight policies, 45 percent were characterized as having enforcement policies, and 34 percent were characterized as having both.[13]

A report by the Council on Government Relations (COGR; an association of research universities) also suggested inadequacies in the procedures used to promote compliance with conflict of interest policies. It concluded:

> While virtually all research universities and organizations have written policies governing individual financial conflicts of interest in research-related areas, most institutions are still developing formal and informal education programs to assure that the policies are well understood and that compliance by affected faculty and researchers is fully in place. (COGR, 2002, unpaged)

[12] As described in footnote 1, two independent, trained reviewers read the policies that the medical schools submitted (without identifying information) and then rated them according to specified criteria. For the administration and oversight categories, the reviewers gave yes or no answers to these two questions: Is it clear that there is a party responsible for general oversight to ensure compliance? Is it clear that there are sanctions for noncompliance?

[13] Some schools that at first failed to provide relevant policies have since supplied or indicated that they will supply additional information (personal communication, Gabriel Silverman, AMSA Scorecard Director, AMSA, June 6, 2008).

Effectiveness of Disclosure Policies

A physician's or researcher's disclosure of financial relationships, either to the institution or to a broad audience, is a necessary step for identifying and avoiding or managing conflicts of interest, but it also has important limitations. First, disclosure alone does not resolve conflicts of interests or prevent the harms that may result from a conflict. Second, some evidence suggests that the disclosure of a conflict of interest may have little effect or may even be counterproductive in some circumstances.

Experimental studies in psychology Several experimental studies in psychology raise general questions about the effectiveness of disclosure of a conflict of interest and even suggest the potential for unintended adverse consequences. For example, in two sets of experimental studies of disclosure by individuals in an advice-giving role, researchers concluded that the disclosure of conflicts of interest significantly benefited the advice givers but hurt the interests of those to whom the disclosure was made (Cain et al., 2005). Although the authors of those studies noted that the findings should be treated as no more than evidence that disclosure can potentially have unintended consequences, they caution that most of the mechanisms that produce the effects found are likely to exist except when the recipients of the advice are savvy and experienced.

The disclosure of financial relationships can also be ineffective for reasons unrelated to those discussed in the studies just cited. For example, when a large amount of information is disclosed (e.g., on prescription inserts or in certain informed-consent forms), critical points can get lost among less important details. That is, the disclosure of more information may, in some situations, be counterproductive. (Appendix D provides an additional review of the relevant psychological research.)

Journal readers Two randomized studies suggested that the disclosure of an author's financial interests can reduce journal readers' perceptions of the believability and importance of research reports. One study found that journal readers found an article to be less "interesting, important, relevant, valid, and believable" when the authors were disclosed to be employees of a (fictitious) pharmaceutical company instead of employees of an ambulatory care center (Chaudhry et al., 2002, p. 1392). The other study found that readers rated "importance, relevance, validity, and believability" lower if it was disclosed that the authors had stock holdings rather than nothing to disclose and if it was disclosed that the authors had received a research grant from a company rather than nothing to disclose (Schroter et al., 2004).

Research participants Several studies have suggested that disclosures to prospective research participants of investigators' financial relationships have little impact on decisions to participate in research (see, e.g., Kim et al. [2004], Hampson et al. [2006], Weinfurt et al. [2006a, 2008a,b]), and Gray et al. [2007]. In a survey of participants in clinical trials for the treatment of cancer, more than 70 percent of the respondents would still have enrolled in the clinical trial even if the researcher had financial ties to the pharmaceutical company sponsoring the trial or had received royalty payments (Hampson et al., 2006). Only 31 percent wanted the researcher's financial interests to be disclosed.

Other studies have described hypothetical clinical trials to individuals with chronic diseases and varied the kind of information presented about the researchers' financial relationships with the sponsors of the trial (Weinfurt et al., 2008a,b). The respondents' willingness to participate in a hypothetical clinical trial varied substantially, depending on the type of financial relationships. The respondents were more concerned when the researchers held equity in the sponsoring company than when the researchers received a payment to cover the cost for each participant in the study. Trust in the researchers decreased somewhat after the disclosure of equity interests. Other factors, such as the benefits and the risks of the clinical trial, had more of an impact on the respondents' decision to participate in the trial.

These studies of research participation can be criticized on methodological grounds for not explaining the risks of conflicts of interest (e.g., bias in the conduct of research and the failure to publish negative findings) or not linking the responses to actual decisions about research participation. It is not known whether the respondents might have been more concerned about researchers' financial relationships with sponsors if they had been given background information about the risks.

Patients Several surveys in the 1990s suggested that many patients were not aware of industry gifts to physicians but were relatively tolerant of most gifts. One study suggested that, overall, patients were considerably more likely than physicians to believe that gifts from pharmaceutical companies influenced physician practice, but only 54 percent of patients were aware of such gifts (Gibbons et al., 1998; see also Blake and Early [1995] and Mainous et al. [1995]). On a different but related issue, one study of the disclosure of information about physician payment mechanisms in managed care plans found that disclosure did not reduce patients' trust in their physicians and might even have "a mild positive impact" on trust (Hall et al., 2002, p. 197; see also Pearson et al. [2006]). Other studies have suggested that patients are interested in information about how their physicians were paid or, more generally, what financial incentives the patients' health plan imposes on participating physicians (Kao et al., 2001; Levinson et al., 2005). (Chapter 6 briefly discusses conflicts of interests created by physician payment methods.)

PROHIBITING OR ELIMINATING CONFLICTS OF INTEREST

Prohibition as a Preventive Strategy

Some institutions have conflict of interest policies that prohibit certain financial relationships outright because their risks are considered to greatly outweigh any potential benefits. As described further in Chapter 5, a 2008 report by AAMC recommended that academic medical centers prohibit a wide range of financial relationships with industry. Several medical schools (e.g., the University of Pittsburgh, the University of Texas Medical Branch at Galveston, and the University of California system) have policies prohibiting gifts, and some prohibit participation in company speakers bureaus (e.g., the University of Massachusetts, the Mayo Clinic, and the University of Louisville).[14]

Also in 2008, the Pharmaceutical Research and Manufacturers of America revised its *Code on Interactions with Healthcare Professionals* to state that companies should not offer pens, notepads, and other non-educational items to health care professionals. In Massachusetts, recent legislation gives these guidelines legal force by requiring the public health department to establish "regulations for a marketing code of conduct . . . that shall be no less restrictive than the most recent version" of the codes on interactions with health care providers of the Pharmaceutical Research and Manufacturers of America and the Advanced Medical Technology Association (see Chapter 111N, section 2, Massachusetts Senate No. 2863). Thus, policies may forbid both the giving and the receiving of certain gifts. (Implementing regulations were published in March 2009 [see Lopes, 2009; see also Chapter 6].)

Some conflict of interest policies prohibit certain relationships but allow exceptions. For example, federal policies covering NIH and other employees of the U.S. Department of Health and Human Services state that its employees may not have an "employment relationship" with drug, medical device, or biotechnology companies; grantees; health care providers; or health insurers. They also may not be paid to teach, speak, write, or edit for such organizations. The policies allow for prior approval of certain

[14] Except for the information for the University of California system (University of California, 2008), this information comes from policies summarized by AMSA (2008b) and then checked by reference to documents on the AMSA website or through links to those documents.

exceptions if prohibition of a relationship is not "necessary to ensure public confidence in the impartiality or objectivity with which HHS programs are administered" (HHS, 2005, p. 51572).

To cite another example, AAMC recommends that medical schools set a "rebuttable presumption that an individual who holds a significant financial interest in research involving human subjects may not conduct such research . . . [except when] the circumstances are compelling" (AAMC, 2001, p. 7). (The "rebuttable presumption" concept is taken from the law and refers to assumptions that are taken to be true unless they are explicitly and successfully challenged in a particular case.) A compelling circumstance would exist, for example, if a researcher with a conflict of interest has unique expertise or skill with implanting and adjusting a complex new medical device and this expertise is needed to carry out an early-stage clinical trial safely and competently. Generally, some kind of management plan would then be devised. This approach is discussed further in Chapter 4.

Prohibition or Elimination as a Management Strategy

The options for managing conflicts of interest discussed in the next section all permit the continuation of a relationship in some situations in which a conflict exists. In certain cases, however, continuation of the relationship is not acceptable because of the severity of the threat that it poses to the primary interest. In that case, an individual with a conflict of interest may agree to end the relationship that creates the conflict, for example, by selling company stock, resigning from a company governing or advisory board, or ceasing to consult for a company. Alternatively, an individual with a conflict of interest may decide to forgo participation in such an activity rather than eliminate the financial relationship in question. Some relationships with conflicts of interest may be difficult to eliminate, for example, the relationship with a spouse because of a conflict of interest involving the spouse's employment.

The committee found no systematic assessment of the adoption, implementation, or effectiveness of policies prohibiting certain financial relationships with industry. Somewhat more information is available on the management of conflicts of interest.

EVALUATING AND MANAGING CONFLICTS OF INTEREST

The management of a conflict of interest is necessary when an assessment of an individual's financial relationships identifies a conflict of interest and when disclosure alone is inadequate but elimination of the conflict is a requirement that is too severe. AAMC has recommended that medical schools create conflict of interest committees to make these assessments and propose management strategies, when appropriate. Professional societies may rely on senior staff or members (e.g., chairs of guideline development panels) for assessments of relationships and responses.

The management options will vary depending on the nature of the conflict and the activity under consideration. Examples of management options follow:

- asking an individual with a conflict of interest to reduce the value of a financial relationship so that it falls below a threshold amount;
- requiring that an individual forgo participation in committee votes, deliberations, or decisions about a topic related to that individual's conflict of interest;
- modifying the design of a research project or having a researcher with no conflict of interest serve as the principal investigator; or
- providing an observer to monitor and evaluate the content of a continuing education course conducted by an individual with a conflict of interest for bias.

What Is Known About Management Policies, Practices, and Consequences

The available data suggest that institutions vary considerably in how they oversee and manage conflicts of interest. Ehringhaus and Korn (2004) reported that 76 percent of medical schools responding to the 2003 AAMC survey had established, as recommended by AAMC, a standing committee to evaluate conflict of interest disclosures, and 21 percent included at least one committee member from outside the institution, also as recommended by AAMC. Eighty-one percent of the medical schools responding to the AAMC survey allowed investigators with a significant financial interest to conduct research involving human participants when compelling circumstances exist. Only 61 percent of the respondents indicated that they had adopted the rebuttable presumption or a similar strategy, and only 26 percent indicated that they had a definition of the compelling circumstances or similar conditions that would allow rebuttal of the presumption.

Even within a single university system, conflict of interest practices may vary (see, e.g., several studies of the University of California system reported by Boyd et al. [2004], Lipton et al. [2004], and Boyd and Bero [2007]). For example, within the University of California system, some campuses have standing committees that meet at least monthly, whereas others convene committees on an ad hoc basis (Boyd et al., 2004). Some but not all campuses include committee members from outside the campus community. Some committees are structurally linked through centralized computer systems to other oversight bodies, such as the campus institutional review board, whereas others do not share financial information within the university unless they are asked to do so.

Assessing Risks of Disclosed Relationships

If an organization's policy requires more than just disclosure, the next step is a review to assess whether a disclosed relationship constitutes a conflict of interest and what risks or potential benefits the relationship presents. As described earlier, a department chair or similar individual may review disclosures and identify conflicts of interest or may refer potential conflicts of interest for further review by a conflict of interest committee or other group or official.

The IOM committee found little systematic investigation of the institutional practices and or criteria used to assess financial relationships and conflicts of interest. One small qualitative study of a university system found that individual conflict of interest committees made decisions on a case-by-case basis, taking into account multiple considerations (e.g., the extent and the nature of the financial relationship and the type of research and research design) and following no rigid formula (Boyd and Bero, 2007). The committees rarely made a direct assessment of the likelihood that an investigator would act improperly.

Some specific advice on assessing the severity of conflicts of interest is available. The AAMC-AAU report on conflict of interest in research involving human subjects describes several considerations that should be taken into account when the risks and possible benefits of allowing an investigator with a conflict of interest to participate in such research are assessed (AAMC-AAU, 2008) (Box 3-2).[15] It also discussed the application of these questions to 10 illustrative cases.[16]

The FDA has developed guidance on whether an individual with a conflict of interest should be allowed to serve on one of its advisory committees (FDA, 2008b). Some of the questions roughly correspond to the considerations identified in Chapter 2. For example, one question is whether a "particular matter" under consideration by a committee

> will have a direct and predictable effect on the financial interests of any organization? . . . A "predictable" effect . . . is a real, as opposed to a

[15] In general, this report follows the practice of recent IOM reports in referring to research participants rather than research subjects (see, e.g., IOM [2001, 2003, 2004]; see also NBAC [2001]). When quoting and sometimes when referring to AAMC and other reports that employ the latter usage, the report follows their practice.

[16] The 2002 report by COGR also included an analysis of cases, and some university educational materials likewise feature analyses of case studies as a means of providing an understanding of the risks presented by financial relationships (see, e.g., Columbia University [undated]).

BOX 3-2
Risks and Potential Benefits to Consider in Assessing the Severity of a Researcher's Conflict of Interest

- Risks to human subjects: to what extent could the conflict of interest increase the risk (considering the role specified for the researcher with the conflict of interest in recruiting or treating research participants)?
- Risks of bias in data collection, analysis, and reporting: to what extent could the researcher with the conflict of interest compromise the integrity of the data?
- Risks to reputation: to what extent could the reputation of the researcher with the conflict of interest or the researcher's institution be damaged, even if the institution establishes a plan to manage the conflict?
- Expected benefits to medicine, science, and public health: how do the expected benefits of allowing the research to proceed compare with the risks?

SOURCE: Adapted from AAMC-AAU, 2008.

> speculative, possibility that the matter will affect the financial interest. It is not necessary, however, that the magnitude of the gain or loss be known, and the dollar amount of the gain or loss is immaterial. . . . [M]ost potential advisory committee recommendations pertaining to marketing status, labeling, post-marketing requirements, and device classification or reclassification would ordinarily have a "direct and predictable effect" on financial interests. . . . Financial interests that ordinarily will not be affected in a direct and predictable manner include a grant or contract between an organization and the employee's university to conduct research on a product that is not the subject of the particular matter before the advisory committee or a competitor product. (FDA, 2008b, pp. 10–14)

FDA rules involving clinical investigators also take into consideration aspects of the study design—for example, the use of objective end points, blinding, or the participation of multiple investigators—that might reduce the potential of an investigator's interests to bias the study results (21 CFR 54.5). (The rules cover financial disclosures and the management of the relationships of clinical investigators in studies that companies plan to use to support FDA approval of the marketing of a medical product.)

Management Strategies

Survey data indicate that medical schools employ various strategies to manage conflicts of interest in research (Table 3-2). Disclosure to some outside party seems to be a common and preferred response to an identi-

TABLE 3-2 Percentage of Medical Schools Citing Different Management Policy Options When Researchers Have a Significant Financial Interest in Their Research

Policies Suggested or Required by Organizations Permitting Participation After a Conflict of Interest Is Identified	Percentage of Medical Schools
Monitoring the research project	87
Eliminating the investigator's significant financial interest	83
Disclosing significant financial interests to human subjects on the consent form	86
Using either internal or external data safety monitoring boards	54
Regularly auditing the informed consent and research subject enrollment process	51
Involving a patient representative during the consent and enrollment process	26
Involving a patient representative during recruitment of research subjects	22

SOURCE: Adapted from Ehringhaus and Korn, 2004.

fied conflict of interest (see, e.g., Boyd and Bero [2000] and Ehringhaus and Korn [2004]).

One analysis of cases in which researchers disclosed their financial relationships found that university conflict of interest committees determined that 26 percent of the cases reviewed involved conflicts of interest that needed management (Boyd et al., 2004).[17] The three most commonly applied management strategies were requiring disclosure in publications and presentations (40 percent of the managed cases), appointing an oversight committee to protect the interests of students involved in the project (21 percent of the managed cases), and eliminating the relationship during the period of the project (22 percent of managed cases). The least common management approach was eliminating the conflict of interest or prohibiting the research.

The IOM committee is not familiar with any evaluations of the implementation or the consequences of different management strategies. This is a significant deficit. At one of the committee's public meetings, an experi-

[17] Financial ties were most often with pharmaceutical companies or biotechnology companies. Across the seven campuses involved in the analysis, payment for consulting activities accounted for 54 percent of the financial disclosures, equity holdings accounted for 38 percent of the disclosures, payment for talks accounted for 14 percent, scientific advisory board membership accounted for 13 percent, membership on a company's board of directors accounted for 12 percent, and being a company founder accounted for 7 percent. Over this period, investigators became more likely to have multiple financial ties with a single company, such as financial ties through the receipt of consulting income, honoraria, and stock.

enced clinical researcher questioned the strategy of appointing an oversight committee to monitor research involving an investigator with a conflict of interest (Benet, 2008). In that scientist's view, so many decisions need to be made in the course of a research project that it is not realistic to expect a faculty member to want to or have time to participate in the close and effective monitoring of another faculty member's research. In addition, monitoring imposes costs that might be judged in some cases to exceed the potential benefits.

In Chapter 9, the committee recommends the development and funding of a program of research on conflict of interest. The outcomes of conflict of interest policies, both positive and negative, would be a key issue for consideration in such a program of research.

Knowledge and Attitudes Regarding Conflict of Interest Policies

A few studies suggest that many investigators do not understand their institution's conflict of interest policies and may be skeptical about them. In one in-depth qualitative study of clinical investigators, less than half of the respondents could accurately describe their institution's policies (Boyd et al., 2003). In addition, many respondents believed that the individual investigator, the professional society, and the public at large—not the university—were the appropriate monitors of conflicts of interest. Although many respondents recognized the general risks associated with conflicts of interest, they believed that they were personally not at risk for bias resulting from financial relationships, a common finding in the research reviewed for this report.

In another, web-based survey of researchers at a single medical center (response rate of less than 40 percent), 17 percent of the respondents were not aware of the institution's conflict of interest policies and 60 percent could correctly describe at least one (but not all) of the policies (Lipton et al., 2004). With respect to consequences, 43 percent of the respondents believed that the policies discouraged a faculty member's ability to start new companies, 31 percent believed that the policies discouraged consultation with companies, and 21 percent believed that the policies discouraged sponsored research but another 21 percent thought that they encouraged such research. Although 14 percent believed that the school's policies hindered their own research agenda, 82 percent believed that it had no effect. Among the respondents who actually had a financial relationship that was subject to committee review, 91 percent said that they were satisfied with how the review was handled, but some of the remaining 9 percent who were not satisfied had very negative attitudes toward the process.

Policy Dissemination and Education Strategies

AAMC has advised academic medical centers to provide education and training about their conflict of interest policies to all faculty, staff, students, and trainees (AAMC, 2001). In 2002, NIH reported that the policies of some research institutions were difficult to locate and were sometimes interspersed in various other institutional policies on issues such as ethics, purchasing, and consulting. It recommended that institutions present their conflict of interest policy "as a complete, self-contained document with citations and web links to supporting policies, procedures, and Federal and state regulations, as appropriate" (NIH, 2002, unpaged). The Office of Extramural Research at NIH recently created an online tutorial on conflict of interest and other materials intended to help investigators understand and comply with NIH policies (the tutorial is available at http://grants.nih.gov/grants/policy/coi/).

The IOM committee's review of the policies and other information on conflict of interest from academic medical centers and universities showed that they vary considerably in the informational resources that they make available to their faculty and staff. Some schools provide online resources that are intended to help people easily find relevant institutional policies and resources (including individuals who can answer questions about the policies). Examples include the University of Minnesota, which has a web-based training module on conflict of interest (University of Minnesota, 2008), and Stanford University, which has frequently asked question units on conflict of interest and related university policies, as well as a quiz and other resources (Stanford University, undated).

A professional society may publicize its policies by publishing them in the society's journal(s). It may also make the policies accessible to the public on its website.

Compliance and Enforcement

The earlier discussion of compliance with and the enforcement of disclosure policies reviewed information about compliance with and the enforcement of policies as they apply to individuals. The discussion in this section focuses on the extent to which research institutions follow applicable PHS rules.

A 2002 review of a sample of grantee policies undertaken by the NIH Office of Extramural Research found that institutional policies often did not reflect the requirements of the PHS regulations (NIH, 2002). In 2007, NIH reported on 18 targeted site reviews regarding grantee compliance with PHS conflict of interest policies. It found no instances of intentional noncompliance and concluded that the institutions that it visited generally had "implemented the Federal regulation thoughtfully and with diligence" (NIH, 2007). It did, however, report some problems with timely and consistent reporting and suggested the need for improvements in several areas, including educational and enforcement procedures, the clarity of the forms used to report conflicts of interest, and definitions.

A 2008 report by the OIG of the U.S. Department of Health and Human Services criticized NIH's oversight of grantee institutions (OIG, 2008). Although NIH accepted some of the report's suggestions, it rejected taking a more active oversight role, particularly requiring and reviewing detailed conflict of interest reports from institutions. Doing so would "effectively, if not legally, transfer the locus of responsibility for managing [financial conflicts of interest] from the grantee institution to the Federal Government" (Zerhouni [2008] in OIG [2008, pp. 20–21]). The OIG disagreed that collection of the information would usurp grantee responsibilities, and it argued that without some details about the nature (and not just the existence) of the conflicts that were identified, NIH lacks important information that it needs to oversee and enforce PHS regulations.

Also in 2008, NIH announced the development of and began testing an electronic reporting and tracking tool that that would allow grantee institutions to prepare and submit required conflict of interest reports and search past reports. Consistent with one of the OIG report's recommendations, the tool would also provide a central web-based location for grantee conflict of interest reports received across NIH (Bravo, 2008; see also NIH [2008b]). In addition, NIH has initiated procedures and training to ensure proper NIH staff oversight of conflict of interest issues involving grantees.

The IOM committee identified some publicly reported instances of NIH enforcement of PHS policies. For example, in October 2008, after congressional inquiries and reports of apparent major inaccuracies in a researcher's financial disclosures to Emory University, NIH suspended a $9 million grant for a study led by the researcher and instituted special conditions for the institution's other studies conducted with the support of NIH grants (Harris, 2008; Kaiser, 2008). Subsequently, the university removed the individual from his post as department chair and significantly restricted his outside activities (Shelton, 2008).

RECOMMENDATIONS

Empirical data on conflict of interest policies are limited, have methodological shortcomings, and tend to focus on academic institutions. Some institutions do not make their policies easily accessible. Institutions also revise their policies, which limits the usefulness of older studies. Nonetheless, the available evidence points to substantial variations in institutional requirements for the disclosure of financial relationships or conflicts of interest.

Variations exist in who is required to report on a conflict of interest, when reporting is required, and what relationships and what details about these relationships are to be reported (e.g., the exact amounts of payments rather than payments above a threshold or within dollar categories). Variations also exist in what relationships are prohibited, what criteria are considered in evaluating financial relationships, what strategies are employed when a conflict of interest is identified, and what is done to monitor and promote adherence to policies. These extensive variations raise concerns that some institutions may not have sufficient data to make determinations about the extent and the nature of an individual's financial relationships or to judge the severity of a conflict of interest. Some institutions may also lack adequate procedures for evaluating and eliminating or managing identified conflicts.

The committee expects that there are many explanations for the variations in policies, including the press of other issues demanding attention, a reluctance to propose changes that may spark controversy and dissension, and cultural traditions that vary in how restrictions on the pursuit of personal gain are viewed. Absent outside pressures and oversight, variation in conflict of interest policies may encourage an unhealthy competition among institutions to adopt weak policies and shirk enforcement. It may also aid investigators who want to avoid restrictions on their pursuit of secondary financial interests.

The recommendations presented in this chapter and in this report are intended to discourage such undesirable institutional and individual behavior but not to damage beneficial collaborations. If institutions do not act voluntarily to strengthen their conflict of interest policies, such inaction may prompt government regulation. (The recommendations below focus on individual conflicts of interest. Chapter 8 presents recommendations on conflicts of interest at the institutional level.)

Adopting Conflict of Interest Policies

The committee's first recommendation deals with institutional basics: the adoption of a policy and the creation of a conflict of interest committee. The details of the policies may vary, depending on an institution's mission and other characteristics, but certain features are fundamental to credible and meaningful conflict of interest policies.

> **RECOMMENDATION 3.1 Institutions that carry out medical research, medical education, clinical care, or practice guideline development should adopt, implement, and make public conflict of interest policies for individuals that are consistent with the other recommendations in this report. To manage identified conflicts of interest and to**

monitor the implementation of management recommendations, institutions should create a conflict of interest committee. That committee should use a full range of management tools, as appropriate, including elimination of the conflicting financial interest, prohibition or restriction of involvement of the individual with a conflict of interest in the activity related to the conflict, and providing additional disclosures of the conflict of interest.

Recommendation 3.1 calls on all institutions that conduct medical research, offer medical education, provide clinical care, or develop practice guidelines to adopt comprehensive conflict of interest policies for their employees. These policies should cover all those whose decisions and judgments affect their institution's missions and primary interests. Consistent with the committee's charge, the recommendation refers only to relationships with pharmaceutical, medical device, and biotechnology companies. In practice, individual institutions will design their policies to cover other relevant relationships. These might include consulting or speaking arrangements with health insurance companies, leadership positions with professional organizations, teaching at other institutions, and service on government advisory committees. (As described in Chapter 2, some of these relationships may present conflicts of commitment.)

So that those who rely on academic medical centers, medical journals, professional societies, patient advocacy groups, and other institutions may assess an institution's conflict of interest policies, the policies should be publicly available, for example, on the institution's website. Although the details will vary, it is also important for institutions to disseminate and explain their policies to those who are subject to them. Strategies might include the provision of an education module and the inclusion of a set of frequently asked questions.

Recommendation 3.1 also calls on academic medical centers and other institutions to create conflict of interest committees to manage conflicts of interest involving individuals. This reiterates a recommendation of AAMC, which found in its 2003 survey that not all medical schools reported that they had such committees. Professional societies and other institutions would also benefit from conflict of interest committees that would implement their policies. For example, a conflict of interest committee for a professional society would review conflicts that arise in different aspects of the society's work, including the development of clinical practice guidelines and the conduct of society meetings and educational programs. (For some very small institutions, the formation of a formal committee may not be necessary if the relevant responsibilities are clearly defined and assigned to appropriate staff or, possibly, volunteers.) A conflict of interest committee should bring experience and consistency to evaluations of financial relationships with industry and decisions about those relationships, although the specific details (e.g., how risks and potential benefits are assessed and what management options are considered) may vary, depending on the activity in question. The recommendation mentions monitoring as an activity of the conflict of interest committee, but in practice, the details of monitoring may best be handled by an administrative unit, with the conflict of interest committee providing more general oversight.

Improving Information for Identifying and Evaluating Conflicts of Interest

Disclosure as an Element of Policy

The disclosure of financial relationships with industry is only one part of a comprehensive conflict of interest policy, but it is nonetheless an essential step. Unless institutions know about these relationships, they cannot assess them and determine whether additional steps—such as the elimination or management of a relationship—are necessary. Recommendation 3.2 identifies key features of policies on disclosure. Recommendations in Chapters 4, 5, 6, and 7 provide guidance about the elimination or management of conflicts of interest in the contexts of medical research and education, patient care, and practice guideline development, respectively.

RECOMMENDATION 3.2 As part of their conflict of interest policies, institutions should require individuals covered by their policies, including senior institutional officials, to disclose financial relationships with pharmaceutical, medical device, and biotechnology companies to the institution on an annual basis and when an individual's situation changes significantly. The policies should

- **request disclosures that are sufficiently specific and comprehensive (with no minimum dollar threshold) to allow others to assess the severity of the conflicts;**
- **avoid unnecessary administrative burdens on individuals making disclosures; and**
- **require further disclosure, as appropriate, for example, to the conflict of interest committee, the institutional review board, and the contracts and grants office.**

Conflict of interest policies should cover individuals who have discretion in the conduct of research and educational activities, the provision of clinical care, and the development of clinical practice guidelines. (Senior officials are also covered by Recommendation 8.1 in Chapter 8, which examines institutional conflicts of interest.) Disclosures should be made at least annually and more often if an individual's situation changes. They should also be updated during the year if an individual's situation changes significantly, for example, because an existing relationship expands (e.g., a faculty member who is a company consultant is also appointed to the company's governing board) or because a new relationship (e.g., a new consulting arrangement) is created that is relevant to a specific activity (e.g., participation in a panel developing a clinical practice guideline). In addition to requiring disclosure of conflicts of interest to the institutional review board and the other entities listed in the recommendation, policies may also cover additional disclosures, for example, to entities responsible for continuing medical education program oversight.

Elements of a disclosure policy may vary depending on the institution, but the disclosures should be sufficiently specific to support the identification of conflicts of interest and an evaluation of their severity. For example, if information on the dollar value of relationships is reported in categories rather than specific amounts, the highest categories should reach into the hundreds of thousands of dollars. The committee recommends the elimination of minimum thresholds for individual reporting of financial relationships. As discussed earlier in this chapter, the 1995 PHS regulations specify a $10,000 threshold, which applies to the individual and his or her spouse and dependent children. Most PHS grantees have adopted this threshold, although approximately one-quarter require reporting regardless of the dollar value of the relationship. The committee recognizes that elimination of the minimum threshold would add to the burden both for those reporting and for those reviewing relationships but believes that it is important to increase the accuracy of reporting and provide institutions with a more complete picture of an individual's financial relationships across different reporting categories (e.g., consulting, advisory committee service, and speaking). The committee also notes research that suggests that even small payments may put an individual at risk of unconscious bias. In their joint report on conflict of interest in human subjects research, AAMC and AAU also recommended removing minimum (de minimis) thresholds (AAMC-AAU, 2008). NIH should seek revisions in the PHS regulations to eliminate the threshold, but NIH grantees should act without waiting for such revisions.

Greater Consistency in Disclosure Policies

The committee recognizes that the objective of achieving sufficient specificity in disclosures may sometimes be in tension with the objective of minimizing the administrative burdens of disclosure. To the extent that the consensus process proposed in Recommendation 3.3 is successful, it may help resolve these tensions by promoting greater consistency across institutions. Greater consistency should simplify the demands on those who must understand and comply with the disclosure requirements of multiple institutions.

RECOMMENDATION 3.3 National organizations that represent academic medical centers, other health care providers, and physicians and researchers should convene a broad-based consensus development process to establish a standard content, a standard format, and standard procedures for the disclosure of financial relationships with industry.

To achieve greater consistency in institutional disclosure requirements, Recommendation 3.1 calls for a broad-based national consensus development process. This undertaking would be convened by national organizations representing academic medical centers, other health care providers, physicians, and researchers and would also include representatives of professional societies; consumer and patient advocacy groups; accreditation, certification, and licensing agencies; medical journals and organizations of medical journal editors; health plans and insurers; government agencies, including NIH and the FDA; and organizations with expertise in database development and management. The process used by AAMC to develop its recent recommendations on relationships with industry in medical education offers one model for the process, although the task would be narrower and more detailed in its focus on definitions of the financial relationships to be disclosed, reporting formats, and similar matters.

The committee appreciates that different disclosures may be required for different purposes. For example, the information that a medical journal needs from the authors of a manuscript differs from the information that a government agency may require for members of an advisory panel. For similar institutions (e.g., for medical journals as a category and for similar government advisory panels as a category), the objective would be to develop a consensus on a common format.

A major task for the consensus development process would be to agree on the categories of relationships that need to be disclosed and the type of information about each relationship that is needed to evaluate it. Consulting is an example of a category that needs further specification. That term can cover relationships that range from the provision of promotional or marketing support to a company to the offering of objective technical advice on scientific advances, products in development, or research study design. The institution of standard categories, definitions, and similar agreements should reduce confusion, misunderstandings, and misinterpretations.

In technical terms, the task for the consensus group would be to specify the elements for a relational database, including the definitions and attributes of these elements. Once the elements are specified, the expectation is that software developers would create programs that physicians and

TABLE 3-3 Candidate List of Categories of Financial Relationships with Industry to Be Disclosed

Research grants and contracts
Consulting agreements
Participation in speakers bureaus
Honoraria
Intellectual property, including patents, royalties, licensing fees
Stock, options, warrants, and other ownership (excepting general mutual funds)
Position with a company
Company governing boards
Technical advisory committees, scientific advisory boards, and marketing panels
Company employee or officer, full or part time
Authorship of publications prepared by others
Expert witness for a plaintiff or a defendant
Other payments or financial relationships

researchers could use on their computers to enter, store, and update information on their financial relationships. The software would then format the information as needed for disclosures for various purposes (e.g., submission to an academic medical center or a medical journal). It would be similar to reference software that allows authors to format references to meet the specifications of different journals.

As a starting point, Table 3-3 presents a candidate list of basic categories of the relationships to be disclosed. Each requires further definitions, and some might require subcategories. The committee did not propose a specific format for the provision of information about these relationships. It is important, however, that any format promote completeness and specificity, for example, by requiring individuals to check one box if they have a particular relationship, to check another box to declare explicitly that they do not have the relationship, and to provide certain details about an indicated relationship (e.g., its value, the company involved, and the nature of the work).

In addition to the categories of relationships to be disclosed, the consensus process needs to address several other key questions. For example, what details of relationships need to be reported (e.g., the amount of income and the name of the company)? How should amounts be reported? Would it be preferable to have individuals making disclosures check a box indicating the range of income from a relationship or should they provide specific dollar amounts? Will a single time frame (e.g., the relationships in existence during the previous 12 months) be adequate for all purposes? How should the financial relationships of close family members (e.g., spouses or domestic partners, dependent children, and parents) be considered?

Company Reporting of Payments to Individuals and Institutions

Recommendations 3.2 and 3.3 involve disclosures by individuals to organizations. The next recommendation proposes requirements for companies. Several state laws and proposals for additional state or federal rules reflect concerns about inaccurate and incomplete disclosures. As discussed earlier, these laws and proposals vary, for example, in the types of companies and payments or relationships that they cover and in provisions for public reporting. In response to proposals for additional state and national legislation, several industry groups and individual companies have supported some form of company disclosure while seeking to minimize the administrative burdens of such reporting and to protect information that might reveal business strategies to competitors (Finance Committee, U.S. Senate, 2008). Recommendation 3.4 calls for a broad national reporting program.

> **RECOMMENDATION 3.4 The U.S. Congress should create a national program that requires pharmaceutical, medical device, and biotechnology companies and their foundations to publicly report payments to physicians and other prescribers, biomedical researchers, health care institutions, professional societies, patient advocacy and disease-specific groups, providers of continuing medical education, and foundations created by any of these entities. Until the Congress acts, companies should voluntarily adopt such reporting.**

A national law covering company payments to physicians, researchers, and medical institutions would be a useful supplement to policies that require individual physicians, researchers, and others to disclose financial relationships to institutions. It should provide that company-reported payments be readily available on a searchable public website that allows the aggregation of all payments made to an individual or organization, although some personal identifying information might be restricted to protect individuals against, for example, identity theft. Such a database could help institutions and potentially others to monitor adherence to institutional disclosure policies. It would not substitute for institutional conflict of interest policies. It also would not eliminate conflicts of interest. One objective of drafting and implementing legislation and explaining it to the public and those affected would be to discourage the inference that all reported relationships are bad and to avoid harm to constructive collaborations.

The committee did not investigate program options and administration in detail, but it generally supports the approach to company reporting discussed by MedPAC during several public sessions in 2008 and presented in MedPAC's March 2009 report (MedPAC, 2008a,b,c,d, 2009). Consistent with the committee's recommendation but in contrast to state policies and some other proposals for federal policy, MedPAC's proposal covers not only payments to physicians but also payments to a range of organizations, including medical schools, professional societies, and providers of continuing medical education. The committee's proposal would add payments to biomedical researchers. The MedPAC recommendation would add payments to pharmacies and pharmacists, health plans, and pharmacy benefit managers as well as payments by medical supply companies. Companies could include clarifying details about the context of a payment (e.g., specifying whether the payment is a research grant that covers all project costs and not just the investigator's salary). The committee considers these to be reasonable provisions for a company reporting program.

Implementing regulations would need to specify clear definitions and exact categories for the reporting of payments. The consensus-building activity proposed in Recommendation 3.3 could contribute to this specification and promote consistency with institutional disclosure policies.

As proposed by MedPAC, the database of company-reported information would be public, but the physician's National Provider Identifier (NPI) would not be given.[18] The entire database would be available to researchers who enter into confidentiality and data use agreements with the secretary of the U.S. Department of Health and Human Services. The database would be searchable by manufacturer; recipient name, location, and specialty (if applicable); type of payment; name of related product (if applicable); and year. The MedPAC report did not include an estimate of the costs to the government of creating and maintaining the systems but notes that the costs would be higher than those of state systems, only one of which makes the data public, but not in a searchable database.

In MedPAC's proposal, company reporting would be required annually, but reporting for a clinical trial could be delayed until the trial was publicly registered or until FDA approval related to the development of a new product was granted (but not later than 2 years after the payments were made). The national policy would preempt state policies, to the extent that they cover the same categories of payments and recipients, and would provide for civil penalties for noncompliance. Legislation introduced in the U.S. Congress in 2009 includes similar provisions on these points (Grassley, 2009).

In addition to the proposal on company reporting, MedPAC has also proposed that the Congress require hospitals and other providers to report (and the government to post on a public website) on physicians' direct

[18] The NPI is a unique number mandated by the U.S. government for most U.S. physicians that is available in a publicly accessible database that links it to the physician's name, practice location, business office location, license numbers, and other identifiers.

or indirect ownership shares in the facility (MedPAC, 2009; see further discussion in Chapter 6). The provision of recommendations on conflicts of interest arising from physician ownership of facilities was outside this committee's charge. The reporting program proposed by MedPAC would make considerable additional information available to researchers, patients, and others.

A discussion of the pros and cons of establishing a broader system of disclosure is presented in Appendix F.

Recommendations in the Following Chapters

The recommendations in this chapter call for institutions to adopt conflict of interest policies consistent with the recommendations in this report and for individual and cooperative institutional efforts and legislative actions to strengthen policies on the disclosure of individual and institutional financial relationships with industry. The next four chapters of this report offer additional recommendations related to policies and practices in the specific areas of medical research, medical education, patient care, and the development of clinical practice guidelines. Chapter 4 calls for institutions to generally bar researchers with a conflict of interest from conducting research with human participants except when the investigator's expertise is essential to the safe and rigorous conduct of the research. Chapters 5 and 6, among other recommendations, call for physicians and researchers to forgo and institutions to prohibit or end certain relationships with industry that present unacceptable risks of undue influence over professional decision making or a loss of public trust.

Chapter 7 includes recommendations for reducing industry influence in the development of clinical practice guidelines and increasing the levels of disclosure of organizational and individual financial relationships. Chapter 8 recommends that institutions establish policies at the board level to identify, limit, and manage institution-level conflicts of interest. The final chapter calls for a range of organizations to develop incentives to promote the institutional adoption and implementation of the policies recommended here. It also calls for the development of a research agenda to evaluate and guide improvements in conflict of interest policies and procedures.

4

Conflicts of Interest in Biomedical Research

Biomedical research provides discoveries that may lead to new or better tests and treatments that improve individual and public health. Patients, patients' families, physicians, other researchers, and policy makers need to trust that the design, conduct, and reporting of such research are unbiased and that the time and effort that they contribute to research will be used to advance science. Participants in clinical trials need to trust that they are not exposed to unnecessary risk. Conflict of interest policies should not only address concerns that financial relationships with industry may lead to bias or a loss of trust but should also consider the potential benefits of such relationships in specific situations.

Research partnerships among industry, academia, and government are essential to the discovery and development of new medications and medical devices that provide improved means for the prevention, diagnosis, and treatment of health problems. Historically, the federal government has taken the lead in supporting discoveries in basic science, whereas commercial firms have focused on the discovery of specific medicines and then their development through clinical trials to the regulatory approval of marketable products. (As discussed below, the development pathway for medical devices often differs from the pathway for pharmaceuticals.) Before 1980, the federal government held the patents resulting from publicly funded basic research, but very few patents were licensed for commercial development. In 1980, the U.S. Congress passed the Patent and Trademark Amendments of 1980 (P.L. 96-517, commonly known as the Bayh-Dole Act, after its sponsors). The law allowed institutions to patent discoveries resulting from federally funded research and to grant licenses for others to develop those discoveries. Universities may retain licensing and royalty fees, which they generally share with their scientists who developed the patented discovery. Since the law's passage, patent licensing and other financial relationships linking medical researchers and research institutions with industry have expanded substantially (Schacht, 2008). Some scholars, however, have pointed to factors in addition to the legislation that may be associated with the historical increase in the numbers of patents, including a broadening of the criteria that allow materials to be patentable (particularly for life forms) and advances in biomedical research (see, e.g., Mowery et al. [2001, 2004] and Sampat [2006]; see also *Diamond v. Chakrabarty*, 447 U.S. 303 [1980]).

This chapter starts with a brief overview of some dimensions of university-industry collaborations in biomedical research and then summarizes data on the extent of the relationships between pharmaceutical, device, and biotechnology companies and academic research institutions and individual researchers. The next sections review concerns about these relationships and responses to those concerns. (Appendix E provides an additional discussion of the nature and importance of academic-industry collaboration in medical research.) Because many conflicts of interest at the institutional level emerge from research discoveries, the discussion of these conflicts and the responses to them presented in Chapter 8 is also relevant. The final section of this chapter offers recommendations.

COLLABORATION AND DISCOVERY IN BIOMEDICINE

The path from a scientific discovery to the marketing of a new drug, device, or biological product is typically long and complex and involves a diversity of expertise and resources. For example, basic researchers, often at academic medical centers and other research institutions, can identify new potential targets for therapies and new strategies for treatment, suggest additional diseases that may be able to be treated by existing and newly developed compounds, and suggest both how to target therapies to the patients who are the most likely to benefit and how to avoid particular treatments for patients at high risk for adverse events from those treatments. Scientists at the National Institutes of Health (NIH) also contribute to the discovery process, and important clinical research is undertaken at the NIH Clinical Center. In addition, basic scientists at biotechnology and pharmaceutical companies have made fundamental discoveries that have led to new therapies.

Scientists at pharmaceutical companies can help identify or develop drugs that may be active against new biological targets that have been identified by individuals who conduct basic research. These companies also have the critical ability to use good manufacturing practices to produce a candidate drug in sufficient quantities for clinical trials and then for large-scale commercial distribution, if the product is approved for marketing.

Furthermore, they have experience with the Food and Drug Administration (FDA) drug approval process, which includes extensive requirements for preclinical and clinical testing and for manufacturing. Finally, pharmaceutical companies also supply or raise the capital needed to fund the lengthy process of bringing a product to market. Medical device companies and biotechnology companies play analogous roles in translating discoveries made through basic research into products or services for medical and public health practice, although the specific details differ from those involved with the drug approval process. (Appendix E provides a more detailed discussion of the discovery and development process.)

The committee heard testimony that collaboration between academic and industry researchers in the drug discovery process can be mutually beneficial (Benet, 2008; Cassell, 2008). When a new disease mechanism is discovered, academic and industry scientists can work together to identify promising therapeutic targets and treatment approaches. Furthermore, academic researchers can inform industry when they identify potential new targets for chemical intervention. Drug companies can then quickly scan their chemical libraries to search for compounds with potential biological activity and describe what problems they have encountered as they have tried to identify the specific targets of those compounds. This begins the long process of applied chemistry, which is needed to identify a candidate drug.

Many examples illustrate that academic collaboration with pharmaceutical and biotechnology companies can lead to dramatic therapeutic advances that save lives and improve the quality of life. Particularly dramatic are those related to therapies for human immunodeficiency virus (HIV) infection. Collaborations contributed to delineation of the pathophysiology of the disease and the development of successive new classes of drugs, including reverse transcriptase inhibitors, protease inhibitors, and entry inhibitors (Braunwald et al., 2001). These advances have transformed a uniformly fatal illness into a chronic disease that people are now generally able to survive for decades. A few other examples include the following:

- an anticoagulant (abciximab), which is a monoclonal antibody against the platelet glycoprotein IIb/IIIa, that has been shown to prevent thrombotic complications of coronary angioplasty (EPIC Investigators, 1994; Tcheng et al., 2003);
- pulmonary surfactant, which improves survival in neonates with respiratory distress syndrome and which was developed by a number of academic researchers at different universities working in close collaboration with several pharmaceutical companies (personal communication, Jeffrey A. Whitsett, Chief, Section of Neonatology, Perinatal and Pulmonary Biology, Cincinnati Children's Hospital Medical Center, December 9, 2008);

- rituximab, a monoclonal antibody against the CD20 marker on B cells, which is effective in patients with certain types of lymphoma and leukemia, rheumatoid arthritis, and multiple sclerosis and in preventing the rejection of transplanted organs (Maloney et al., 1997; Edwards et al., 2004; Hauser et al., 2008);
- bortezomib, a proteasome inhibitor, which improves survival in patients with multiple myeloma (San Miguel et al., 2008); and
- imatinib, a tyrosine kinase inhibitor, which has greatly prolonged the survival of patients with chronic myelogenous leukemia (Druker et al., 2006).

Compared with the drug development process, the development of complex medical devices tends to be a more continuous process of innovation and refinement that involves frequent alterations in device design, materials, manufacturing processes, or other characteristics. Examples of medical devices that have been developed as a result of close academic-industry collaborations include implanted defibrillators (Jeffrey, 2001), prosthetic heart values (Gott et al., 2003), and mechanical ventilators (Keszler and Durand, 2001). Advances in many technologies, such as pulse oximetry for the monitoring of anesthesia and phototherapy for the treatment of disease, highlight the results that may accrue from a combination of research collaboration and communication with senior clinicians about their experiences (Mike et al., 1996; Dicken et al., 2000; McDonagh, 2001; Severinghaus, 2007; Vreman et al., 2008).

Nevertheless, advances in medical devices may result in conflicts of interest. For example, the process of device refinement (particularly when the refinements are minor or are not associated with well-designed clinical studies) is at the center of controversies over whether some consulting arrangements between orthopedic surgeons and the manufacturers of orthopedic devices represent fair payments for technical services or are inducements for the surgeons to use the device.

To promote further progress in moving discoveries from basic science into successful products, NIH has developed major initiatives to strengthen early translational research, which focuses on transforming specific discoveries into clinically useful products or services (see, e.g., NIH [2008d] and CTSA [2009]). At academic centers, this research may involve populations of individuals with rare diseases or biological agents that do not have obvious commercial potential. Such research may, nonetheless, lay the foundation for companies to develop successful products or at least for company licensing of compounds or agents for which university research has provided proof-of-concept data but for which companies must take the next steps.

INDUSTRY FUNDING AND RELATIONSHIPS IN BIOMEDICAL RESEARCH

Growth and Magnitude of Industry Funding

Industry funding for biomedical research has been growing in recent decades and is now the largest source of funding for such research in the United States. Between 1977 and 1989, the proportion of the total funding for clinical and nonclinical research supplied by industry grew from 29 to 45 percent (Read and Campbell, 1988; Read and Lee, 1994). Between 1995 and 2003, the yearly figures (which are based on sources of information somewhat different from those for 1977 to 1985) ranged from 57 to 61 percent (Moses et al., 2005; see also Hampson et al. [2008]). This funding supports work in the laboratories of pharmaceutical, device, and biotechnology companies; contracts for research conducted by universities and other nonprofit research institutions; and contracts with commercial contract research organizations that carry out clinical trials in academic and private practice settings.

Extent of Academic-Industry Relationships

Industry relationships with academic biomedical researchers are extensive. A 2006 national survey of department chairs in medical schools and large independent teaching hospitals found that 67 percent of academic departments (as administrative units) had relationships with industry (Campbell et al., 2007b). In addition, 27 percent of nonclinical departments and 16 percent of clinical departments received income from intellectual property licensing. Among the department chairs, 60 percent had relationships with industry, including serving as a consultant (27 percent), a member of a scientific advisory board (27 percent), a paid speaker (14 percent), an officer (7 percent), a founder (9 percent), or a board member (11 percent) for a company. In some universities, companies fund individual departments, multidisciplinary research centers, or campuswide research programs (Bero, 2008).

For individual academic researchers, studies from the 1990s show that they have widespread relationships with industry. In a 1996 survey, 28 percent of life sciences faculty who conducted research received support from industry sources (Blumenthal et al., 1996a,b). The prevalence of support was greater for researchers in clinical departments (36 percent) than for those in nonclinical departments (21 percent). In a 1998 study, 43 percent of academic scientists in the 50 most research intensive universities reported receiving research-related gifts (independent of a research grant or contract) during the preceding 3 years (Campbell et al., 1998). The most widely reported gifts received from industry were biomaterials used in research (24 percent),[1] discretionary funds (15 percent), research equipment (11 percent), and trips to professional meetings (11 percent). Among those receiving gifts, 66 percent viewed them as important to their research.

A study of disclosures at the University of California at San Francisco found that by 1999, approximately 8 percent of principal investigators at the institution reported personal financial ties to the sponsor of a particular research project (Boyd and Bero, 2000). Thirty-four percent of these involved temporary speaking engagements, 33 percent involved consulting relationships, 32 percent involved paid positions on a scientific advisory board or board of directors, and 14 percent involved equity in a firm (more than one type of involvement for a single research project was possible).

Although evidence is limited and not recent, some research suggests that faculty members who have research relationships with industry are more productive in certain respects than faculty who do not have such relationships. One study found that researchers in the former group are significantly more likely than researchers in the latter group to report that they are involved with a start-up company (14 versus 6 percent) or that they have applied for a patent (42 versus 24 percent), have had a patent granted (25 versus 13 percent), have a patent licensed (18 versus 9 percent), have a product under review (27 versus 5 percent), or have a product on the market (26 versus 11 percent) (Blumenthal et al., 1996a). That study also reported that these faculty reported that they had published significantly more articles in peer-reviewed journals in the previous 3 years than faculty without industry funding (15 versus 10 articles) (Blumenthal et al., 1996a). In general, a greater number of biomedical patents should benefit society, since patents are usually a key step in the development of new therapies or diagnostic tests. Likewise, greater publication productivity should, in general, advance scientific knowledge.

The associations reported above do not prove causality. Industry may fund scientists who are more productive or whose research has more commercial potential. Alternatively, industry may provide funding that allows scientists to be more successful commercially and academically, or such support may encourage funded scientists to be more active commercially.

CONCERNS ABOUT RELATIONSHIPS WITH INDUSTRY

Despite their benefits, relationships with industry create conflicts of interest that can undermine the primary goals of medical research. Where

[1] One reviewer of the report observed that companies view the provision of these proprietary materials as a service to the academic community and that they may, in any case, not have a mechanism for charging for them.

there are conflicts, legitimate and serious concerns can be raised about the openness of research and potential bias in the design, conduct, and reporting of research (see, e.g., Gross [2007]). Whether or not the conflicts actually lead to unwarranted secrecy or biased results in particular cases, they have the potential to threaten the reputation of the research enterprise if they are not avoided or identified and managed responsibly.

The review below does not cover marketing activities disguised as research, in particular, so-called seeding trials that companies design to change the prescribing habits of participating physicians rather than to gather scientifically valid information. These studies, which potentially expose study participants to risk without investigating scientifically significant questions, are discussed in Chapter 6.

Industry Funding of Research and Reduced Openness in Science

A fundamental tenet of academic science is that information, data, and materials should be shared. Such sharing could be at risk in academic-industry collaborations. A 2003 National Research Council report identified "the commercial and other interests of authors in their research data and materials" as major obstacles to information sharing (NRC, 2003, p. 1).

A 1995 survey of life sciences faculty in the 50 most research intensive institutions found that 14 percent of those with funding from industry reported that trade secrets had resulted from their research, whereas 5 percent of those without funding from industry did so (Blumenthal et al., 1996a). Trade secrets were defined as information that is kept secret to protect its commercial value. In some cases, this finding may represent the normal and necessary protection of key information prior to the filing of a patent on intellectual property, with the resulting enhanced opportunity for successful commercialization. (Unlike trade secrets, patents require the disclosure of information but protect property interests in a discovery for a defined period.) A 1993 study of academic genetics research found that faculty with research funding from industry were significantly more likely to delay publication of their research results by more than 6 months to allow the commercialization of their research (Blumenthal et al., 1997).

The situation may have changed since the 1993 study cited above because some basic science journals have adopted more stringent policies on data sharing and withholding (see, e.g., NRC [2003], NPG [2007], and Piwowar and Chapman [2008]). In any case, not only journals but also the research institutions themselves could better maintain the integrity of research to the extent that they adopt more stringent policies on data sharing.

A related concern involves access to data. In some industry-supported research, the investigator lacks full access to the study data and depends almost entirely on company statisticians for analysis (Bombardier et al., 2000; Silverstein et al., 2000; Curfman et al., 2005). The conflict in such situations raises reasonable concerns about the integrity of the data. To address this problem, some journals have recently decided not to publish the results of studies funded by industry unless there is full access to the data and independent repetition of the data analyses by academicians or government employees not affiliated with the sponsor (DeAngelis et al., 2001). In addition, many universities have recently added a requirement for access to study data to the terms of their research contracts with industry.

Research Funding from Industry and Pro-Industry Findings in Published Research

Several systematic reviews and other studies provide substantial evidence that clinical trials with industry ties are more likely to have results that favor industry. One meta-analysis found that clinical trials in which a drug manufacturer sponsors clinical trials or the investigators have financial relationships with manufacturers are 3.6 times more likely to find that the drug tested was effective compared to studies without such ties (Bekelman et al., 2003).[2] Another meta-analysis that included non-English-language studies found that studies that favored a drug were four times more likely to be funded by the maker of the drug than any other sponsor (Lexchin et al., 2003). A more recent literature review found that 17 of 19 studies published since the preceding two meta-analyses reported "an association, typically a strong one, between industry support and published pro-industry results" (Sismondo, 2008, p. 112). Similarly, another review found that industry-funded studies were more likely than other studies to conclude that a drug was safe, even for studies that found a statistically significant increase in adverse events for the experimental drug (Golder and Loke, 2008).

In addition, a study of materials submitted to the FDA in support of successful new drug applications found that clinical trials with statistically favorable results were almost twice as likely to be published as industry-funded studies that did not have favorable results (Lee et al., 2008). Overall, the results of more than half of clinical trials submitted to the FDA in support of a new drug application remained unpublished more than 5 years

[2] "A study was included if it met the following criteria: (1) its stated primary or secondary purpose was to assess the extent, impact, or management of financial relationships among industry, investigators, or academic institutions; (2) it contained a section describing study methods; (3) it was written in English; and (4) it was published following the passage of the Bayh-Dole Act of 1989" (Bekelman et al., 2003, p. 455). "The main outcomes were the prevalence of specific types of industry relationships, the relation between industry sponsorship and study outcome or investigator behavior, and the process for disclosure, review, and management of financial conflicts of interest" (p. 454).

after approval of the drug. Furthermore, comparisons of information submitted to regulatory agencies with information on the same trials published in the medical literature have found changes in the ways that the results of the trials were reported so that the published results appeared to be more favorable than the results reviewed by regulatory agencies. Such selective reporting of trial results includes additions of favorable outcomes, deletions of unfavorable outcomes, and changes in the statistical significance of the outcomes reported (Hemminki, 1980; Melander et al., 2003; Chan et al., 2004a; Rising et al., 2008; Turner et al., 2008). Recent requirements for web-based reporting of clinical trial results are described below.

Other studies have found that research funded by industry was more likely to report conclusions that favored the sponsor's drug, even if the results did not in fact support such conclusions. For example, studies that have examined clinical trials involving specific clinical specialties or particular clinical problems have found an association between industry sponsorship and results that favor industry. Examples include clinical trials of statins for the treatment of elevated cholesterol levels (Bero et al., 2007), breast cancer studies (Peppercorn et al., 2007), clinical trials of new antipsychotic drugs (Heres et al., 2006), and various nutrition-related studies (Lesser et al., 2007; see also Perlis et al. [2005]).

Several possible explanations can be offered for the association between industry support and results that are favorable to the sponsor. First, pharmaceutical and biotechnology companies seek to invest in products that will be shown to be effective and safe; hence, compounds that enter clinical trials have been selected as being likely to succeed. (That is, for-profit companies may be more risk adverse than nonprofit sponsors and fund mostly studies that seem likely to produce favorable results.) Second, investigators might have become persuaded by their own research that a drug is efficacious and, as a result, develop financial relationships with trial sponsors to help promote the future clinical development or use of the drug. Third, industry studies might be less rigorously designed or designed in a way that will bias the findings in favor of a drug, leading to false-positive conclusions that an intervention is effective, or they might be well designed but not actually conducted according to the protocol (Bero and Rennie, 1996; Steinman et al., 2006). Fourth, sponsors may be more likely to fully publish the results of studies with favorable findings (Rising et al., 2008).

The findings of three systematic reviews do not support the suggestion that industry-sponsored trials are poorly designed. They concluded that the quality of industry-sponsored trials is comparable to that of studies funded by other sources (Bekelman et al., 2003; Lexchin et al., 2003; Hampson et al., 2008). The methodologies used in those assessments of the quality of trials did not, however, take into account such issues as the appropriateness of the control intervention, the clinical relevance of the research question, and whether the findings of the studies were fully published (Lexchin et al., 2003; Hampson et al., 2008).

In addition, it is sometimes suggested that journals prefer to publish articles that report positive findings rather than equivocal or nonexistent relationships. Several studies, based on self-reports from the authors of unpublished studies, suggest instead that authors' decisions to not submit manuscripts with the findings of their studies account for the majority of unpublished studies (Dickersin et al., 1987, 1992; Dickersin, 1990; Easterbrook et al., 1991). Similarly, a more recent study—based on inquiries to investigators about trial results that were not published—suggested that "studies were not published because they were not submitted" (Rising et al., 2008, p. 1568).

Box 4-1 summarizes several incidents that have added to concerns about bias in the reporting of industry-funded studies. Most involve an alleged failure to publish negative findings from industry-sponsored clinical trials or long delays in publication. These incidents involved a number of pharmaceutical companies and different types of drugs. Sometimes the information became known only after legal proceedings led to the disclosure of confidential internal industry documents.

In addition, systematic reviews that look at meta-analyses rather than individual clinical trials as the unit of analysis also find an association between industry funding and conclusions that favor the sponsor's product. One study found that industry-supported reviews had more favorable conclusions, noted fewer reservations about the methodological limitations of the trials included, and were less transparent than reviews conducted by the Cochrane Collaboration.[3] All seven industry-sponsored reviews recommended the experimental drug without reservation, whereas none of the Cochrane Collaboration reviews did (Jorgensen et al., 2006). Another study, a review of meta-analyses of clinical trials of treatments for hypertension, found that meta-analyses conducted by individuals with financial ties to a single drug company were not more likely than meta-analyses conducted by individuals who received funding from other sources to have results that favored the sponsor's drug. Financial ties to a single company were, however, associated with favorable conclusions by the authors of the meta-analyses. Among meta-analyses conducted by individuals with financial ties to one drug company, 27 of 49 (55 percent) reported favorable *results* from the meta-analysis, but 45 of 49 (92 percent) reported favorable

[3] The Cochrane Collaboration describes itself as "an independent, nonprofit, international organization that develops and disseminates systematic reviews of health care interventions and promotes the creation and use of evidence to guide clinical and policy decisions" (see http://www.cochrane.org/docs/descrip.htm). It relies primarily on volunteers who conduct reviews according to specific standards. It has policies intended to limit bias and restrict financial conflicts of interest in its activities.

BOX 4-1
Examples of Biased Reporting in Clinical Research

In a pivotal trial of celecoxib for treatment of arthritis, only data on outcomes at 6 months were presented, even though the original protocol called for the trial to be of a longer duration and the outcomes at 12 months were available when the manuscript was submitted (Hrachovec and Mora, 2001). The outcomes at 6 months showed an advantage for the study drug, but the outcomes at 12 months showed no advantage compared with the use of the control drugs (Wright et al., 2001).

Published clinical trials suggest that selective serotonin reuptake inhibitors have a favorable benefit-risk profile in children with depression. When unpublished data were considered, the evidence indicated that the risks appeared to outweigh the benefits for all but one drug in this class (Whittington et al., 2004).

The results of trials of paroxetine that demonstrated an increased risk of teenage suicide or a lack of efficacy were not published. The data were revealed only after a lawsuit was brought against the manufacturer (Gibson, 2004).

The manufacturer of aprotinin, an antifibrinolytic drug used in cardiac surgery to decrease bleeding, withheld data that use of the drug increased the risk of renal failure, heart attack, and congestive heart failure (Avorn, 2006).

The results of a clinical trial that compared the use of ezetimibe plus a statin with the use of a statin alone in individuals with elevated cholesterol levels were not published until 2 years after the conclusion of the trial. The results showed no difference in carotid artery wall thickness in the two groups (Kastelein et al., 2008).

The results of a pivotal clinical trial of a blood substitute (PolyHeme) in patients undergoing elective vascular surgery were not released for 5 years after the trial was stopped by the sponsor. The trial showed significant increases in the rates of mortality and heart attacks in the group receiving the experimental intervention (Burton, 2006; Northfield Laboratories, 2006).

The manufacturer of an implantable cardioverter-defibrillator allegedly failed to report critical, potentially fatal design defects for more than 3 years (Hauser and Maron, 2005).

The manufacturer of a novel immune modulator for the treatment of HIV infection refused to provide a complete set of data to the investigators in a randomized clinical trial that showed that the investigational agent was ineffective (Kahn et al., 2000).

The manufacturer of a brand-name thyroid hormone attempted to block the publication of an article showing that a generic thyroid replacement therapy had bioavailability similar to that of the brand-name preparation (Rennie, 1997).

conclusions. The authors of the review suggested that there was a "discordance between the data that underlie the results and the interpretation of these data in the conclusions" (Yank et al., 2007, p. 1204).

Thus, although there is little direct evidence that industry sponsorship has led to deliberate skewing of the results or reporting, there are multiple cases in which industry sponsors have withheld important study results and in which the conclusions presented in the reports appear to overstate the study findings. The risk of undue influence in research exists. The risk is particularly relevant in clinical trials, when the prospect of direct harm to patients (as well as research participants) is a more immediate concern than is the case for most nonclinical research. In this case, conflict of interest policies may help prevent an erosion in public confidence beyond that which may result from research that documents bias or the withholding of data.

Ghostwritten research articles also raise concerns about bias as well as the ethics of author attribution. A conflict of interest is inherent in this practice when the industry sponsor has more control over the article than the nominal authors. Chapter 5 discusses ghostwriting and also participation on speakers bureaus and recommends that academic medical centers forbid faculty from accepting the authorship of ghostwritten articles and participation in speakers bureaus.

Terms of Research Contracts

Some academic health centers allow provisions in research contracts that give industry sponsors important control over the reporting of research findings. In a 2004 survey involving academic medical centers, 7 percent of respondents reported that their institution would allow industry sponsors to revise manuscripts or decide whether results should be published, and more than 5 percent reported that they were unsure about the answers to both questions (Mello et al., 2005a). Half allowed the sponsor to draft the manuscript, whereas only 40 percent prohibited that practice. Seventeen percent of the responding institutions reported disputes over control or access to the data from research. Such disputes also figured in some of the incidents cited in Box 4-1 (see, e.g., Rennie [1997] and Kahn et al. [2000]).

Funding arrangements with contract research organizations have also raised concerns about inappropriate control by industry sponsors (Bodenheimer, 2000; Mirowski and Van Horn, 2005; Shuchman, 2007; Lenzer, 2008). For example, the International Committee of Medical Journal Editors (ICMJE) has expressed concern about the role of contract research organizations that conduct the majority of industry-funded trials, often without the protections that many university research contracts require, including rights of access to the source data and rights to publication (Davidoff et al., 2001). Although the committee found no systematic assessments or comparisons of bias in research conducted by these organizations, any lack of such controls over unilateral industry influence raises concerns.

Issues Involving Research Participants or Students

As Chapter 3 discussed, academic medical centers vary in their policies on disclosure to research participants of investigator's conflicts of interest. It also noted that several surveys suggest that participants in clinical trials currently are not highly concerned about investigators' financial conflicts of interest. Most respondents report that their decision to enroll in a clinical trial would not be greatly affected by learning that the researcher had a financial relationship with the sponsor. Some respondents even believed that "a greater financial interest would make the investigator do a better job" (Weinfurt et al., 2006a, p. 903).

It is not clear, however, whether participants in clinical trials understand how conflicts of interest could potentially compromise study designs and the protection of research subjects or how they could contribute to bias in the reporting of the results—with the possible consequence being harm to future patients. Furthermore, it is not clear that it is reasonable to expect the average participant to understand these issues. In any case, even if research subjects are not worried about conflicts of interest, other important members of the public may be concerned. As noted in earlier chapters, the political and economic support of the research enterprise depends critically on the confidence of the opinion leaders in government, the media, and academia. When they have doubts about the integrity of the enterprise, that essential support may begin to erode.

Concerns have also been raised about how researcher conflicts of interest might affect their advice about or supervision of the research of medical students, residents, fellows, and junior faculty (AAMC, 2008b; AAMC-AAU, 2008). For example, in their recent report on conflict of interest policies in human subjects research, the American Association of Medical Colleges (AAMC) and the Association of American Universities (AAU) noted the potential for the exploitation of these individuals by conflicted senior investigators or advisers. Such exploitation is unethical and also has the potential to bias the design, conduct, and findings of research. Areas that may raise problems with undue influence include decisions about an individual's inclusion or exclusion from a research project; the focus, design, and conduct of a study; the publication of research findings (including the suppression of publication); and the treatment of intellectual property interests.

RESPONSES TO CONCERNS ABOUT CONFLICTS OF INTEREST IN RESEARCH

Limits on Conduct of Research by Investigators with Conflicts of Interest

As discussed in Chapter 1, much of the impetus for conflict of interest policies in universities stems from concerns about industry-funded biomedical research and investigators who have financial stakes in the outcomes of their research. In 1995, the U.S. Public Health Services (PHS) issued regulations that require institutions receiving PHS research funding to develop conflict of interest policies that require the disclosure and management of certain financial relationships between researchers and industry (see Appendix B). Chapter 3 noted reviews by NIH and others that questioned the adequacy of policy adoption and the implementation of the PHS regulations by research institutions, which in turn, raised additional concerns about the adequacy of government oversight of institutional compliance.

Because the PHS regulations were not specific on many issues and because some studies indicated shortfalls in their implementation, AAMC issued a report in 2001 with recommendations to help academic medical centers develop sound conflict of interest policies for research involving human subjects (AAMC, 2001).[4] A key policy recommendation called for institutions to establish a "rebuttable presumption" that researchers may not conduct research involving human participants when they have a financial stake in its outcome. This presumption can be rebutted when compelling circumstances justify the researchers' involvement.[5]

A 2003 AAMC survey indicated that only 61 percent of medical schools had adopted the rebuttable presumption in their policies (Ehringhaus and Korn, 2004). In addition, only a minority of the medical schools with such a policy had defined the compelling circumstances that would support an exception.

To further promote the adoption of conflict of interest policies governing research involving human participants, AAMC joined with AAU to issue a second report that offered additional guidance and support for

[4] As noted in Chapter 1, this report generally follows the practice of recent Institute of Medicine reports in referring to research participants rather than to research subjects.

[5] In the words of the AAMC report, the rebuttable presumption means that an "institution will presume, in order to assure that all potentially problematic circumstances are reviewed, that a financially interested individual may not conduct the human subjects research in question" (AAMC, 2001, p. 12). The report goes on to say that the "rule is not intended to be absolute: a financially interested individual may rebut the presumption by demonstrating facts that, in the opinion of the COI [conflict of interest] committee, constitute compelling circumstances . . . [and] would then be allowed to conduct the research under conditions specified by the COI committee and approved by the responsible IRB [institutional review board]" (p. 12).

policy development and implementation (AAMC-AAU, 2008). The report reemphasized the importance of the rebuttable presumption. It also presented informative case studies and a template for analyzing these cases to illustrate how different situations can be evaluated for the existence of a conflict of interest, the risks presented by the conflict, the options for eliminating or managing a conflict, and the compelling circumstances that might justify the participation of an investigator with a conflict of interest in research with human participants. Among the examples of risks cited in the template is the extent to which the reputation of the researcher with a conflict of interest or his or her institution could be damaged, even if a plan for managing the conflict is created and implemented.

Unlike the PHS regulations that cover both clinical and nonclinical research, the 2008 AAMC-AAU recommendations focused on clinical research. One recommendation did, however, call for medical center conflict of interest committees to review investigator conflicts of interests in certain nonclinical studies. Examples include those that can be "reasonably anticipated . . . to progress to research involving human subjects within the coming 12 months" (p. 9).

The committee found much less information and analysis about conflict of interest policies affecting nonclinical biomedical research than about policies affecting clinical research. Universities and medical schools may have different policies for different kinds of research or may apply different criteria to evaluate conflicts of interest in research that does not involve humans (as reported in Chapter 3). One university, however, recently adopted a conflict of interest policy that explicitly states that "[t]o protect against the risks that may accompany relationships with Interested Businesses, it is not ordinarily allowable for an Individual who has a Significant Financial Interest in an Interested Business to Conduct Research involving that Interested Business" (Columbia University, 2009).

Although an immediate risk to research participants does not exist in basic research, the potential for bias in basic research does exist. The result could be the initiation of clinical trials based on flawed basic science. In general, a weighing of risks against expected benefits should allow conflict of interest committees to apply policies while taking into account differences in clinical and nonclinical research, including differences in what constitutes a reasonable justification for researchers to be involved in research in which they have a financial stake.

Terms for Research Contracts

AAMC has not proposed comprehensive formal recommendations on the terms of research contracts with industry, but it has issued two reports with suggestions and recommendations that respond to concerns about the integrity of clinical trials (Ehringhaus and Korn, 2004, 2006). The first report provides a checklist of topics, including publication rights and intellectual property, to be covered in research contracts. Among other elements, one or both reports call for contracts to explicitly grant researchers free access to study data, to include no restrictions on publication (except for a slight delay for sponsor review and possible filing of a patent application), and to require a good faith and timely effort to publish the results of research in a peer-reviewed journal.

Requirements to Register and Report on Clinical Trials

Congressional, journal editor, and other requirements for the registration of clinical trials are, in part, a response to concerns about conflict of interest in industry-sponsored research and research reporting. The registration of clinical trials and the provision of key details about the trial protocol and the data analysis plan ensure that basic methods for the conduct and analysis of the findings of a study as well as the primary clinical end points to be assessed and reported are specified before the trial begins and before data are analyzed. The substitution of ad hoc or secondary end points for primary end points and other important departures from the protocol can thus be detected in reports of the findings of a trial. Clinical trials registries also allow others to determine whether the results from a trial have not been presented or reported at all. Researchers carrying out critical literature reviews can then contact the investigators to try to obtain unpublished results. After ICMJE stated that clinical trial registration should be considered a prerequisite for the publication of research articles, the numbers of trials registered increased substantially (Zarin et al., 2005).

In 2007, the U.S. Congress expanded the types of clinical trials of drugs, biologics, and devices—and the kinds of information about these trials—that must be registered (P.L. 110-85). To further address the problem of withholding negative findings, it also required the creation of a link from the ClinicalTrials.gov registry to a database of reports of basic results for applicable trials.[6] The reported results are to include basic demographic and baseline information, findings for primary and secondary outcomes, and a point of contact.

[6] In addition, the Pharmaceutical Research and Manufacturers of America has coordinated the creation of a voluntary online resource to provide information to physicians about the results of clinical trials (see http://www.clinicalstudyresults.org/).

Study Methodology, Data Analysis, and Research Reporting

To the extent that the design of clinical trials is standardized and publicized, the implementation of conflict of interest policies is also assisted. Abuses and patterns of abuses can be more readily detected, which may make more evident the need for changes or reforms in the policies. Efforts to improve the design of clinical trials and other types of research stretch back decades and include a range of techniques, including the random assignment of subjects to intervention and control groups and the blinding of investigators and participants to treatment assignment. In addition, NIH has supported programs to train physician investigators to conduct rigorous clinical research. Experts in research methodology, statistics, and evidence-based medicine have developed techniques to limit bias in research and have codified standards and checklists for reporting research findings. These standards and checklists cover various types of studies, including clinical trials (see, e.g., Moher et al. [2001]), evaluations of clinical tests (Bossuyt et al., 2003), epidemiological studies (see, e.g., von Elm et al. [2007], but see also the comments of the editors of *Epidemiology* [Editors, 2007]), and meta-analyses (see, e.g., Moher et al. [1999] and Stroup et al. [2000]).

ICMJE now specifies a format for the reporting of results and refers authors to the CONSORT checklist for the reporting of the findings of randomized clinical trials (see, e.g., Moher et al. [2001], CONSORT Group [2007], and von Elm et al. [2007]) (Table 4-1). Standards for the reporting of methods and results help editors, reviewers, and readers assess the validity of a research paper. Studies suggest that these standards also improve the design and conduct of the research itself (see, e.g., Plint et al. [2005]).

In addition to these standards for the conduct and reporting of the results of clinical trials, the FDA has suggested that it is desirable for the data-monitoring committees for clinical trials to have statistical reports prepared by statisticians who are independent of the trial sponsors and clinical investigators (FDA, 2001). For industry-funded clinical trials "in which the data analysis is conducted only by statisticians employed by a company sponsoring the research," the *Journal of the American Medical Association* requires that a statistical analysis also be conducted by an independent statistician at an academic institution, such as a medical school, academic medical center, or government research institute, that has oversight over the person conducting the analysis and that is independent of the commercial sponsor (Fontanarosa and DeAngelis, 2008, p. 95; see also a review of opinions about this requirement in Rockhold and Snapinn [2007]).

TABLE 4-1 Checklist for Reporting Clinical Trials from CONSORT 2001 Statement

Item	Description
1	How participants were allocated to interventions (e.g., random allocation, randomized, or randomly assigned)
2	Scientific background and explanation of rationale
3	Eligibility criteria for participants and the settings and locations where the data were collected
4	Precise details of the interventions intended for each group and how and when they were actually administered
5	Specific objectives and hypotheses
6	Clearly defined primary and secondary outcome measures and, when applicable, any methods used to enhance the quality of measurements (e.g., multiple observations and training of assessors)
7	How sample size was determined and, when applicable, explanation of any interim analyses and stopping rules
8	Method used to generate the random allocation sequence, including details of any restrictions (e.g., blocking or stratification)
9	Method used to implement the random allocation sequence (e.g., numbered containers or central telephone), clarifying whether the sequence was concealed until interventions were assigned
10	Who generated the allocation sequence, who enrolled the participants, and who assigned the participants to their groups
11	Whether or not participants, those administering the interventions, and those assessing the outcomes were blinded to group assignment; if done, how the success of blinding was evaluated
12	Statistical methods used to compare groups for primary outcome(s); methods for additional analyses, such as subgroup analyses and adjusted analyses
13	Flow of participants through each stage (a diagram is strongly recommended); specifically, for each group, report the numbers of participants randomly assigned, receiving intended treatment, completing the study protocol, and analyzed for the primary outcome; describe protocol deviations from study as planned, together with reasons
14	Dates defining the periods of recruitment and follow-up
15	Baseline demographic and clinical characteristics of each group
16	Number of participants (denominator) in each group included in each analysis and whether the analysis was by intention to treat; state the results in absolute numbers when feasible (e.g., 10/20, not 50%)
17	For each primary and secondary outcome, a summary of results for each group, and the estimated effect size and its precision (e.g., 95% confidence interval)
18	Address multiplicity by reporting any other analyses performed, including subgroup analyses and adjusted analyses, indicating those that were prespecified and those that were exploratory
19	All important adverse events or side effects in each intervention group

TABLE 4-1 Continued

Item	Description
20	Interpretation of the results, taking into account study hypotheses, sources of potential bias or imprecision, and the dangers associated with multiplicity of analyses and outcomes
21	Generalizability (external validity) of the trial findings
22	General interpretation of the results in the context of current evidence

SOURCE: CONSORT Group, 2001 (see also Moher et al. [2001]).

Peer Review and Journal Policies on Disclosure

Peer review is a key step used to detect and reduce bias in publications and improve the quality of research reporting. Effective review depends on independent reviewers who are not biased by their own financial relationships with industry. As described in Chapter 3, journals vary in the extent to which they apply conflict of interest policies to reviewers. Meaningful peer review is also assisted by the previously described standards for the reporting of methods and data in manuscripts.

In response to concerns about the reporting of research results described earlier in this chapter, medical journals have moved toward increasingly specific requirements for disclosure of authors' financial interests (see ICMJE [2008] and WAME [2008] for the statements of two associations of medical journal editors). Still, as described in Chapter 3, journal policies remain variable. The completeness and accuracy of disclosures are continuing issues for medical journals as well as for academic medical centers and other institutions. These concerns have led to action in some states and recommendations for the federal government to establish a policy that requires companies to report payments to physicians, researchers, and institutions, as outlined in the preceding chapter. Chapter 3 includes a committee recommendation supporting such a program.

Issues Involving Research Participants and Students

As described in Chapter 3, AAMC recommended in 2001 and again in 2008 policies that require some form of disclosure of investigator conflicts of interest to research subjects, and many medical schools have adopted those policies. Chapter 3 also reviewed some of the findings from a set of coordinated research projects and activities to investigate the views of research participants and ways of informing them. This research is itself a major response to concerns about practical and ethical issues in managing conflicts of interest in research, for example, balancing the disclosure of information with the design of an informed consent form and process that does not overwhelm research participants.

AAMC has also recommended the disclosure of investigator conflicts of interests to other members of the research team. It also advised that schools prohibit "agreements with sponsors or financially interested companies that place restrictions on the activities of students or trainees or that bind students or trainees to non-disclosure provisions" (AAMC, 2001, p. 20). In a later statement about the responsibilities of biomedical graduate students and their advisers, AAMC states that advisers should "recognize the possibility of conflicts between the interests of externally funded research programs and those of the graduate student" and should commit that those conflicts will not be allowed to interfere with the student's thesis or dissertation research (AAMC, 2008b, p. 6). The research adviser also agrees to discuss authorship policies and intellectual property policies related to disclosure, patent rights, and publication. In addition, in a series of questions that should be asked when assessing the risks of allowing an investigator with a conflict of interest to conduct research with human participants and the possibility that a conflict can be appropriately managed, the AAMC-AAU report includes questions about whether the "the roles of students, trainees, and junior faculty and staff [are] appropriate and free from exploitation" and whether special protections are needed for "vulnerable members" of the research team (AAMC-AAU, 2008, pp. 25 and 28, respectively). One protection might be to provide such individuals with access to independent senior faculty members for independent review and guidance when questions and concerns arise.

RECOMMENDATIONS

Relationships between industry and research institutions and researchers are common and are often mutually beneficial. They also serve society by generating valuable preventive, diagnostic, and therapeutic products. At the same time, these individual and institutional relationships have risks that could jeopardize the integrity of scientific research and conflict with the ethical conditions for the conduct of research with humans. Analyses indicate that they are associated with decreased openness in sharing data and findings, and cases in which negative findings are not published in a timely fashion or at all raise concerns. Some studies also suggest that meta-analyses sponsored by a single company tend to present conclusions favorable to industry sponsors even when the actual findings of the analyses are not favorable. Moreover, when investigators themselves have a financial stake in the outcomes of their research, it creates conflicts of interest, which may lead to bias and the erosion of confidence in the research enterprise.

Chapter 2 discussed why conflicts of interest matter even if they do not actually lead to undue influence or bias in a particular case. Correlations or associations in studies such as those reported here are enough to support concerns over potential conflicts of interest. The purpose of conflict of interest policies is preventive: the policies are intended to remove or reduce relationships that create a risk of undue influence or erosion of confidence in the research enterprise.

As described in this chapter and in Chapter 3, research institutions vary in their conflict of interest policies, including the extent to which they have adopted and implemented PHS conflict of interest regulations and policies recommended by AAMC and AAU. Government and press investigations and payment data reported by companies have revealed failures of individual researchers to fully and accurately disclose their financial relationships with industry, as required by institutional or government policies.

The preceding section of this chapter provided an overview of recommendations for action that should be taken by research institutions, research sponsors, investigators, and medical journals to protect the integrity of biomedical research, safeguard research participants, and preserve public trust. The recommendation below focuses on one specific concern: the conduct of research with human participants by investigators with a financial interest in the outcome of that research. The discussion of the recommendation is followed by a review of standards for nonclinical research and a suggestion that NIH take a lead role in further examination of the involvement of conflicted investigators in this kind of research.

Clinical Research

It is critical that the public trust that research institutions are protecting the integrity of the medical research on which clinical practice and education depend. Such protection is especially important in clinical research because bias in the design, conduct, or reporting of the findings of such research may expose human participants to risks without the prospect of gaining valid, generalizable knowledge and may ultimately expose much larger numbers of patients to ineffective or unsafe clinical care.

Recommendation 4.1 calls for research institutions to allow researchers with a conflict of interest to conduct research involving human participants only when a researcher's participation is truly essential and is also managed to limit risk. This recommendation is similar to the AAMC "rebuttable presumption" described earlier in this chapter.

RECOMMENDATION 4.1 Academic medical centers and other research institutions should establish a policy that individuals generally may not conduct research with human participants if they have a significant financial interest in an existing or potential product or a

company that could be affected by the outcome of the research. Exceptions to the policy should be made public and should be permitted only if the conflict of interest committee (a) determines that an individual's participation is essential for the conduct of the research and (b) establishes an effective mechanism for managing the conflict and protecting the integrity of the research.

This recommendation covers principal investigators and others who share substantial responsibility for the design, conduct, or reporting of the findings of clinical studies. Relevant financial interests often involve stock or other ownership in a company making a product that could be affected by the results of a study, including not only a product under study but also a product that is an alternative to the intervention under study. (Although AAMC recommended no minimum threshold for the initial disclosure of financial interests, it suggested that "significant interest" should generally be defined as a financial interest of $10,000 or more.)

In exceptional cases, a clinical investigator may be judged to be essential if his or her participation is determined—after careful assessment—to be necessary for the safety, reliability, or validity of the research, circumstances that AAMC described as compelling. Often cited as examples are situations in which inventors of a medical device or investigators responsible for certain kinds of breakthrough scientific discoveries are crucial to research, especially early-phase studies, because of their "insights, knowledge, perseverance, laboratory resources" or access to "special patient populations" (AAMC-AAU, 2008, p. 6; see also Witkin [1997] and Citron [2008]).

A specific example of a compelling situation might involve the participation in a pilot study of the inventor of an implanted medical device that requires a complex, new surgical procedure that has not been mastered by others. The reasons for allowing a researcher with a conflict of interest to participate in a pilot or early-phase study or other investigation in a particular situation should be persuasive to others who are presented with the facts of the case. In most cases of a conflict of interest, no compelling argument that the investigator's participation is essential can be made. Even if the investigator's participation is essential, the elimination of the conflict of interest (e.g., through the sale of stock) is the preferred step. If an exception is granted, it should be made public.

If an exception is made for an investigator with a conflict of interest, the next step is for the conflict of interest committee to establish a strategy for managing the conflict and a plan for monitoring the strategy's implementation during the course of the research. For instance, the plan might specify that the researcher with the conflict of interest not serve as the principal investigator. It might also restrict the researcher recruiting subjects; obtaining informed consent; assessing the clinical end points; analyzing data; or writing the results, conclusions, and abstracts for publications reporting the findings of the study. The plan might, however, allow the researcher to participate in aspects of study design, fund raising, and manuscript review.

Nonclinical Research

Most of the discussion of conflicts of interest in research has focused on clinical research. This emphasis reflects concerns that research participants might be harmed or that bias might contribute to the making of incorrect decisions about approving new drugs and devices or changing clinical practice. Because conflicts of interest in various kinds of nonclinical research have been little investigated, the committee found it difficult to evaluate arguments about the extent and the consequences (or the lack of consequences) of investigator and institutional conflicts of interest in this sphere of research. It thus did not make a formal recommendation about conflicts of interest in nonclinical research. The committee did, however, hear testimony that new models of academia-industry collaboration are needed to promote basic scientific discoveries and the development of new therapies while also addressing concerns about conflicts of interest (Moses, 2008; see also Moses and Martin [2001]).

No matter the type or stage of research, certain fundamentals still apply. All researchers should be subject to an institution's disclosure policies, as described in Chapter 3, and the institution's conflict of interest committee or its equivalent should be notified when investigators have financial stakes in the outcomes of their research. Similarly, following the conceptual framework presented in Chapter 2, once a financial relationship or interest has been disclosed, it should be evaluated for determination of the likelihood that it will have an undue influence that will lead to bias or a loss of trust. If a risk is judged to exist, a conflict of interest committee might conclude that the implementation of safeguards is necessary. Such safeguards could consist of a management plan that includes the involvement of a researcher without a conflict of interest in certain aspects of the research and disclosure of the conflict to coinvestigators and in presentations and publications.

Additional studies on the extent of financial relationships in nonclinical research and their consequences, as well as the consequences of conflict of interest policies, are needed to establish a sounder base of evidence for future policies. Given its extensive and direct relationships with basic scientists, NIH could play a central role in gathering such evidence. As discussed in Chapter 9, NIH could fund research on conflicts of interest in nonclinical scientific research. Furthermore, NIH could convene working groups and public meetings to promote a fuller understanding—empirical, conceptual, and practical—of conflicts of interest in nonclinical research and propose responses. Such meetings might identify good practices in developing academia-industry relationships in nonclinical research and suggest how such relationships might be developed in ways that promote constructive collaboration while appropriately addressing concerns about conflicts of interest. The development of illustrative case studies might help institutions better understand and manage conflicts of interest in nonclinical research.

Other Relevant Recommendations in This Report

The adoption of the recommendations made elsewhere in this report would also affect researchers, research institutions, and companies. These recommendations call for standardization of the procedures used to disclose conflicts of interest to harmonize the requirements of different institutions and reduce the disclosure burdens on individuals (Recommendation 3.3), implementation of methods for the easier verification of certain financial disclosures (Recommendation 3.4), limitations on certain relationships with industry (e.g., acceptance of gifts and participation in promotional activities) for academic medical center personnel (Recommendation 5.1), and promotion of reforms in industry policies on consulting and research grants (Recommendation 6.2).

Chapter 8 includes a recommendation that responsibility for the oversight of institutional conflicts of interest be lodged in the governing boards of institutions (Recommendation 8.1). Many conflicts of interest at the institutional level involve research or proposed research in which a university or medical school has a financial stake related to its interests in patents or start-up companies.

In addition, the committee recommends that other public and private organizations create incentives to support the adoption of the recommendations made in this report (Recommendation 9.1). As one example, NIH could expand its recent efforts to provide more guidance and oversight to grantee institutions covered by the PHS regulations, issue regulations directing grantees to adopt institutional conflict of interest policies (Recommendation 8.2), and take a lead role in the development of a research agenda on conflict of interest (Recommendation 9.2). NIH could also consider requiring investigators funded by NIH awards to be trained on conflict of interest principles and policies. (NIH has a new training module on conflict of interest that could be tailored for investigators.) Other public agencies that support academic biomedical research, for example, the U.S. Department of Defense, could also provide guidance compatible with that presented in this report.

Taken together, the changes recommended here should not burden socially valuable collaborations between academic researchers and industry. Rather, they should help justify and maintain public trust in their integrity.

5

Conflicts of Interest in Medical Education

Medical education prepares physicians for a lifetime of professional work. Education that is objective and that teaches students how to critically evaluate the evidence prepares physicians to keep current with scientific advances throughout their professional lives.

This chapter is organized around the concept of the learning environment, which shapes and reinforces the professional attitudes and behavior of physicians throughout the continuum of learning that begins in medical school and extends through residency training and to lifelong learning. Learning environments in medicine are diverse. They include conference rooms and lecture halls, patient care locales (such as inpatient service and outpatient practice locations), laboratories, and the Internet. Some continuing education programs take place at restaurants or resorts.

If the learning environment provides the stage for education, the curriculum provides the script. Reviews of undergraduate and graduate medical education often emphasize the "formal curriculum" (i.e., required courses and explicit educational objectives).[1] That formal curriculum aims to help students develop the core competencies that are defined by accreditation agencies. Each educational activity has learning objectives, and the totality of educational sessions must address all the core competencies.

The learning environment also includes two other elements: the informal curriculum (i.e., ad hoc interactions among teachers and students) and

[1] The committee follows the convention in medical education of referring to the years of medical school as "undergraduate medical education" and the post-M.D. years of residency and fellowship as "graduate medical education." Unless otherwise described (e.g., research fellows), fellows are physicians in subspecialty training programs. This report refers to "residents" and "fellows" rather than "trainees" (a description commonly used by medical educators).

the hidden curriculum (i.e., institutional practices and culture) (see, e.g., Hafferty [1998], Ratanawongsa et al. [2005], Cottingham et al. [2008], and Haidet [2008]). Ideally, these two elements convey messages that are consistent with the formal curriculum, but in practice they may not. For example, the formal curriculum might include course work on medical ethics, research methodology, and appropriate relationships with industry. Concurrently, the informal and hidden curricula might be characterized by disparaging faculty comments on their institution's conflict of interest policies and the failure of institutions to adopt and implement sound policies.

Unfortunately, some aspects of each curriculum may contribute to undesirable attitudes or practices. The Association of American Medical Colleges (AAMC) observed in a 2008 report that the conflicts created by a range of common interactions with industry can "[f]or medicine generally, and for academic medicine in particular . . . have a corrosive effect on three core principles of medical professionalism: autonomy, objectivity, and altruism" (AAMC, 2008c, p. 4). Members of the U.S. Congress have also expressed concern about commercial relationships in medical education, primarily continuing medical education (see, e.g., Finance Committee, U.S. Senate [2007]). In contrast to the requirements for recipients of U.S. Public Health Service research awards, the federal government does not require the recipients of direct or indirect funds for medical education to establish and administer conflict of interest policies.

This chapter next provides a brief background on the current context of medical education. It then examines the literature on conflict of interest issues and responses in the learning environments of undergraduate, graduate, and continuing medical education. The discussion covers access to educational environments by sales representatives of medical product companies (e.g., drug detailing, which is a visit to a doctor by a sales representative for a pharmaceutical company), the provision of drug samples and other gifts to faculty and students, and industry-sponsored scholarships and fellowships. A separate section considers a concern that cuts across all phases of education: intellectual independence in presentations and publications and the risks associated with speakers bureaus and ghostwritten publications. (Chapter 4 discussed concerns about how researcher conflicts of interest might affect their advice or supervision involving the research of medical students, residents, fellows, and junior faculty.)

The committee concluded that, in general, industry financial relationships do not benefit the educational missions of medical institutions in ways that offset the risks created. The chapter thus ends with recommendations that are intended to protect the integrity and limit the potential for undue industry influence in medical education. As explained in Chapter 1, the committee focused on conflicts of interest involving physicians and biomedical researchers; but much of the core rationale for the recommendations may be relevant to nursing, pharmacy, dentistry, and other professions, even though some of the specifics might differ. Chapter 6 considers many of the same issues in the context of physicians in practice outside academic settings.

BACKGROUND AND CONTEXT

Scale and Oversight of Medical Education

American medical education evolved during the 19th and early 20th centuries from pure apprenticeships to proprietary medical schools of variable quality to a reformed and formal educational system that stresses both science and professionalism. During the middle decades of the 20th century, an increasingly elaborate structure of graduate (post-M.D.) medical education emerged, characterized by multiyear residencies in medical specialties beyond the traditional internship year. The latter half of the century saw the growth of requirements by state licensing boards and specialty certification boards for demonstrated participation in accredited continuing education activities (Caplan, 1996).

Today, the scale of American medical education is impressive. The United States has

- 130 accredited medical schools (AAMC, 2008d),[2] approximately 400 major teaching hospitals (Salsberg, 2008), more than 100,000 faculty members (Salsberg, 2008), and approximately 75,000 medical students (AAMC, 2008e);
- 8,355 accredited residency programs for 126 specialties and subspecialties (2006–2007) and more than 107,000 active full-time and part-time residents (2005–2006) (ACGME, 2007b); and
- 740 national providers of accredited continuing medical education (and 1,600 accredited state providers)[3] that reported more than 7 million physician participants in their programs (ACCME, 2008a, 2009), a number that includes multiple registrations among the nation's more than 800,000 active physicians (a count that includes medical residents) (Salsberg, 2008).

[2] The count includes four schools granted preliminary accreditation in 2008. It does not include accredited Canadian schools or the 20 accredited U.S. schools of osteopathic medicine.

[3] These providers are accredited by state medical societies under the rules of the Accreditation Council on Continuing Medical Education.

The Liaison Commission on Medical Education (LCME) is the oversight agency that is responsible for the accreditation of the nation's medical schools. Its members are appointed by AAMC and the American Medical Association (AMA). The Accreditation Council for Graduate Medical Education (ACGME) accredits residency training programs in the United States. The sponsoring institution for a residency program may be a hospital, medical school, university, or group of hospitals (ACGME, 2008). Accreditation bodies define the core competencies for students, residents, and fellows and ensure that the formal curriculum covers all essential aspects of medical education. ACGME board members are appointed by AAMC, AMA, the American Board of Medical Specialties, the American Hospital Association (AHA), and the Council of Medical Specialty Societies (CMSS). Accredited continuing medical education providers are accredited by the Accreditation Council for Continuing Medical Education (ACCME). Its member organizations are AHA, AMA, AAMC, CMSS, the Association for Hospital Medical Education, and the Federation of State Medical Boards. State medical societies may also accredit providers within a state.[4] In addition, AMA, the American Academy of Family Physicians, and certain other groups set standards and certify credits for specific courses that physicians can take (from accredited providers) to meet state licensure board and other requirements for accredited continuing medical education (see, e.g., AMA [2006, 2008b]).[5] Accredited providers usually issue certificates to document that a physician has completed a certified course. Consistent with common usage, this report uses the phrase accredited continuing medical education to refer to education that is (1) presented by accredited providers and (2) certified for course credits.

Changing Environment and Fiscal Challenges

Academic medical centers dominate the provision of undergraduate and graduate medical education. The institutions consist of two related enterprises: a medical school that trains physicians and conducts research and a system that provides health care services. The latter system may include teaching hospitals, satellite clinics, and physician office practices. Academic health centers include other health professions schools, such as a school of dentistry, nursing, or pharmacy (Wartman, 2007).

[4] As described by ACCME, "ACCME has two major functions: the accreditation of providers whose CME [continuing medical education] activities attract a national audience and the recognition of state or territorial medical societies to accredit providers whose audiences for its CME activities are primarily from that state/territory and contiguous states/territories" (ACCME, 2005).

[5] AMA also authorizes credits for other activities, such as publishing an article in a peer-reviewed journal or achieving and maintaining specialty board certification.

In recent years, academic medical centers have struggled financially because of low levels of payment for poor and uninsured patients, reductions in the Medicare indirect medical education adjustment for hospital payment rates, and lower profit margins for the provision of hospital services to Medicare patients. (In the late 1990s, medical schools also faced declining admissions, but admissions increased from 2003 to 2007 [AAMC, 2008a].) At the same time, teaching hospitals have faced rising costs because of the incorporation of new medical informatics systems and expensive medical technologies and restrictions on the numbers of hours that residents may work. The Medicare Policy Advisory Commission has characterized 53 percent of major teaching hospitals as being under high financial pressure—compared to 28 percent of hospitals overall (MedPAC, 2009). Given these circumstances, financial support from industry may seem attractive.

Physicians in training also face financial challenges. In 2006, the median levels of debt of medical students graduating from public and private medical schools were $120,000 and $160,000, respectively (Jolly, 2007). Medical school graduates can expect to pay approximately 9 to 12 percent of their after-tax income after graduation for educational debt service (Jolly, 2007). This level of indebtedness and the delayed gratification of a profession that requires years of training before independent practice is permitted can contribute to a sense of entitlement, which, in turn, may position medical students, residents, and fellows to be strongly influenced by gifts and attention from representatives of pharmaceutical and medical device companies (see, e.g., Levine [2008]). Sierles and colleagues (2005) found that 80 percent of the medical students that they surveyed believed that they were entitled to gifts. In addition, as discussed in Chapter 6, once they are in practice, limits on reimbursements for physician services make debt repayment more of a burden than in the past and may make gifts and other financial relationships with industry more appealing.

Industry Funding of Medical Education

During most of the 20th century, medical product companies were not major participants in medical education. The exception was sales representatives, who provided information to residents and faculty as well as to nonacademic physicians. In the latter decades of the century, however, medical product companies became increasingly involved in sponsoring continuing medical education, including grand rounds and other academic-based programs. In a 2008 report on industry funding of medical education, a task force of AAMC observed generally that

> Over recent decades, medical schools and teaching hospitals have become increasingly dependent on industry support of their core educational mis-

> sions. This reliance raises concerns because such support, including gifts, can influence the objectivity and integrity of academic teaching, learning, and practice, thereby calling into question the commitment of academia and industry together to promote the public's interest by fostering the most cost-effective, evidence-based medical care possible. (AAMC, 2008c, p. iii)

The committee found no data on the amount or proportion of undergraduate or graduate medical education supported by industry. It also found little systematic information on specific categories of financial support, for example, grants for residencies or fellowships, direct or indirect financial support for grand rounds, or donations for buildings or other capital items. The most extensive information on academic institutions' ties with industry comes from a 2006 survey of department chairs at medical schools and the 15 largest independent teaching hospitals (67 percent response rate). The responses indicated that 65 percent of clinical departments received industry support for continuing medical education, 37 percent received industry support for residency or fellowship training, 17 percent received industry support for research equipment, and 19 percent received unrestricted funds from industry for department operations (Campbell et al., 2007b). The committee did not categorize industry payments for meals, gifts, and visits by sales representatives as support for medical education because these activities do not fit the learning objectives in the formal curriculum.

Information on industry funding for accredited continuing medical education comes from yearly surveys by ACCME. Figure 5-1 shows that commercial sources (excluding advertising and exhibits at programs organized by accredited providers) provide a substantially larger share of income for education providers today than they did in 1998. By 2003, about half of all funding for accredited continuing medical education programs came from commercial sources. The fees paid by program attendees once provided the majority of provider income, but today industry-supported programs are often provided free or at reduced cost to physicians (Steinbrook, 2008a).

LEARNING ENVIRONMENTS IN MEDICAL SCHOOLS AND RESIDENCY PROGRAMS

The ultimate mission of medical education is to prepare physicians to provide effective, safe, high-quality, efficient, timely, affordable, and patient-centered care to patients. In revising the standards that provide the framework for essential aspects of medical education, both LCME and ACGME have recently emphasized how the learning environment can affect the development of core professional values and core competencies, includ-

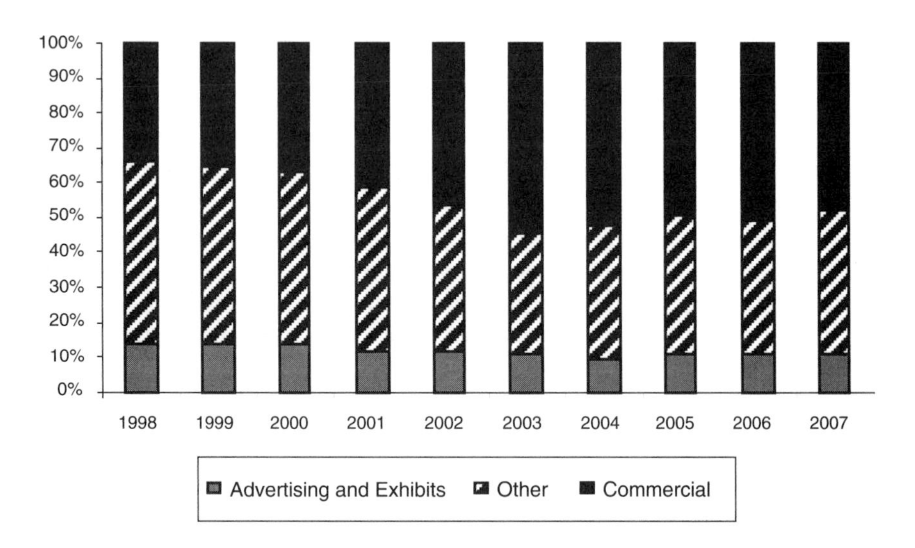

FIGURE 5-1 Sources of income reported by respondents (accredited providers of continuing medical education) to ACCME annual survey, 1998 to 2007. SOURCE: Compiled from ACCME, 2008a.

ing how to critically review the evidence and to commit to lifelong learning about scientific advances.

Both LCME and ACGME recognize the power of the local learning environment to shape the knowledge, skills, behaviors, and attitudes of the next generation of physicians. To achieve accreditation, institutions providing undergraduate or graduate medical education must have curricula and resources that, among other requirements, (1) promote the development of appropriate professional attributes; (2) help learners at all levels think critically and appraise the evidence base for research reports, practice guidelines, and marketing materials; and (3) provide appropriate role models and mentoring. In addition, a standard on the creation of the appropriate learning environment must be implemented (LCME Standard MS-31-A). Recently, ACGME has required institutions to have a statement or institutional policy that addresses interactions between vendor representatives or corporations and residents and their programs (Requirement III. B.13 [ACGME, 2007a]).

The Learning Environment in Undergraduate and Graduate Medical Education as a Target of Industry Influence

Scope of Relationships Between Industry and Students, Medical Schools, and Teaching Hospitals

Interactions between medical students and industry are common. Table 5-1 summarizes the results from a survey of third-year medical students at eight major medical schools. Almost all students had received an industry-provided lunch or other gift. More than one-third had attended a social event hosted by a drug company.

Information from two surveys of residency directors similarly documents frequent interactions with pharmaceutical companies. For example, a 2002 survey of emergency medicine residency program directors found that approximately 40 percent allowed industry to fund social activities, and a similar percentage allowed pharmaceutical representatives to teach residents (Keim et al., 2004). Twenty-nine percent said that industry travel support could be made contingent on residents attending an industry event. Only 50 percent said that they always or very frequently followed ACGME recommendations for industry funding of core lectures, and 10 percent said that they always or very frequently allowed pharmaceutical representatives unrestricted access to residents. In a 2002 survey of psychiatric residency program directors, 88 percent reported that they allowed industry to provide lunches for their residents, and among this group, the mean was about five lunches per week (Varley et al., 2005). Approximately a third of the programs solicited travel funds from industry (31 percent) or allowed residents to seek such funding from industry on their own (34 percent).

Value of Relationships

Some interactions with industry can have educational value, for example, when an industry scientist participates in a seminar on drug development strategies or when a device company representative provides supervised training on a complex and innovative medical device that has recently been approved for marketing. Other examples may include unrestricted grants to academic medical centers that support student or resident research stipends or participation in scientific conferences. On a much larger scale, universities have benefited from company gifts for buildings, research programs, and auditoriums.

Pharmaceutical companies argue that their representatives provide information on new drugs. Yet, medical students, residents, and fellows have ready access to the latest scientific information through faculty members, information technologies that allow them to search the medical literature,

TABLE 5-1 Third-Year Medical Students' Interactions with Drug Companies

Type of Event	No. of Students. (N = 826)	No. (%) of Students Who Received a Gift or Participated in at Least One Event	Exposure Frequency per Month[a]	
			Mean (SD)	Range
A lunch provided by a drug company	793	768 (96.8)	1.08 (0.76)	0–4.2
A small, noneducational gift (e.g., pen or coffee mug)	801	754 (94.1)	0.87 (0.69)	0–3.5
A journal reprint or a glossy brochure from a pharmaceutical representative	800	716 (89.5)	0.53 (0.52)	0–3.5
A snack (e.g., donut, candy, coffee) provided by a pharmaceutical representative	800	713 (89.1)	0.75 (0.72)	0–8.5
A grand rounds sponsored by a drug company	798	690 (86.5)	0.54 (0.57)	0–2.4
A dinner provided by a drug company	801	405 (50.6)	0.13 (0.21)	0–2.4
A drug sample from a pharmaceutical representative	799	435 (54.4)	0.10 (0.20)	0–2.1
Another social event (e.g., party) sponsored by a drug company	799	272 (34.0)	0.06 (0.11)	0–0.8
A book donated by a drug company[b]	826	421 (51.0)		
Attendance at a workshop sponsored by a drug company[b]	826	214 (25.9)		
Registration fee for a conference paid for by a drug company[b]	826	37 (4.5)		
Participation in a market survey sponsored by a drug company[b]	826	29 (3.5)		
Participation in a research project sponsored by a drug company[b]	826	22 (2.7)		
Travel expenses for a conference paid for by a drug company[b]	826	15 (1.8)		
Nominated for an award sponsored by a drug company[b]	826	5 (0.6)		
Obtained a fellowship sponsored by a drug company[b]	826	4 (0.5)		

[a]For each student, an exposure index was calculated as the sum of the monthly frequencies for the first eight items.
[b]Monthly frequency data were not requested.
SOURCE: Sierles et al. Medical students' exposure to and attitudes about drug company interactions: a national survey. *Journal of the American Medical Association* 294(9):1034–1042 (September 7, 2005).

and open-access sources of evidence-based literature reviews and summaries. The committee recognizes that some medical students and residents who have become accustomed to interactions with representatives may value the meals that they receive as a respite and may view the gifts that they bring as either inconsequential or as an appropriate reward for their demanding schedules and economic sacrifices.

The discussion below focuses on several different types of academic-industry relationships and the literature about their consequences. Each section includes a discussion of private- and public-sector responses to concerns about the extent and consequences of these relationships. In addition to consulting reports by AAMC and other groups, the committee examined the policies of a number of medical schools. It found many of these policies at or available through links from the websites of the American Medical Student Association (AMSA) and the Institute on Medicine as a Profession (IMAP). The AMSA website also includes the organization's scorecard, which presents school-by-school ratings of various policy elements (e.g., the policy on the acceptance of gifts) and which has received considerable attention from the media.[6]

The committee notes that the recommendations in the 2008 AAMC report on medical education apply off campus as well as on campus. The report calls for academic medical centers to "communicate to off-site training facilities their expectation that the off-site venues will adhere to the standards of the academic center regarding interactions with industry" (AAMC, 2008c, p. 10).

Site Access by Drug and Device Company Representatives

Issues and Evidence

Drug detailing, that is, a visit to a doctor by a sales representative for a pharmaceutical company, is a common way that companies promote their products and establish relationships with physicians in academic and community settings. In 2004, an estimated 36 percent of the $57.5 billion that pharmaceutical companies spent on product promotion went for detailing (Gagnon and Lexchin, 2008).

Medical device companies also employ sales representatives to promote their products to physicians and hospitals, although the responsibilities of

[6] The AMSA ratings, the methodology, and other information can be found at http://amsascorecard.org/. The IMAP information can be found at http://www.imapny.org/coi_database/. Both groups use information and policies received in response to a survey conducted under the auspices of the Prescription Project with funding from the Pew Charitable Trust. Some schools did not respond initially, and others refused to supply their policies.

some of these representatives may be more complex. They may provide training, equipment calibration, and additional services or advice related to implants and other sophisticated technologies used in the operating room and elsewhere (see, e.g., ECRI Institute [2007]). In one instance, the Food and Drug Administration (FDA) has required physicians to be trained by company representatives as a condition for the approval of a device (see, e.g., FDA [2004b] and Dawson [2006]).

The committee did not locate any information about how drug or device detailing activity differs between academic and nonacademic settings or how specific tactics of detailing and their effects may vary by setting or type of physician (e.g., resident versus faculty member versus community physician). Interactions with drug company representatives are common in academic settings. Medical students average about one interaction with drug company representatives a week, and 80 to 100 percent of students report interactions (see, e.g., Bellin et al. [2004], Sierles et al. [2005], and Fitz et al. [2007]). As described by one faculty member,

> [d]rug company representatives are a major presence. They sponsor Journal Club (where trainees learn to review new data and research), they pay for many of our weekly speakers and regularly offer free dinners for the residents and faculty. They enjoy free access to our mailboxes and regularly detail our trainees in their offices, hallways and in our little kitchen. (Shapiro, 2004, p. F5)

Medical students and residents reported that they received insufficient training in interacting with drug representatives. Studies also indicate that students and residents believe that their own prescribing behavior is not affected by drug company gifts, although they believe that the prescribing behavior of their colleagues is (Sierles et al., 2005; Zipkin and Steinman, 2005). Limited evidence suggests that educational interventions "show some promise" in affecting the attitudes and behaviors related to relationships with industry (Carroll et al., 2007).

Overall, research suggests that drug company representatives may influence prescribing patterns and requests for additions to hospital formularies. The effects appear to be modest but consistent across various kinds of research and disciplines. One review concluded that the "pharmaceutical industry has a significant presence during residency training, has gained the overall acceptance of trainees, and appears to influence prescribing behavior" (Zipkin and Steinman, 2005, p. 777). Another review (which was not limited to educational settings) concluded that detailing "affects physician prescription behavior in a positive [i.e., the more detailing that there is, the more of an effect that it has] and significant manner" (Manchanda and Honka, 2005, p. 787).

Taken together with the information reviewed below on the role of drug samples and gifts (which typically accompany sales visits), the literature suggests that academic medicine and the public have reason to be concerned about the easy access of sales representatives to medical students, residents, and faculty. In addition, the committee could find no evidence that the exposure of students and residents to drug and device sales representatives—without additional training and supervision—contributes to the achievement of learning objectives or the development of core competencies, for example, increasing an individual's ability to critically evaluate presentations or promoting adherence to evidence-based clinical practice guidelines.

Responses

AAMC has recommended tight limits on site access by sales representatives from medical product companies, particularly uninvited and unscheduled visits and unsupervised access to individual students and residents (see Box 5-1) (see, e.g., AMSA [2008a] and AAMC [2008c]). The recommended rules for device representatives are somewhat less stringent than those for drug representatives and allow limited exceptions for training on the use of complex new devices and the other activities mentioned above. A number of medical schools and teaching hospitals have adopted policies consistent with the AAMC recommendations.

A quality assurance and risk management document prepared by the ECRI Institute (2007) recommends several additional safety and administrative provisions for device representatives who are allowed access to the operating room.[7] The recommendations include training requirements for device representatives as well as procedures to ensure patient safety, privacy, and informed consent and to prevent kickbacks (ECRI Institute, 2007). In addition, the ECRI Institute document suggests that medical schools have not provided adequate training in the use of devices. It emphasizes that hospitals and physicians are responsible for seeing that personnel have the appropriate training on the use of the devices that they regularly use, so that reliance on device representatives is limited and appropriately supervised.

[7] ECRI Institute is a technology assessment organization that has a long history of providing advice to health care institutions and government on medical device safety. It is one of the Evidence-Based Practice Centers designated by the Agency for Healthcare Research and Quality and is a Collaborating Center of the World Health Organization.

BOX 5-1
AAMC Recommendations on Site Access by Sales Representatives

Site Access by Pharmaceutical Representatives

- To protect patients, patient care areas, and work schedules, access by pharmaceutical representatives to individual physicians should be restricted to non-patient care areas and nonpublic areas and should take place only by appointment or invitation of the physician.
- Involvement of students and trainees in such individual meetings should occur only for educational purposes and only under the supervision of a faculty member.
- Academic medical centers should develop mechanisms whereby industry representatives who wish to provide educational information on their products may do so by invitation in faculty-supervised structured group settings that provide the opportunity for interaction and critical evaluation. Highly trained industry representatives with M.D., Ph.D., or Pharm.D. degrees would be best suited for transmitting such scientific information in these settings.

Site Access by Device Manufacturer Representatives

- Access by device manufacturer representatives to patient care areas should be permitted by academic medical centers only when the representatives are appropriately credentialed by the center and should take place only by appointment or invitation of the physician.
- Representatives should not be allowed to be present during any patient care interaction unless there has been prior disclosure to and consent by the patient, and then only to provide in-service training or assistance on devices and equipment.
- Student interaction with representatives should occur only for educational purposes under faculty supervision.

SOURCE: AAMC, 2008c.

Drug Samples

Issues

Physicians and patients often value drug samples provided as gifts because they allow physicians to send a patient home with a medication that can be evaluated for its short-term effects and side effects without requiring the patient to fill and pay for a full prescription. For low-income patients, many of whom are treated at academic medical centers and teaching hospitals, samples can provide access to needed medications (Daugherty, 2005).

Some research has, however, suggested that poor or uninsured patients are somewhat less likely than higher-income or insured patients to receive a drug sample (Cutrona et al., 2008). Drug samples may also be used by physicians themselves or their families. In a 1997 survey of residents, 32 percent of all medications used by residents were obtained from drug sample cabinets or directly from drug representatives (Christie et al., 1998). As discussed in Chapter 6, some professional societies approve such use.

Other research points to risks associated with physician acceptance of drug samples. In academic medical centers, drug samples may be associated with the prescription of new brand name drugs in situations in which the sample drugs are different from the physician's preferred drug or are not recommended by evidence-based practice guidelines or in situations in which less expensive drugs or generic equivalents are available for the same indication. One study of a sample of university-based physicians' responses to several clinical scenarios found that from 17 to 82 percent of the physicians would dispense a drug sample, and, in two of three scenarios, a great majority would do so instead of using their usually preferred drug—largely on the grounds that use of the sample would avoid costs to the patient (Chew et al., 2000). Residents were more likely than attending physicians to report that they used drug samples. In a second study, which involved residents in an inner-city clinic, half were randomized to forgo the use of available free drug samples. They were more likely than the control group to choose unadvertised drugs and were more likely to use over-the-counter drugs. The authors concluded that access to drug samples influences residents' prescribing decisions (Adair and Holmgren, 2005). A third study found that physicians who prescribed angiotensin-converting enzyme inhibitors or calcium channel blockers (a departure from the recommendations of the Joint National Commission on High Blood Pressure Treatment) were more likely than other physicians to report that they provided patients with samples of antihypertension medications (Ubel et al., 2003). This relationship persisted even after physician and practice variables were taken into account.

Responses

Concerns about the possible negative effects of drug samples have led some academic health centers to restrict or ban their provision. For example, some medical schools require drug samples to be received and distributed by a medical center pharmacy and prohibit their direct provision to individual physicians (see, e.g., University of Massachusetts [2008]). Other policies may allow donation of products only for purposes of evaluation or education and not to support "patient care purposes on an ongoing basis" (University of California, 2008, p. 4). When the University of Michigan

Health System (2007) prohibited the distribution of drug samples in patient care and non-patient care areas, it provided committee-approved vouchers for starter medications for clinic patients and for limited exceptions if a clinic director believed that a sample of a specific drug was clinically necessary. The most common provision among the policies reviewed by the committee was a prohibition on the personal use of samples by physicians or their family members.

AAMC (2008c) recommends that samples—if their distribution is by the institutions—should be centrally managed, when feasible (e.g., when timely access to the medications is possible). It warns that the "acceptance and use of drug samples transmits the message to students and trainees that information about samples received from industry sales personnel is sufficient without independent critical evaluation" (p. 16). The recommendation does not mention the personal use of samples by physicians or their family members or staff.

In a March 2009 report, the Medicare Payment Advisory Commission recommends that the U.S. Congress require manufacturers and distributors of drugs to report their distribution of drug samples. It also recommends that the secretary of the U.S. Department of Health and Human Services make the information available for analysis through data use agreements.

Gifts from Medical Product Companies

Issues

As noted earlier in this chapter, surveys indicate that almost every medical student has received a meal and a small noneducational gift from a drug company and that other interactions are common as well (see, e.g., Sigworth et al. [2001], Bellin et al. [2004], Sierles et al. [2005], and Fitz et al. [2007]). In one study, residents were asked to empty their pockets of pens, penlights, calipers, and other items (Sigworth et al., 2001). Ninety-seven percent of the residents had at least one item marked by a pharmaceutical insignia, and about half of the items carried by residents were so branded. More than 90 percent of the residents said that they thought that interactions with drug company representatives influenced their prescribing.

The committee found no studies documenting an educational benefit of these kinds of gifts from industry. Although medical students or residents may find the gift of an expensive textbook welcome, nothing similar to the benefits of academic-industry collaboration in biomedical research has been argued for gifts from industry in medical education.

In contrast, studies of medical personnel combined with social science research provide reasons for concern about the risks of industry relationships and gifts, even small gifts. The paper by Jason Dana in Appendix D reviews this literature. It suggests that even small gifts can be influential. Furthermore, because influence may operate at an unconscious level, it can distort the choices of people who believe that they are objectively making decisions. Disclosure of interests and education about bias may be useful, but they cannot be relied upon to overcome the potential for undue influence and bias associated with conflicts of interest. A number of studies suggest that medical residents, faculty, and other physicians tend to think that they themselves are less likely than others to be influenced by gifts or other interactions (see, e.g., McKinney et al. [1990], Steinman et al. [2001], Halperin et al. [2004], Zipkin and Steinman [2005], and Morgan et al. [2006]).

Few studies have specifically investigated the effects of industry relationships on teaching. One study compared the attitudes of internal medicine residents and faculty about the impact of gifts or income from industry on teaching within and outside the institution (Watson et al., 2005). In general, students were more likely than faculty to perceive industry influence in association with gifts or income. Both students and faculty perceived visiting attending faculty as more susceptible to such influence than regular faculty, and both perceived off-site teaching as more subject to influence than on-site activities. For example, residents were more likely than faculty to believe that gifts or income from industry influences how attending physicians teach on rounds (47 versus 34 percent), during in-hospital lectures and journal clubs (58 versus 30 percent), and during out-of-hospital dinner lectures and journal clubs (80 versus 57 percent). For responses about the effects on visiting attending physicians, the numbers were even higher, with 89 percent of residents and 72 percent of faculty reporting that they believed that gifts or income from industry affected teaching by this group during out-of-hospital dinner lectures and journal clubs. Moreover, 62 percent of residents and faculty believed that annual income or gifts of less than $10,000 could influence an attending physician's teaching. Sixty-five percent of residents and 74 percent of faculty preferred that speakers disclose all financial relationships with industry rather than just report relationships that speakers considered relevant to the educational topic. Although these findings are from a single study in a single institution, they do raise particular concerns about presentations given outside the medical school setting.

Responses

AAMC (2008c) recommends that schools ban the acceptance of industry-supplied food or meals, except in association with ACCME-accredited educational programs. This ban should apply both on and off campus. A few universities (e.g., the University of Michigan and Yale University by 2005) initiated restrictions some years before the AAMC statement. Schools that ban vendor-provided meals on campus (e.g., Stanford University) may not be explicit about the acceptance of meals at off-site locations, although several schools (e.g., Yale University) also discourage this.

As discussed in more detail in Chapter 6, AMA allows gifts of modest value that are viewed as having some benefit to patients (e.g., meals as part of an educational activity) or the physician's practice (e.g., notepads). The policies of several medical centers (e.g., Wake Forest University, Case Western Reserve University, and the University of Minnesota) are similar to this policy.

In addition to policy changes within the academic community, the Pharmaceutical Research and Manufacturers of America (PhRMA) recently revised its voluntary *Code on Interactions with Healthcare Professionals* (PhRMA2008, effective 2009). Except for the section on scholarships and education funds, the document does not refer specifically to interactions in academic settings. As discussed further in Chapter 6, the revised code more strongly discourages "noninformational" physician-company relationships, such as the provision of tickets to sporting events, token consulting arrangements, speaker training programs at resorts, and meals by sales representatives outside a physician's office or other medical setting.

Industry-Sponsored Scholarships and Training Positions

Issues

Little information on the extent of industry funding for undergraduate and graduate medical education is available, although AAMC has stated that medical schools have become increasingly dependent on such funding for such major activities. The committee is aware of industry-funded residencies or fellowships in a few areas, for example, dermatology residencies funded by companies making dermatologic products (Kuehn, 2005); industry-funded fellowships in rheumatology (Goldblum and Franzblau, 2006); and industry support for psychiatry resident fellowships, awards, and the Chief Resident Leadership Conference (APA, 2008).

The rationale for industry funding of residencies and fellowships seems to rest on physician or researcher shortages in certain specialties and the desire to attract more individuals to these areas through additional industry-supported training positions. For example, the American Academy of Dermatology (AAD) launched an initiative in 2004 to fund 10 dermatology residency positions (Kuehn, 2005). The AAD created a fund to accept donations from the academy, pharmaceutical companies, and other interested parties. Awards were assigned to 10 university programs ($60,000 per year for 3 years), and no recipient would be identified as having been funded by a particular company or companies.

Responses

AAMC (2008c) recommends that academic medical centers establish and implement policies requiring that industry funds for scholarships and similar purposes be given centrally to the administration of the medical center. In addition, industry should have no involvement in the selection of recipients, and no "quid pro quo [should] be involved in any way" (p. 21). The objective is to "prevent the establishment of one-on-one relationships between industry representatives and students and trainees" and minimize "the possibility that these funds will be perceived or used as direct gifts" (p. 21). The committee supports the AAMC recommendations. AMA and PhRMA both permit industry funding of scholarships for medical students, residents, or fellows to attend carefully selected educational conferences when the selection of recipients is made by the academic or training institution.

Changing the Environment or Creating Educational Interventions

To the extent that industry influence operates at an unconscious level, the most effective strategies for reducing the risk of undue influence may involve changing the environment in ways that eliminate or reduce the source, especially when the source offers little or no countervailing educational benefit. That is a major rationale for the policies cited above that eliminate gifts, meals, and other noneducational interactions from the learning environment. Some evidence suggests that the learning environment influences attitudes. Two studies have reported that residents who trained in environments that restricted interactions between industry representatives were less likely than residents who trained in environments without such restrictions to view promotional interactions as being beneficial (Brotzman and Mark, 1993; McCormick et al., 2001). One literature review found weak evidence that trainees who were exposed to educational interventions may be "less accepting of pharmaceutical industry marketing tactics" than those who are not (Carroll et al., 2007, p. e1533). The review noted that two studies that involved industry personnel in the design of the educational intervention found that the participants were more positive toward industry and industry representatives than they were before the intervention.

Some research—including research in academic medical centers as well as community settings (see, e.g., Solomon et al. [2001])— suggests the value of "academic detailing" or educational outreach programs provided by clinical pharmacists or other experts as an objective educational alternative to the activities of medical product companies. Because these programs are aimed at physicians outside academic institutions, this research is reviewed in Chapter 6.

THE LEARNING ENVIRONMENT IN ACCREDITED CONTINUING MEDICAL EDUCATION

Physicians commit to life-long learning to keep pace with new knowledge and skills and to maintain their current skills. Most state licensing boards, specialty boards, and hospitals require accredited continuing medical education for relicensure, recertification, or staff privileges. Thus, it is important to promote a constructive learning environment in this arena as well as in undergraduate and graduate education. This discussion focuses on accredited continuing medical education. (As noted earlier, this report uses the phrase accredited continuing medical education to refer to education that is presented by accredited providers and is certified for course credits.)

Providers of accredited continuing medical education are more numerous and diverse than providers of undergraduate and graduate medical education. The major ACCME-accredited providers are physician membership organizations (n = 270), publishing/education companies (n = 150), medical schools (n = 123), and hospitals and health care delivery systems (n = 93). In 2008, ACCME had 740 accredited providers of continuing medical education, and state medical societies accredited approximately 1,600 additional providers (ACCME, 2008a, 2009). What ACCME calls "publishing/education companies" are often described as "medical education and communication companies," or MECCs, and that term is used here. According to data reported by the Society for Academic Continuing Medical Education (SACME) for 2006, about 40 percent of medical schools held commercially sponsored "satellite" meetings in conjunction with national professional society meetings, and 70 percent of these meetings were managed by communications companies (SACME, 2007).

Table 5-2 shows the shares of total income, participants, hours of instruction, and activities (all providers) accounted for by several types of accredited continuing medical education providers. Medical schools accounted for a considerably larger share of total hours of instruction than might be expected from their share of the total income received by education providers. In contrast, MECCs (publishing/education companies) account for a considerably smaller share of all instructional hours than of total income.

Accredited continuing medical education programs embedded in medical schools are shaped in part by the missions, culture, and challenges of the larger institution. The programs' members are represented by SACME,

TABLE 5-2 Share of Total Accredited Continuing Medical Education Income, Instruction Hours, Participants, and Activities Accounted for by Major Types of ACCME-Accredited Providers

	Share (as %)			
Provider Organization Type	Total CME[a] Income	Total Hours of CME Instruction	Total CME Participants	All CME-Sponsored Activities
Medical school	17	45	31	30
Publishing/education company	33	9	30	30
Physician membership organization (nonprofit)	35	23	26	20
Other providers	15	23	13	20
TOTAL	100	100	100	100

[a]CME = continuing medical education.
SOURCE: ACCME, 2008a, Tables 2, 3, 4, 7.

which describes its mission as promoting "research, scholarship, evaluation and development" of educational and professional development programs "to enhance the performance of physicians . . . for purposes of improving individual and population health" (SACME, 2008a, unpaged). Professional society programs are also shaped by the missions, culture, and resources of the society. Most MECCs are for-profit organizations. They are represented by the North American Association of Medical Education and Communication Companies, which is "dedicated to providing representation, advocacy, and education for its members" (NAAMECC, 2009).

The curriculum for accredited continuing medical education is also diffuse. All states except Colorado, Indiana, Montana, New York, South Dakota, and Vermont have some requirements for accredited continuing medical education for physicians who want to maintain (reregister) their license (AMA, 2008a). The policies are generally not specific about the content of the accredited continuing medical education, although a number of states have certain content requirements, for example, palliative and end-of-life care or patient safety (AMA, 2008a). Medical specialty boards have more specific and coherent requirements. They have also recently adopted a "maintenance of certification" model for ensuring continuing physician competence, and this model has implications for the future content of accredited continuing medical education.[8] Approximately 85 percent of U.S.

[8] The American Board of Medical Specialties and its 24 member boards have been moving from a process of recertification based on an examination taken once every several years to

physicians are board certified, so recertification requirements affect the majority of physicians (ABMS, 2007).

In addition to accredited continuing medical education, physicians also have access to an array of nonaccredited education programs sponsored by a wide range of public and private organizations. Many conferences sponsored by the National Institutes of Health and other government agencies do not offer credit, although some do. Hospitals sponsor a range of medical staff education programs that do not offer credits. The committee heard testimony that a professional society may organize a scientific meeting of research presentations for which it controls the selection of topics and speakers (ASH, 2008; Kaushansky, 2008). The organization may then seek financial support from industry, often small grants from several companies. Because of limited budget and staff, a small society may not pursue the provision of continuing medical education credits even when it provides safeguards against commercial bias consistent with accreditation standards. When medical product companies organize nonaccredited continuing medical education, the offerings may range from dinner seminars to training on the use of a medical device and satellite symposia at professional society meetings (some satellite symposia offer credit). Some nonaccredited programs controlled by companies may be little more than marketing. Others, such as programs that provide training on the use of a complex new medical device, may meet legitimate education needs, although the presentations may still be more positive about the device than presentations by an independent educational source would be. The committee lacked the resources to investigate nonaccredited activities.

Some medical schools have policies that require their faculty to limit participation in industry-supported programs to programs that meet certain conditions. These conditions may be similar or identical to the standards for accredited continuing medical education (see, e.g., Boston University [2007] and the University of Pittsburgh [2007]).

As noted earlier, the committee commissioned a paper on conflict of interest concerns, policies, and practices in other professions. That paper, which is presented as Appendix C, examines conflicts of interest in law, accounting, engineering, and architecture. In general, other professions differ from medicine in that they have no authority similar to that of physicians to prescribe regulated products for client's personal use and, except to various degrees for law, do not have vulnerable clients.

In some respects, the current system of continuing legal education

---

a maintenance of certification program that emphasizes continuing self-evaluation of practice and knowledge and other activities to maintain competence. Boards may develop self-assessment programs that also offer continuing medical education credit that will meet state licensing board and other requirements.

resembles the system of continuing medical education in decades past. Much continuing legal education is provided by law schools as part of their service mission, although law firms and commercial companies also offer programs. Programs may be offered at no charge or may be paid for by individual lawyers or their firms or employers. Programs sometimes have corporate sponsorship, but the sponsors' products tend to be resources for the lawyer (e.g., software and information resources) rather than for the lawyer's clients and thus do not present the same concerns about bias in presentations that occur in medicine. Although legal continuing education cannot be seen as an exact model for medicine, it does suggest that alternatives (e.g., higher fees and employer subsidies) to the major role of industry funding for continuing medical education may exist.

Industry Funding in Accredited Continuing Medical Education

Survey data from ACCME show that industry funding of accredited continuing medical education increased by more than 300 percent between 1998 and 2007 (ACCME, 2008a, Table 7).[9] Moreover, profit margins increased substantially, from 5.5 percent in 1998 to 31 percent in 2006 (Steinbrook, 2008b). For the many providers of accredited continuing medical education, this combination of increased reliance on industry funding and increased profitability provides strong incentives to resist efforts to curtail such funding.

The contribution of funding from industry (primarily from drug, medical device, and biotechnology companies) varies by the type of provider of accredited continuing medical education (Table 5-3). Funding from industry provides more than half of the total income for medical schools and almost three-quarters of the total income for MECCs. Professional societies (i.e., physician membership organizations) as well as MECCs show a significant margin of income over expenses.

Although professional societies are not as dependent on industry funding for their accredited educational programs as MECCs or medical schools, they receive nearly equal amounts of funding from commercial sources (24 percent) and advertising and exhibit income (25 percent). ACCME's survey does not count the latter as commercial support.

SACME surveys provide additional data on the significance of industry

---

[9] One widely cited analysis estimated that every $1.00 of industry spending on physician meetings and events generated an average of $3.56 in increased revenue (cited in Walker [2001]; see also CEJA [2008] and NAAMECC and Coalition for Healthcare Communication [2008]). Descriptions of the reported analysis do not indicate the relative weight of accredited versus nonaccredited activities in the estimate or whether accredited continuing medical education was distinguished from other types of meetings, such as promotions. Nonetheless, it suggests a rationale for industry support of a range of educational activities.

TABLE 5-3 Income, Expenses, and Source of Support as Percentage of Income, by Type of Accredited Provider of Continuing Medical Education, 2007

Organization Type (No. of Organizations)	Total Income	Expenses as % of Total Income	Total Commercial Support (% of Total Income)	Advertising and Exhibits Income (% of Total Income)
Nonprofit (physician membership organization) (270)	$887,181	68	$215,388 (24)	$217,907 (25)
Publishing/Education Company [MECC](150)	830,811	74	594,420 (71)	10,831 (1)
School of medicine (123)	427,668	88	245,790 (57)	23,203 (5)
Hospital/health care delivery system (93)	105,014	95	47,498 (45)	7,407 (7)
Nonprofit (other) (38)	160,397	79	78,412 (49)	11,852 (7)
Not classified (33)	55,188	79	29,263 (53)	2,423 (4)
Government or military (15)	69,452	100	255 (0)	376 (0)
Insurance company/managed care company (14)	3,489	193	318 (9)	35 (1)

NOTE: Monetary data for 2007 are in 1,000s of dollars. Data for a third category of income (other) are not shown here. As categorized by ACCME, other income represents income other than commercial support and advertising and exhibit income. Data for providers accredited by state medical societies are not included, but ACCME survey data show that commercial sources accounted for about 25 percent of their income.
SOURCE: ACCME, 2008a (Table 7).

funding for medical school programs. In 2006, the typical (median) medical school received some commercial support for about 45 courses, which represented almost 70 percent of its educational activities (SACME, 2007). About 7 percent of schools reported that the majority of their courses were supported by a single commercial source, and the mean number of such courses across all respondents was two. Respondents also reported that "if commercial support were no longer provided, the typical school would no longer hold 11 courses, representing 23% of the school's courses" (p. 3).

Because they depend on industry for almost three-quarters of their income, MECCs could be severely challenged by an end to direct commercial funding, which some have proposed (Fletcher, 2008), or by a decision by medical product companies to shift their support to academic institutions, as one company recently did (Loftus, 2008). They could still have a role if academic medical centers continued to contract with them to manage or administer some of their continuing medical education programs.

Providers of accredited continuing medical education may solicit industry support for their programs. For example, a medical education company described opportunities to provide educational grants for a large meeting sponsored jointly with an academic medical center, as shown in Box 5-2. Other organizations sell sponsorship opportunities for everything from meeting coffee breaks to hand sanitizers and flash drives.

In addition to support for organizational programs, industry also provides support to individual physicians. On the basis of the findings from a 2004 survey, Campbell and colleagues (2007a) found that 26 percent of physicians reported that industry paid for their admission to continuing medical education meetings and 16 percent reported payments for serving as a speaker or on a speakers bureau.

Conceptually, industry support may be direct or indirect. Direct funding is from the company to the program provider. Indirect funding may occur in several ways. The company may set up a foundation that it substantially controls to provide the funding, or the provider may set up a foundation to receive the funds. Such arrangements may not provide any protection against the company influencing the content of the accredited continuing medical education. Alternatively, the company may provide funds to an intermediary, such as a central continuing medical education office in an academic health center. These arrangements are intended to separate the funding from decisions about the course content. The committee has heard criticisms that despite ACCME requirements that course directors review the course content for bias, the recipient of industry funds may have an implicit understanding that additional industry funds will not be offered in the future if the course does not present topics of interest to the company and use speakers who are favorable to the company's products.

BOX 5-2
Example of a Solicitation of Industry Support (Educational Grants) for a Large Accredited Continuing Medical Education Program

Several support levels are listed below. Please note that educational support is appreciated at any dollar level. Please contact our office for further details. We appreciate that our supporters recognize the need for [the organization] to maintain authority and autonomy in decisions regarding program format, content, and faculty.

Cornerstone Supporter
Total: $195,000
Foundation Supporter
Total: $135,000
Leadership Supporter
Total: $80,000

Satellite Symposia
Open to Cornerstone and Foundation Supporters

1 Breakfast Symposium	Fee: $15,000
1 Lunch Symposium	Fee: $20,000
1 Breakfast Symposium	Fee: $15,000
1 Lunch Symposium	Fee: $20,000
1 Breakfast Symposium	Fee: $15,000

Symposium fee includes:

- Program listing on the [meeting] website, linking to the program provider's online registration site for the satellite symposium.
- Program listing and schedule in the meeting materials distributed to all meeting attendees.
- One complimentary email to the preregistration mailing list for use in promotion of the satellite symposium.
- One time complimentary use of the preregistration mailing list for use in promotion of the satellite symposium (restrictions apply).
- One insert into the delegate literature bag for use in promotion of the satellite symposium.

SOURCE: Excerpted from Oncology Congress, 2008, 2009.

Concerns About Industry Support for Accredited Continuing Medical Education

The substantial support that industry provides for accredited continuing medical education indirectly subsidizes physicians who pay less for many accredited continuing medical education programs than they otherwise would. As the preceding section indicates, industry support also contributes to the financial well-being of many educational providers that depend on it for the major part of their income for the provision of accredited continuing medical education.

The committee found little systematic research on other consequences of industry-supported continuing medical education, for example, whether it promotes bias in individual programs or in overall educational offerings. One study published before the adoption of the first ACCME standards for commercial support compared programs funded by rival pharmaceutical companies and found that the programs favored the products of their funders (Bowman, 1986). A study by Orlowski and Wateska (1992) focused on a kind of industry-sponsored activity that provoked considerable criticism and that now is not permitted for accredited education, that is, a program held at a resort with all expenses paid for attendees and with limited time actually devoted to the educational content. The authors found, using actual prescribing data obtained before and after the activity, that this "elaborate promotional technique . . . was associated with a significant increase in the prescribing of the promoted drugs at one institution" (p. 273). The investigators also found that the physicians involved did not believe that the activity would affect their practices.

Another study found that courses on primary care directed by academic faculty covered a broader range of topics than symposia sponsored directly by industry (Katz et al., 2002). Moreover, 91 percent of the industry-sponsored symposia were sponsored by a company that had recently obtained FDA approval for a drug related to the symposium topic. The industry-sponsored symposia did not cover prevention screening, dermatological diagnoses, child abuse, alcoholism, or the technology resources available for clinicians, which were considered important in the academic program. In that study, the university-based accredited continuing medical education courses received funding from multiple companies through a MECC to the university. University faculty determined the content of their courses, and the MECC handled marketing and meeting logistics. During meal breaks at these courses, symposia funded by industry were also offered.

Unfortunately, much information about accredited continuing medical education, particularly that offered by for-profit providers, is not based on good data but, rather, is based on personal experiences with covert relationships with providers or inferences made on the basis of the nearly total dependence of these providers on pharmaceutical, medical device, and biotechnology companies. One 2008 article, based on personal experience, describes how accredited continuing medical education providers can tailor programs to secure company grants (Gilbert, 2008, unpaged). A commercial provider selected a program concept to "provide a platform for one of the sponsors," which was working on a drug covered by the program. The provider also organized informal workshops with experts who were hired on the basis of their support for the sponsor's message.

Using a checklist that they developed to assess bias in education programs, Takhar and colleagues (2007) concluded that 9 of the 17 continuing medical education programs that they assessed were biased (e.g., by limiting the discussion to the sponsor's product and ignoring alternatives). Work is needed to validate this and other instruments that are intended to be used to assess bias in presentations retrospectively or identify presentations at risk of bias during the planning stage (see, e.g., Barnes et al. [2007]).

The Senate Finance Committee staff report on the use of educational grants by pharmaceutical manufacturers noted that ACCME's reports documented numerous cases of undue influence by companies over "supposedly independent educational programs" (Finance Committee, U.S. Senate, 2007, p. 2). For example, during 2005 and 2006, 18 of 76 program providers were found to be out of compliance with at least one of the ACCME standards related to independence, and some were cited for being under the improper influence of industry.

More specific information on industry practices comes from litigation. Prompted in many instances by whistleblower complaints, the U.S. Department of Justice as well as state attorneys general have filed charges against a number of pharmaceutical and medical device companies for illegal practices related to purported educational activities as well as speaking and writing arrangements. In some cases, one focus of litigation has been the giving of educational grants as an inducement to use the company's products, which can be illegal under the Medicare law. In other cases, the focus has been on industry efforts to bias the content of educational programs and presentations, particularly as part of efforts to promote the off-label use of drugs (i.e., for purposes not approved by the FDA), which is also illegal.[10]

Box 5-3 lists some of the cases in which settlements have been reached. Internal company documents that were made public as a result of the first case described in the box provided insights into the use of speakers bureaus (which included chairs of neurology departments), "educational" teleconferences, and grants to medical education companies (with multiple ties to the company) to further marketing objectives for the drug Neurontin (gabapentin) (Steinman et al., 2006; see also Landefeld and Steinman [2009]).

[10] In 1997, the FDA provided guidance on the characteristics of industry-supported educational activities that distinguish them from promotional activities, which are subject to the labeling and advertising provisions of the Federal Food, Drug, and Cosmetic Act (FDA, 1997). This guidance stresses the role of voluntary oversight, for example, through accreditation; it explicitly disavows an interest in regulating programs.

BOX 5-3
Settlements Involving Educational Activities and Speaking and Writing Arrangements

In 2004, Warner-Lambert paid $430 million to settle U.S. Department of Justice charges that the company promoted off-label uses of the drug Neurontin in violation of the Food, Drug, and Cosmetic Act. "This illegal and fraudulent promotion scheme corrupted the information process relied upon by doctors in their medical decision making, thereby putting patients at risk." Tactics included "[paying] doctors to attend so-called 'consultants meetings' in which physicians received a fee for attending expensive dinners or conferences during which presentations about off-label uses of Neurontin were made; . . . [and sponsoring] purportedly 'independent medical education' events on off-label Neurontin uses with extensive input from Warner-Lambert regarding topics, speakers, content, and participants. . . . In at least one instance, when unfavorable remarks were proposed by a speaker, Warner-Lambert offset the negative impact by 'planting' people in the audience to ask questions highlighting the benefits of the drug" (DOJ, 2004, unpaged).

In 2007, Orphan Medical, Inc., agreed to pay $20 million and accept a corporate integrity agreement to settle charges that it had illegally promoted the drug Xyrem (sodium oxybate) for off-label uses. Among other charges, the company was accused of using unrestricted "educational grants" as an inducement for off-label use and paying tens of thousands of dollar in speaker fees to physicians for their promotion of these uses. One of these physicians has been charged criminally for his behavior (DOJ, 2007b). The associated corporate integrity agreement required, among other provisions, that the company create procedures to ensure that sponsored continuing medical education and educational activities be independent and nonpromotional (OIG, 2007).

In 2008, in a stipulated agreement filed in Oregon, Merck & Co, Inc., agreed to pay $58 million to 30 states and to end certain deceptive practices used to promote the drug Vioxx (rofecoxib). The stipulation prohibits, among other practices, company use of ghostwriting of published journal articles and the nondisclosure of promotional ties with speakers at independent continuing medical education programs (Oregon DOJ, 2008a).

The conditions associated with the settlement in the case specified requirements for the company's reporting of its support for continuing medical education and its financial relationships with speakers and participants (OIG, 2004).[11]

[11] The corporate integrity agreement was signed by Pfizer, which had purchased Warner-Lambert, which, in turn, was the parent company of Parke-Davis, the company named in the case.

Responses to Concerns About Bias in Industry-Funded Accredited Continuing Medical Education

Responses by Private Organizations

Expanded industry support for accredited continuing medical education and the involvement of commercial firms began to become a significant concern in the 1980s and led to ACCME-developed guidelines on commercial support in 1987 and then ACCME-developed standards in 1992. These standards have been criticized as doing little to curb industry influence over the content of accredited continuing medical education (see, e.g., Relman [2001, 2003]; see also Ross et al. [2000], Krimsky [2003], and Brody [2007]). In 2004, ACCME issued new, more restrictive standards.

The accreditation standards now require the disclosure of conflicts of interest by meeting planners as well as speakers. They also require the review of the educational content for bias and the resolution of conflicts of interest in some fashion (e.g., by finding an alternative speaker or identifying and eliminating biased content in a presentation). In addition to the standards, ACCME has developed tools (e.g., definitions, frequently asked questions, and slide presentations) to help educational providers with program implementation.

The SACME survey mentioned above reported that academic providers found the 2004 standards to be difficult to implement (SACME, 2007). Only 5 percent of the respondents considered the standard related to resolving conflicts of interest to be easy to implement. Slightly less than half of the respondents thought that the standards had reduced bias a little or somewhat.

In 2008, the ACCME board of directors adopted a statement that indicated that accredited continuing medical education providers "cannot receive guidance, either nuanced or direct, on the content of the activity or on who should deliver that content" (ACCME, 2008b, p. 3). The organization also announced that it was devoting more resources to implementation and enforcement, which would eventually require an increase in member fees (ACCME, 2008b). In addition, ACCME issued a request for comments on a proposal related to commercial support, which included as options the elimination of commercial support, the continuation of the current situation, and the development of a new paradigm (ACCME, 2008d). The executive summary for the November 2008 board of directors meeting states that analysis of the comments is continuing and that action is not anticipated before the end of 2009 (ACCME, 2008c).

Notwithstanding the changes in ACCME standards, criticisms of industry funding and influence continue (see, e.g., Steinbrook [2005, 2008b] and Fletcher [2008]). ACCME's limited resources for monitoring adherence to its standards (as of early 2008, it had approximately a dozen staff members) are also a concern (Kopelow, 2008).

Other issues involve the monitoring of the content of presentations. Program-by-program and presentation-by-presentation assessments for bias are labor-intensive activities, and instruments for the systematic assessment for bias need further development and validation. The committee found no studies describing or evaluating the effectiveness, burdens, and adverse consequences of such monitoring for bias overall or by category of accredited continuing medical education provider. ACCME requirements for monitoring may stimulate research in this area.

Some critics raise broader questions about the value, goals, and structure of the current system of accredited continuing medical education (see, e.g., Fletcher [2008]). Some have also proposed ending direct industry support for continuing medical education (see, e.g., Brennan et al. [2006], Fugh-Berman and Batt [2006], CEJA [2008], and Fletcher [2008]). In 2008, the AMA House of Delegates referred back to its Committee on Ethical and Judicial Affairs a proposal that physicians and organizations not accept industry funding for professional medical education (AMA, 2008c; see also Relman [2008]). The summary of a 2008 consensus conference held at the Mayo Clinic describes a conclusion that continuing medical education requires a "strategic management process that focuses on the integrity of an enterprise" and that deals "in a convincing, transparent and accountable manner issues such as commercial interest influence, conflicts of interest, bias, sources of evidence and the quality of product, process and delivery" (Kane, 2008, p. 8). It also stressed the need for research (and funding for research) to guide reforms.

In a 2008 report on industry funding of medical education, AAMC recommended that academic medical centers set up audit procedures to assess compliance with ACCME standards. The report observed that given "the heavy dependence by academic medical centers on industry funding" for continuing medical education, it was essential that they comply with "evolving" ACCME standards and take other steps to ensure the independence of their program offerings (AAMC, 2008c, p. 19). The report also recommended that academic medical centers establish a central office through which all requests for industry support and the receipt of funds for continuing medical education would be coordinated and overseen. It further proposed that institutions should prohibit faculty, students, residents, and fellows from participating in non-ACCME accredited industry events that are labeled as continuing medical education. Also, if medical centers allow faculty participation in industry-sponsored, FDA-regulated programs, they should set standards for appropriate faculty involvement.

In its revised code of conduct, PhRMA includes provisions on industry support for continuing educational programs. With an eye to federal kickback laws, it advises companies to separate decision making about educational grants from sales and marketing units and to "develop objective criteria for making CME grant decisions to ensure that . . . the financial support is not an inducement to prescribe or recommend a particular medicine or course of treatment" (PhRMA, 2008). For nonaccredited educational activities, the code provides that the organizers of the activity should control its content, faculty, materials, and similar details. As noted earlier, one pharmaceutical company announced that it would no longer fund educational programs offered by MECCs.

Most medical school policies reviewed by the committee already state that their programs should meet the standards for commercial support set forth by ACCME. Some have instituted further restrictions. In 2007, Memorial Sloan-Kettering Cancer Center announced a 6-month trial period during which it would no longer accept industry funding for its continuing medical education programs (industry provided about 25 percent of total funding for continuing medical education at that institution). To reduce costs, off-site programs were moved on-site, free lunches were eliminated, advertising was cut, and fewer external speakers were used. Although the fees for external participants were raised by 10 to 20 percent, program attendance stayed the same (Kovaleski, 2008). The ban on industry funding is now permanent. At least one other institution has also announced that it will no longer accept direct industry funding for specific accredited continuing medical education courses either on or off campus, nor will it accept payments from third parties that have received commercial support (Stanford University School of Medicine, 2008). Industry support is, however, permitted if it is not designated to a specific subject, course, or program but is for use in a broadly defined field and is provided through a central university office for continuing medical education.

Responses by Public Agencies

As described above, the U.S. Department of Justice and state attorneys general have charged a number of companies with illegal practices related to the funding of educational programs, including accredited programs in some instances. In addition, in its 2003 compliance guidelines for pharmaceutical manufacturers, the Office of the Inspector General (OIG) of the U.S. Department of Health and Human Services identified the provision of educational grants as an activity that place a company at high risk for violating federal antikickback rules and certain FDA regulations (OIG, 2003). These compliance guidelines advise manufacturers to separate their grant-making activities from their sales and marketing activities to "help insure that grant funding is not inappropriately influenced by sales or marketing motivations and that the educational purposes of the grant are legitimate"

(p. 21). Other activities identified as having a high potential for fraud and abuse include the provision of gifts, entertainment, and personal services compensation arrangements. The OIG guidelines also recommend (pp. 20–21) that manufacturers

1. separate grant-making functions from sales and marketing functions;
2. establish objective criteria for awarding grants that do not take into account the volume or value of the recipient's purchases;
3. establish objective criteria for awarding grants that ensure that the funded activities are bona fide; and
4. refrain from controlling speakers or content of educational activities funded by grants.

The 2007 Senate Finance Committee staff report cited above concluded that most large pharmaceutical companies had established written policies and procedures on educational grants, limited sales representatives from soliciting requests or promising funding, and established a centralized mechanism for administering grants.

GHOSTWRITING, SPEAKERS BUREAUS, AND INDEPENDENCE OF PUBLICATIONS AND PRESENTATIONS

Concerns about Ghostwritten Publications, Participation in Speakers Bureaus, and Other Industry-Controlled Work

Two hallmarks of academic integrity are intellectual independence and accountability for one's work. Certain practices by medical school faculty create a hidden curriculum that subverts the professional values endorsed by the formal curriculum. One example is taking credit as the author of a manuscript prepared by an unacknowledged or inadequately acknowledged industry-paid writer. (An adequate acknowledgment would specify the roles of these writers, for example, as the preparers of the first draft, as well as the roles of the listed authors.) Another example is participating in an industry speakers bureau or other long-term speaking arrangement with a company, regardless of how the relationship is labeled. One concern is that ongoing company payments for presentations (and travel to attractive locations) create a risk of undue influence. A second concern that is frequently tied to the speakers bureau label is that the company exerts substantial control over the content of a presentation. Industry influence in these arrangements may be direct (e.g., when a talk and slides are largely or entirely prepared by someone else or when speakers are instructed to provide the company-prepared responses to questions and avoid the favorable mention of competing products). Influence may also be less direct (e.g., when a company-trained and company-paid physician modifies talks to fit the objectives of the company) (see, e.g., Elliott [2006] and Carlat [2007]). The committee recognizes that companies have an interest in some oversight of presentations for a variety of reasons, including the need to comply with FDA prohibitions on promoting the use of drugs for the treatment of conditions not approved by the agency.

Serving on speakers bureaus appears to be common in clinical medicine. A 2006 survey of academic-industry relationships found that 21 percent of clinical department chairs reported being on a speakers bureau (whereas 2 percent of nonclinical department chairs reported being on a speakers bureau) (Campbell et al., 2007b). As reported earlier, another survey, which was not limited to academics and which asked less specific questions, found that 16 percent of physicians reported serving on a speakers bureau or as a speaker, which could have involved a single presentation (Campbell et al., 2007a). ACGME has expressed concern about "a new variation of a promotional activity in which residents and even medical students receive slides, lecture materials and honoraria and subsequently act as 'experts,' delivering the packaged information at continuing medical education events" (ACGME, 2002, p. 3).

Unacknowledged industry influence over publications is also common. In one study, 13 percent of research articles in major biomedical journals had "ghost" authors, that is, people who filled the criteria for authorship but who were not listed as authors (Flanagin et al., 1998). None of these ghost authors was even acknowledged in the paper. A review of documents obtained during litigation against a major pharmaceutical company concluded that review manuscripts were often prepared by writers for medical publishing companies but authorship was "subsequently attributed . . . to academically affiliated investigators who often did not disclose industry financial support" (Ross et al., 2008, p. 1800). One incident illustrates that such ghostwriting may be discovered only by accident. An academic physician reported that a MECC sent her a draft manuscript of a review article commissioned by a drug company and invited her to be its "author." She declined, but she was subsequently asked by a journal to review an article that was similar to that article and that now had another author (Fugh-Berman, 2005; see also Eaton [2005]). The analysis by Steinman and colleagues (2006) of documents obtained through litigation cited earlier found that those documents describe plans for recruiting academic authors of a series of ghostwritten articles to be prepared by a medical education company. Box 5-3 included examples of company settlements with the Department of Justice related to speaking and writing arrangements.

Another concern about industry relationships is that academic authors of research articles may not have full access to the data from an industry-sponsored study. This issue was discussed in Chapter 4.

In the setting of medical education, the question is not whether assistance by professional writers and others may improve publications and help busy researchers get important, objectively presented findings into print; it may do both. The questions are whether the assistance is hidden, whether it is intended to promote a company's interests rather than present unbiased information, and whether the author takes credit for work that he or she did not do and thus misrepresents the provenance of the article. Such arrangements (which are essentially gifts) send the wrong message about the values of intellectual independence, professional ethics, accountability, and evidence-based medicine. In the context of research, they raise questions about the objectivity of research reports that other researchers as well as practitioners and developers of practice guidelines rely on.

Responses to Concerns About Independence and Accountability in Writing and Speaking

Medical journal editors (including the International Committee of Medical Journal Editors and the World Association of Medical Editors) have taken steps to eliminate ghostwriting (see, e.g., Rennie et al. [1997], Davidoff et al. [2001], ICMJE [2008], and WAME [2008]). As stated by the International Committee of Medical Journal Editors, "[a]ll persons designated as authors should qualify for authorship, and all those who qualify should be listed" (ICMJE, 2008, p. 3; see also Ross et al. [2008]). The objective of authorship policies is to eliminate unethical practices and generally not to preclude legitimate and properly acknowledged writing assistance (see, e.g., Lagnado [2002] and Woolley et al. [2006]).

As described in Chapter 3, one journal has revised its conflict of interest disclosure form to include questions intended to detect commercial sponsorship and unacknowledged authors after concluding that such questions were necessary to detect ghostwritten or promotional submissions (AFMI, 2008). In its disclosure form for continuing medical education programs, the same professional society asks several questions about relationships with speakers bureaus (e.g., whether an individual is acting independently or as an agent) as well as questions about the receipt of assistance with manuscript preparation from commercial entities (AAFP, 2006b).

In its 2008 report on medical education, AAMC recommended, "[a]cademic medical centers should prohibit physicians, trainees, and students from allowing their professional presentations of any kind, oral or written, to be ghostwritten by any party, industry or otherwise" (AAMC, 2008c, p. 22). It noted that properly acknowledged collaborations with industry personnel or medical writers is not ghostwriting. The report also recommends that participation in industry-sponsored speakers bureaus be discouraged.

A few medical school policies reviewed by the committee mention speakers bureaus by name. For example, the University of Massachusetts views speakers bureaus as an "extension of the marketing process" and forbids faculty participation in them. The Mayo Clinic has long prohibited faculty from speaking on behalf of industry, and its current policy prohibits participation in the speakers bureaus of commercial firms because the linkage would imply endorsement by the Mayo Clinic (personal communication, Marianne Hockema, Administrator, Office of Conflict of Interest Review, Mayo Clinic, September 19, 2008). Faculty at the University of Louisville (2008) are "strongly discouraged" from serving as speakers hired by vendors (p. 4). A policy recently adopted by the Johns Hopkins University School of Medicine (2009) states that faculty may not participate on-site or off-site in "activities with any of the following characteristics . . . a company has the contractual right to dictate what the faculty member says; a company (not the faculty member) creates the slide set (or other presentation materials) and has the final approval of all content and edits; the faculty member receives compensation from the company and acts as the company's employee or spokesperson for the purposes of dissemination of company-generated presentation materials or promotion of company products; and/or a company controls the publicity related to the event" (p. 7). The policy notes that some of these activities occur in the context of speakers bureaus but it is the conditions of an activity that determine whether it is permissible.

In addition, a few medical schools (e.g., the University of California at San Francisco, the University of Louisville, and the University of Colorado) forbid ghostwriting (using that term). A few other medical schools (e.g., Stanford University, the University of Missouri, Emory University, and the University of Rochester) cover the practice of ghostwriting by forbidding medical school personnel from publishing, under their own name, articles that are written entirely or in significant part by an industry employee.

The ACCME standards for commercial support require that presenters disclose relevant financial relationships. They provide no explicit guidance or reference to the appropriateness of commercial assistance in the preparation of talks.

The 2008 PhRMA *Code on Interactions with Healthcare Professionals* notes that companies and speakers should understand the difference between (accredited) continuing medical education and company-sponsored speaker programs (PhRMA, 2008). For the latter, "[s]peaker training is an essential activity because the FDA holds companies accountable for the presentations of their speakers" (p. 9). This is a reference to FDA's ban on company promotion of the use of a medication for the treatment of conditions that have not been approved by the agency (FDA, 1997). The

PhRMA code specifies that company policies should provide a cap on the total annual amount that it will pay a speaker and address the "appropriate number of engagements for any particular speaker over time" (p. 10).

RECOMMENDATIONS

Medical Schools and Residency Programs

Policies on Relationships with Industry

This chapter has documented the extensive relationships that exist between industry and medical institutions, faculty, students, and residents and the concerns that have been raised about the risks that these relationships pose to the basic educational missions of academic medical centers and the lack of benefits from such relationships, such as those that support academic-industry collaborations in medical research. It has cited research indicating that even small gifts can be influential and has reviewed the recommendations of organizations such as AAMC and PhRMA. The committee concluded that it is time for medical schools to end a number of long-accepted relationships and practices that create conflicts of interest, threaten the integrity of their missions and their reputations, and put public trust in jeopardy. The risks are substantial and are not offset by meaningful benefits.

RECOMMENDATION 5.1 For all faculty, students, residents, and fellows and for all associated training sites, academic medical centers and teaching hospitals should adopt and implement policies that prohibit

- **the acceptance of items of material value from pharmaceutical, medical device, and biotechnology companies, except in specified situations;**
- **educational presentations or scientific publications that are controlled by industry or that contain substantial portions written by someone who is not identified as an author or who is not properly acknowledged;**
- **consulting arrangements that are not based on written contracts for expert services to be paid for at fair market value;**
- **access by drug and medical device sales representatives, except by faculty invitation, in accordance with institutional policies, in certain specified situations for training, patient safety, or the evaluation of medical devices; and**
- **the use of drug samples, except in specified situations for patients who lack financial access to medications.**

Until their institutions adopt these recommendations, faculty and trainees at academic medical centers and teaching hospitals should voluntarily adopt them as standards for their own conduct.

This recommendation has several targets, most of which focus on promotional relationships. One target is the acceptance by faculty or trainees of items of material value (including small gifts and meals) from industry except in certain situations. These situations, which should be defined in institutional policies, include (1) appropriate payment for legitimate services (such as contracts, grants, and consulting arrangements); (2) charitable donations, which should be given to the institution; and (3) sharing of research materials or data. Under appropriate transfer agreements, the sharing of research materials or data is encouraged, as it promotes medical research. This recommendation covers not only physical gifts, such as pens, notepads, and meals, but also preferences, such as paid speaking engagements that are intended as rewards or inducements. Consulting arrangements and drug samples are discussed further below.

The second target of this recommendation is the involvement of faculty or trainees in presentations or publications for which they cannot ethically claim credit or intellectual independence. Although no physician or researcher should accept authorship of a ghostwritten academic publication (see the discussion earlier in this chapter), failure to meet this standard is particularly troublesome when it involves faculty who have a special obligation to demonstrate intellectual independence and to act as role models. For similar reasons, faculty should not participate in speakers bureaus and similar promotional activities in which they either present content directly controlled by industry or formulate their remarks to win favor and continued speaking fees. If institutions fail to adopt these recommendations, then acceptance of authorship for ghostwritten publications or industry-controlled presentations would constitute a gift to be disclosed to the institution even if the institution's policies do not explicitly mention these arrangements as gifts.

The recommendation's third target is consulting arrangements. Faculty should engage only in bona fide consulting arrangements that require their expertise, that are based on written contracts with specific tasks and deliverables, and that are paid for at fair market value. As part of their administration of conflict of interest policies, university review of faculty consulting and other contracts is prudent and desirable.

The fourth target of this recommendation concerns access to educational environments by sales representatives of pharmaceutical, medical device, or biotechnology companies. Clinical teaching should be done by faculty, not by marketing agents. The recommended restrictions on site access should not discourage appropriate and productive research collaborations between industry and academic researchers. In addition to promoting scientific progress and the development of useful products, collaborations can provide educational benefits to medical students, graduate students, and postdoctoral fellows who might participate in legitimate collaborative research projects with industry under proper supervision.

As described earlier, the AAMC recommendations and some medical school policies set stringent restrictions on access by pharmaceutical sales representatives but establish slightly less restrictive conditions for access by representatives of medical device companies. The recommendations and policies reflect assessments that access by device representatives—if they are properly managed and appropriately limited—can contribute to patient safety. Nonetheless, the expectation is that faculty will quickly learn how to use complex new devices, including relevant surgical techniques, and will then instruct and supervise residents and fellows rather than rely on company representatives to do so. Access under these circumstances would occur after the institutional purchase of a complex device. For the purposes of device evaluation, access by the device representatives would occur before purchase of the device.

The fifth target of this recommendation, which covers drug samples, presents difficult issues. Caring for patients who cannot afford needed drugs is frustrating for physicians who are trying to meet their professional obligations to act in their patients' best interests. Despite the aid provided through Medicaid and Medicare, other public programs, and the patient access initiatives of pharmaceutical companies, many patients are not eligible for such aid and cannot afford to continue to take medications after they have used a sample. Moreover, although physicians and others may believe that drug samples allow low-income patients access to drugs that they could not readily obtain otherwise, this chapter has cited research that suggests that most samples are not, in fact, given to indigent patients and that access to samples may change trainee behavior such that they move away from practicing evidence-based and lower-cost care. Drug samples are not a satisfactory answer to the serious problem of the lack of affordability of medications for many patients, but the committee was reluctant to call on physicians to abandon them completely in the short term.

For academic medical centers, the use of drug samples may often be managed without a direct interaction between a physician and a company representative. Thus, AAMC recommends and this committee agrees that samples (if the institution permits them) should, whenever possible, be centrally managed in ways that allow timely and appropriate patient access.

In the absence of such centralized arrangements, institutions should limit the provision of free drug samples and provide them only to patients who lack financial access to medications in situations in which generic alternatives are not available and the sample medication can be continued at little or no cost to the patient for as long as it is needed. They should also help physicians and patients use alternative public and private resources to obtain the needed medications. The proposal by the Medicare Payment Advisory Commission for company reporting and U.S. Department of Health and Human Services analysis of data about the distribution of drug samples cited earlier in this chapter could, if it is adopted, produce helpful information to guide future policies.

The elements of this recommendation apply both to campus settings and to off-site settings, for example, off-site locations for professional meetings and educational programs. They also apply to volunteer faculty who provide clinical education in their offices or in community hospitals. Chapter 6 presents a parallel recommendation (Recommendation 6.1) for physicians who are not affiliated with academic institutions. That chapter also presents a comprehensive recommendation (Recommendation 6.2) that calls for medical product companies to change their policies to be consistent with these recommendations. The committee recognizes that it takes time for academic medical centers to develop policies. It recognizes the value of policy development processes that involve the assessment of local conditions, the inclusion of those who will be affected, and investigation of the experiences of similar institutions.

Until institutions act, faculty, students, and trainees should still change their own behavior so that it is in line with the recommendations presented above. In addition, consistent with Recommendation 9.1, the committee encourages AAMC, AMSA, and similar membership organizations to continue or initiate survey, monitoring, and other activities to promote the reform of conflict of interest policies in medical education.

Education on Relationships with Industry

RECOMMENDATION 5.2 Academic medical centers and teaching hospitals should educate faculty, medical students, and residents on how to avoid or manage conflicts of interest and relationships with pharmaceutical and medical device industry representatives. Accrediting organizations should develop standards that require formal education on these topics.

Changing the environment within educational institutions is important, but medical schools also need to prepare trainees for practice in environments that may be characterized by more permissive standards of conduct regarding drug and device marketing. Faculty will continue to experience a range of situations in which they will interact with industry representatives and will also need to be prepared to act as educators and role models on industry relationships.

The committee recognizes that the evidence on the effectiveness of educational programs of this sort on physician attitudes and behaviors is not strong, but it believes that a basic level of education supports the development of core competencies and prepares students and trainees for future practice. The establishment of educational standards will help ensure that such education is of high quality and receives appropriate attention.

Accredited Continuing Medical Education

The members of the committee had extensive internal discussions about industry support for accredited continuing medical education. Overall, there was general agreement that continuing medical education has become far too reliant on industry funding and that such funding tends to promote a narrow focus on products and to neglect the provision of a broader education on alternative strategies for managing health conditions and other important issues, such as communication and prevention. Given the lack of validated and efficient tools for preventing or detecting bias, industry funding creates a substantial risk of bias, to the extent that industry-reliant providers want to attract industry support for future programs. Although the committee did not reach agreement on a specific path to reform, it concluded that the current system of funding is unacceptable and should not continue.

RECOMMENDATION 5.3 A new system of funding accredited continuing medical education should be developed that is free of industry influence, enhances public trust in the integrity of the system, and provides high-quality education. A consensus development process that includes representatives of the member organizations that created the accrediting body for continuing medical education, members of the public, and representatives of organizations such as certification boards that rely on continuing medical education should be convened to propose within 24 months of the publication of this report a funding system that will meet these goals.

One option is for this broad-based consensus development process to be convened by the member organizations of ACCME. As described earlier in this chapter, they represent medical specialty boards (American Board of Medical Specialties), hospitals (AHA and the Association for Hospital Medical Education), organized medicine (AMA), medical schools (AAMC), medical specialty societies (CMSS), and state licensure boards (Federation of State Medical Boards). Although these organizations have interests in continuing medical education and in ensuring that continuing education is free of bias and supports core competencies, they do not all have a vested interest in the current system of funding that education.

The consensus development process convened by this or another group should be broad based and should also include representatives of other medical education accrediting bodies (LCME and ACGME), other interested state and federal agencies, public interest and patient advocacy groups, and organizations such as specialty certification boards that rely on continuing medical education. It should also include providers of accredited continuing medical education and industry funders. The deliberations should take into account the findings of other groups that have analyzed funding for continuing medical education or that have made recommendations about improving continuing medical educational methods.

Most committee members believed that a near-term end to industry funding would be unacceptably disruptive for the major providers of accredited continuing medical education, including medical schools and professional societies, which together provide 68 percent of the total number of hours of this type of education (see Table 5-2). A SACME survey found that 77 percent of respondents said that immediate elimination of commercial support would substantially reduce the number of courses at their academic centers and the scope of their programs and could potentially lead to the elimination of programs (SACME, 2008b). Eliminating all industry funding without having in place an alternative model could have other adverse consequences. For example, a surgical society may hold a premeeting accredited workshop involving hands-on teaching of surgical techniques, typically supported by indirect funds from industry. In the committee's experience, the costs of setup and materials for multiple simultaneous workshops can be several million dollars and would be hard to cover by payments from attendees. Furthermore, other innovative educational formats—for example, Internet-based training, simulation-based training, and performance improvement learning activities—also require funding for start-up and updating costs that could be prohibitive for providers to self-fund or fund entirely through nonindustry sources.

A majority of the committee supported the use of a consensus development process to develop a new funding system for accredited continuing medical education that would be free of industry influence but that would leave open the possibility of certain forms of indirect industry funding under conditions that minimized the risk of undue influence on program content. Some committee members supported the use of a consensus development process to develop an alternative funding model but believed that no form of direct or indirect industry funding was acceptable.

Among the options that the consensus development activity could consider are proposals for some kind of pooled funding mechanism. For example, companies could grant funds to some independent central or regional entity that would establish educational priorities and make decisions—perhaps within broad categories—about the distribution of funds on the basis of an independent review of applications from education providers.

Both direct company funding to institutions for specific continuing medical education programs and direct company provision of unrestricted grants to institutions offer clear opportunities for undue influence, particularly for continuing medical education providers that also receive the great majority of their funding overall from companies. A plan for a system free from industry influence would exclude such funding as well as funding from company-controlled foundations.

The committee recognizes that industry willingness to provide funds under a restructured system of funding accredited continuing medical education might be quite limited. Thus, the consensus development process would also need to consider alternative means of financing, steps to reduce program costs, and other strategies that would support high-quality continuing medical education. Options include increased fees for attendees; subsidies from academic medical centers as part of their educational missions; elimination of expensive program locales and amenities; reduced payments to speakers; collaboration among education providers to share the costs of developing certain expensive programs; and rethinking the purpose and methods of continuing medical education, as is already being done in the development of programs for the maintenance of certification by specialty societies. Higher fees might be a particular burden for physicians with lower-than-average professional incomes, including rural physicians and physicians serving disadvantaged populations.

The committee members who opposed any industry funding of continuing medical education through any mechanism believed that physicians (or their employers) should bear the entire cost of accredited continuing medical education that is required for renewal of licensure and specialty certification. Even giving industry funding and program decision-making responsibility to a central office within a medical school, MECC, or other institution would unnecessarily retain conflicts of interest over the choice of course topics, directors, content and speakers, and the leadership of the continuing medical education office. In the view of these committee members, all industry support for accredited continuing medical education should be rejected, just as it is for most undergraduate and graduate medical education.

In the process of hearing testimony relevant to the issue of funding of continuing medical education, many committee members came to the conclusion that a number of other fundamental problems about the focus and the effectiveness of continuing medical education warranted attention. These issues were outside of the purview of the committee. Some will be considered by another committee of the Institute of Medicine, which is charged with making recommendations about the promotion of more effective methods of life-long education for health professionals (IOM, 2009). Analyses of the financing of continuing medical education are planned in conjunction with that project. Those analyses may provide a better understanding of the implications of different proposals about financing in the context of other changes in the system.

The committee focused on accredited continuing medical education. As noted earlier, some nonaccredited activities with industry support are educational rather than promotional and apply safeguards to prevent bias in the selection of topics, speakers, and materials presented. One example is the scientific symposium that is organized and controlled by a professional society and supported by unrestricted grants from companies. Such meetings may be particularly important for fields with many Ph.D. researchers and relatively restricted budgets. Another example is training in the use of complex medical devices provided by medical device companies under the conditions outlined elsewhere in this report (e.g., no gifts or inducements to use the product).

Other Recommendations in This Report

In addition to the recommendations in this chapter, other recommendations in this report would affect institutions that provide undergraduate, graduate, or continuing medical education. The standardization of institutional disclosure policies and formats (Recommendation 3.3) would require work to change policies and information systems, but in the long term, it should make institutional policies less burdensome across all educational institutions—as well as for individuals who must disclose potential conflicts of interest. Academic medical centers, which have repeatedly been embarrassed by revelations of incomplete and inaccurate faculty disclosures of payments from industry, would benefit from a national program of company reporting of payments to physicians and researchers that would allow the verification of certain disclosures (Recommendation 3.4). Because that reporting program would also cover payments to academic medical centers and other providers of medical education, it could provide an incentive for the adoption of institution-level conflict of interest policies, as recommended in this report (Recommendation 8.1). Accrediting organizations, membership groups such as AAMC and CMSS, and government agencies should also develop incentives for institutions to adopt and implement conflict of interest policies (Recommendation 9.2).

Adoption of the recommendation related to the conduct of research in which an investigator has a financial interest would encourage the development of management plans to protect trainees involved in such research if the institution concludes that the participation by the investigator with a conflict of interest in the research is essential (Recommendation 4.1). To the extent that physicians embrace Recommendation 6.1 to reject gifts and similar ties, it would reduce dissonance when students, trainees, and faculty interact with others in the medical community at professional society meetings and in other contexts. Further steps by companies to reform their policies and practices on gifts and payments to physicians (Recommendation 6.2) would allow medical centers to focus more attention on other issues, for example, consulting and other contractual arrangements. Finally, academic institutions can play an important role in implementing a program of research on conflict of interest (Recommendation 9.2).

6

Conflicts of Interest and Medical Practice

A position statement of the American College of Physicians (ACP) observed that "[p]hysicians meet industry representatives at the office and at professional meetings, collaborate in community-based research, and develop or invest in health-related industries. In all of these spheres, partnered activities often offer important opportunities to advance medical knowledge and patient care, but they also create an opportunity for the introduction of bias" (Coyle et al., 2002a, p. 397). This chapter examines these relationships and the sources of conflicts of interest in the context of practicing physicians' primary professional obligations.

Professionals are granted important privileges—including the power to set educational and ethical standards—in return for maintaining competence, being trustworthy and ethical, and working to benefit patients and society. The power to set standards creates certain tensions. As Pellegrino and Relman (1999) have written, "[t]oo often, ethical goals have been commingled with protection of self-interest, privilege, and prerogative. Yet, effacement of self-interest is the distinguishing feature of a true profession that sets it apart from other occupations" (p. 984).

In the realm of patient care, threats to professionalism and questions about conflicts of interest may arise in several situations, some of which involve pharmaceutical, medical device, and biotechnology companies and some of which do not. This chapter focuses on physician financial relationships with industry that usually are not intrinsic to medical practice and that can be avoided. These relationships create conflicts of interest when physicians

- accept company gifts of various kinds, including meals and drug samples;

- act as promotional speakers or writers on behalf of companies; or
- have a financial interest in a medical product company whose products they prescribe, use, or recommend.

In addition, conflicts of interest arise from the ways in which physicians are paid for their services. These conflicts are inherent in any payment system, although each payment method raises different concerns. Physician ownership of health care facilities and self-referral practices also present important and widespread conflicts of interest that have challenged government in its efforts to manage, limit, or eliminate them.

This chapter begins with a brief discussion of physician payment and facility ownership interests as parts of the broader context of medical practice. As planned by the Institute of Medicine, this study was not intended to consider recommendations on physician payment; that is a primary charge of the Medicare Payment Advisory Commission (MedPAC; a body that advises the U.S. Congress). The committee also was not constituted to consider physician ownership and self-referral issues, which would have involved the in-depth examination of a complex regulatory and commercial environment. Therefore, the discussion of these topics is only brief.

The chapter then examines industry promotional activities aimed at practicing physicians and also reviews the responses to concerns about physician financial relationships with industry from private organizations and public agencies. Because the committee considered financial relationships with industry in the context of physicians' professional obligations, the chapter includes a discussion of professional codes of conduct and statements on conflicts of interest in medical practice from professional societies. The chapter concludes with recommendations for the physician community; health care providers; and pharmaceutical, medical device, and biotechnology companies.

THE BROADER CONTEXT: PHYSICIAN PAYMENT, SELF-REFERRAL, AND CONFLICTS OF INTEREST IN MEDICAL PRACTICE

The environment of medical practice has changed significantly in recent decades. Physicians providing patient care have experienced reduced autonomy, increased administrative burdens, and declining incomes. As shown in Figure 6-1, the real income of physicians from medical practice declined about 7 percent from 1995 to 2003, a pattern that contrasts with that for other professional and technical workers. Flat or declining fees from public and private payers appear to be a major contributor to the trend (Tu and Ginsburg, 2006). Although the committee did not locate a

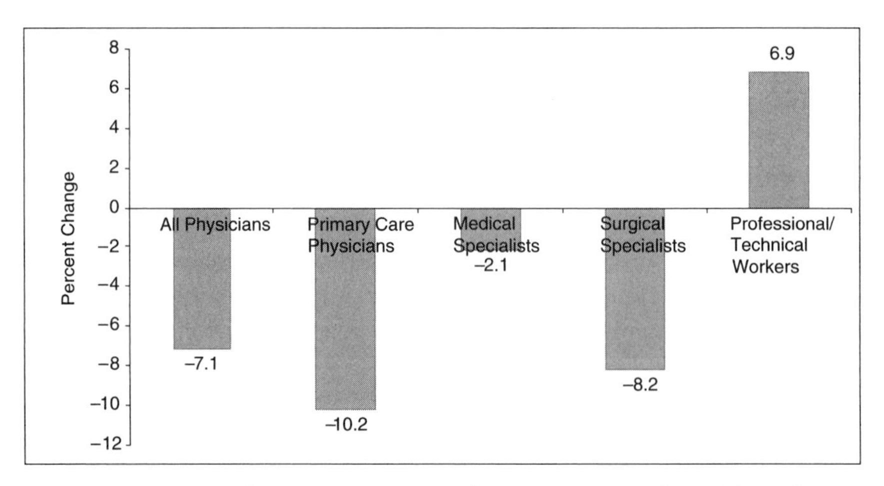

FIGURE 6-1 Percent change in average net physician income, adjusted for inflation, 1995 to 2003. Physician income data are based on reported net income from the practice of medicine (after expenses and before taxes). SOURCE: Tu and Ginsburg, 2006.

more recent analysis of trends, some data (e.g., comparisons of Bureau of Labor Statistics physician and surgeon income data for 2006 and 2007) suggest a more favorable income picture in recent years.

Physician Payment and Conflicts of Interest

Researchers and policy makers have devoted considerable attention to the day-to-day incentives for inappropriate clinical practice related to physician payment arrangements. Each major method of paying physicians has the potential to put physicians' primary interest in promoting the best interests of their patients at odds with their secondary financial interests.

Many studies have concluded that paying physicians for each service that they provide creates incentives for physicians to increase the volume of services, which also increases their income and society's spending for health care (see the reviews by CBO [1986], OTA [1986], PPRC [1987], Smith [1992], and Hsiao et al. [1993]). In addition, the appropriate pricing of specific services and categories of services is a concern (see, e.g., Ginsburg and Grossman [2005] and Bodenheimer et al. [2007]). Higher levels of reimbursement for procedures (e.g., surgeries, invasive procedures, diagnostic imaging, and chemotherapy) compared with the level of reimbursement for non-procedure-related services (e.g., history taking, medical evaluations, and counseling) have contributed to an escalation in the use of procedures and to the shift in the performance of certain lucrative procedural services from hospitals to physicians' offices. One analysis of information from national surveys and long-term, in-depth studies of 12 local markets concluded that physicians' business practices contribute to higher costs and that "policymakers may need to revisit regulation of physicians' conflicts of interest and consider how their financial incentives could be realigned" (Pham et al., 2004, p. 70).

Payments to physicians on a capitated basis (i.e., a fixed, per person payment for a patient population) and managed care restrictions on referrals and certain services raise concerns about the underprovision of needed care (see, e.g., Hillman [1987], GAO [1995], Rodwin [1996], and Sulmasy et al. [2000]). In general, payment methods have become more complex as public and private health insurers have offered incentive payments to physicians related to quality standards, patient satisfaction, and better patient outcomes (see, e.g., Epstein et al. [2004], MedPAC [2005c], Rosenthal et al. [2007], and Nicholson et al. [2008]).

Self-Referral and Physician Ownership of Health Care Facilities

A former editor of the *New England Journal of Medicine* observed that "[p]hysicians have been conflicted about their dual roles as professionals and businessmen for millennia, but this dilemma has sharpened in recent years as income from the practice of medicine has faltered" (Kassirer, 2001, p. 159). The dilemma is particularly evident, first, in the growth of physician ownership of (or other business arrangements with) outpatient diagnostic or treatment centers and specialty hospitals to which they refer patients and, second, in the increase in expensive in-office ancillary equipment (e.g., equipment used for imaging and other diagnostic services ordered by the physician owner). As described by Pham and Ginsburg (2007)

> The allure of profitable services has led to increased physician ownership of ambulatory surgical, imaging, and endoscopy centers and other freestanding facilities such as specialty hospitals. For example, the number of cardiac and orthopedic specialty hospitals serving Medicare patients grew from twenty-one in 1998 to sixty-seven in 2003, the majority of which were for-profit and owned in part by physicians. The number of ambulatory surgery centers (ASCs) grew more than 35 percent between 2000 and 2004, with 83 percent of existing centers partly or wholly owned by physicians. In addition, physicians have brought the capacity for more diagnostic and therapeutic procedures into their practices. (p. 1591)

Physicians' ownership interests in facilities to which they refer patients constitute a conflict of interest. Their secondary interest (i.e., increased income from increased services) has the potential to bias physicians' primary interest in their patients' welfare. Such conflicts of interest may harm patients who receive unnecessary services and may also harm society, which is burdened by excess spending on these services. In fact, some research has contradicted claims that physician ownership improves access for underserved populations (see, e.g., OIG [1989], Hillman et al. [1990], and Mitchell and Scott [1992]).

Concerns about physician self-referral have prompted the passage of complex federal legislation and the implementation of regulations (often collectively referred to as the "Stark laws," after the sponsor of relevant provisions in the Omnibus Budget Reconciliation Act of 1989 and other legislation). In general, federal law prohibits physicians from referring Medicare or Medicaid beneficiaries to entities for "designated health services" if the physicians or their immediate family members have ownership or investment interests in the entities or have compensation arrangements with the entities (42 USC 1395nn and 42 USC 1396b(s)).[1]

In 2008, the Centers for Medicare and Medicaid Services issued a new rule requiring physicians to disclose to patients the physician's ownership of or investment in hospitals (CMS, 2008). It is too early to evaluate the experience with this requirement, although the discussion reviewed in Chapter 3 suggests that the need for caution in assuming the effectiveness of disclosure alone as a safeguard against making biased recommendations. In 2009, MedPAC recommended that Congress require hospitals and other entities that bill Medicare to report physician ownership interests (direct and indirect) and that this information be posted on a public website (MedPAC, 2009). MedPAC also recommended that the secretary of the U.S. Department of Health and Human Services submit a report on the types and prevalence of financial arrangements between physicians and hospitals.

INDUSTRY PROMOTIONAL ACTIVITIES AND PRACTICING PHYSICIANS

Scope and Nature of Marketing Activities

Marketing is a major expense for pharmaceutical companies. A recent analysis estimated that pharmaceutical company expenditures for promotional activities were $57.5 billion in 2004, including $20.4 billion for

[1] "Whole" hospitals are not included under the law, which some suggest has been a factor spurring the growth of physician-owned specialty hospitals (Mitchell, 2008). The law also does not cover the purchase and use of imaging and other ancillary equipment within a physician's office. Designated health services include clinical laboratory services; inpatient and outpatient hospital services; diagnostic radiology services; radiation therapy services and supplies; durable medical equipment and supplies; prosthetics, orthotics, and prosthetic devices and supplies; home health care services; physical therapy services; outpatient prescription drugs; occupational therapy services; and parenteral and enteral nutrients, equipment, and supplies.

detailing (sales visits) by drug company representatives, $15.9 billion for drug samples, and $2.0 billion for meetings (Gagnon and Lexchin, 2008). Little information is available on the marketing of medical devices and biologics.

Pharmaceutical company representatives use a variety of interpersonal techniques, including gift giving, to establish relationships with physicians and promote their products.[2] They may calibrate their approach to their assessments of the physician's personality and intellectual style (see, e.g., Roughead et al. [1998], Fugh-Berman and Ahari [2007], and Greene [2007]). In addition, companies have information on individual physician prescribing practices that they can use to target physicians and then monitor the effects of their relationships (Steinbrook, 2006). As described in Chapter 1 and discussed further in this chapter, some of that information is compiled from physician data sold by the American Medical Association (AMA).

Companies may also use physicians as marketing agents. For example, an article in the *Wall Street Journal* reported data from a market research firm showing that in 2004 pharmaceutical companies sponsored some 237,000 meetings or talks that featured physicians and 134,000 meetings or talks conducted by sales representatives, up from about 60,000 talks of each type in 1998 (Hensley and Martinez, 2005). The same article also cited an internal study conducted by Merck that estimated that discussion groups led by physicians yield almost twice the benefit in terms of additional prescriptions as discussion groups led by sales representatives.

A specific example of the use of physicians for marketing involved a new vaccine for human papillomavirus and cervical cancer. The project signed up "hundreds of doctors and nurses . . . as unofficial spokesmen" who were trained by the pharmaceutical company and were "provided with a multimedia presentation and paid $4,500 for each 50-minute talk, delivered" at company-sponsored meals (Rosenthal, 2008, unpaged).

The scope of pharmaceutical company payments for speeches given by physicians is suggested in a report by the Vermont attorney general based on information received under the state's payment disclosure law (see Chapter 3). Between July 1, 2006, and June 30, 2007, pharmaceutical companies in that state spent almost $3,140,000 on payments to physicians and other providers; 52 percent of the payments were for speaker fees and 30 percent were for food (Sorrell, 2008). As discussed below, companies may

[2] A press release from PeopleMetrics Rx about a study of the influence of drug sales representatives on physician prescribing practices stated that the study found "that sales representatives must develop personal relationships with their physicians to achieve the highest levels of engagement" and that "emotional components such as friendship with the reps are the strongest indicators of Fully Engaged physicians [which] . . . has a positive impact on the duration and frequency of meetings and physician prescribing patterns" (*Business Wire*, 2008).

also market to community physicians through "seeding trials" of medications approved by the Food and Drug Administration.

Surveys of Physician Relationships with Industry

Surveys show that relationships with industry are common among physicians across the nation. In a national probability sample of more than 3,100 physicians, 94 percent reported that they had had some type of relationship with industry during the preceding year. These relationships were primarily the receipt of food in the workplace (83 percent) or drug samples (78 percent) (Campbell et al., 2007a). Thirty-five percent received industry reimbursement for costs associated with professional meetings or continuing medical education; and 28 percent received payments for activities such as consulting, serving on a speakers bureau, or enrolling patients in clinical trials. Cardiologists were more than twice as likely as family practitioners to receive payments, but family practitioners met more frequently with industry representatives than physicians in other specialties. Physicians in solo/dual or group practices met more frequently with representatives than physicians practicing in hospitals and clinics. In sum, relationships between physicians and industry are common and vary by specialty, practice type, and professional activities.

Another national survey of physicians also found that relationships with industry are common: 92 percent of physicians had received free drug samples; 61 percent had received meals, tickets to entertainment events, or free travel; and 12 percent had received financial incentives to participate in drug trials (KFF, 2002). The survey found that 15 percent of respondents thought that drug representatives provided "very useful" information, with another 59 percent describing the information as "somewhat useful." Only 9 percent thought that the information was "very accurate," whereas 72 percent thought that it was "somewhat accurate" (KFF, 2002).

A study of community obstetricians-gynecologists reported that most physicians believed that it was appropriate for physicians to accept drug samples (92 percent), a lunch at which information was provided (77 percent), or an anatomical model (75 percent) (Morgan et al., 2006). Just over half (53 percent) thought that it was appropriate for a physician identified as a "high prescriber" to accept a representative's invitation "to sit in" on a market research meeting as a well-paid consultant. In response to a question about whether interactions with industry should be more strictly regulated, 40 percent disagreed, 34 percent agreed, and 26 percent were neutral. As was found in a number of other studies, the respondents thought that other physicians were more likely (probably or almost surely) to be influenced by receiving a drug sample than the respondents were (38 percent for other physicians versus 33 percent for the respondents). The researchers found no association between the responses and familiarity with the codes of conduct of professional societies.

The studies reported here and in Chapter 5 occurred before the Pharmaceutical Research and Manufacturers of America (PhRMA) revised its *Code on Interactions with Healthcare Professionals* in 2008. These revisions, which set some limits on gift giving and other relationships and which are discussed further below, took effect in January 2009. The Advanced Medical Technology Association (AdvaMed) adopted similar revisions in its *Code of Ethics on Interactions with Health Care Professionals*, effective in July 2009. Thus, it is too early to gauge the effects of these changes on physician relationships with pharmaceutical and medical device companies.

Participation of Community-Based Physicians in Clinical Trials

As mentioned in Chapter 4, physicians in private office settings are increasingly participating in clinical trials that are sponsored by industry and managed by contract research organizations or research site management organizations. The percentage of clinical trials conducted in academic health centers has decreased, and academic health centers are now in the minority among the locations for clinical trials (Klein and Fleischman, 2002). The marketing aspects of some of these trials were described above. The involvement of practicing physicians in clinical trials in the community has potential benefits. For example, their patient pool may be more representative of all patients with the condition being studied than the patient pool of academic physicians, so the results may be more generalizable. Furthermore, the recruitment of participants and the conduct of the study may be more rapid and less expensive in the community setting than in academic medical centers. In addition, such trials may be educational for the participating physicians.

Several concerns have, however, been raised about conflicts of interest in industry-sponsored trials involving community physicians. First, payments to participating physicians may provide incentives to enroll and retain patients, but they may also exceed actual expenses. In guidance provided to pharmaceutical companies, the Office of the Inspector General of the U.S. Department of Health and Human Services has cautioned against payments that exceed fair market amounts for "legitimate, reasonable, and necessary services" (OIG, 2003, p. 21). Second, practicing physicians may have a powerful influence over their patients, perhaps more so than physicians in academic centers, which have high rates of turnover of residents, fellows, and faculty and which allow investigators studying common diseases to recruit participants who are not their personal patients.

In addition, some clinical trials in community practices may be "seeding" trials that companies design to change prescribing habits rather than to gather scientifically useful information (Hill et al., 2008; see also Psaty and Rennie [2006] and Sox and Rennie [2008]). As described in an analysis of documents obtained during litigation, the strategy of such trials is to "target the [clinical] trial to a select group of customers—in this case, primary care physicians; use the trial to demonstrate the value of [the drug] to these physicians; integrate the marketing division and those responsible for trial-related operations in the field with the highest level of precision; and carefully track marketing-related results, that is, rates of [product] prescriptions written by study physicians" (Hill et al., 2008, p. 253). The company in the case under litigation described the physicians as "key customers" (p. 255) and provided them with materials to market their involvement in the study. It also "hid the marketing nature of the trial from participants, physician investigators, and institutional review board members" (Hill et al., 2008, p. 251). As an additional marketing tool, companies may sometimes employ physician opinion leaders as consultants on the use of a drug under study.

A study by Andersen and colleagues (2006) found that general practitioners involved in industry-sponsored studies increased their use of the trial sponsor's drugs, which is consistent with the purpose of using the seeding strategy. Whether the increased use was medically appropriate was not evaluated, but seeding studies subvert ethical standards for research conduct and can put patients at risk.

As part of a broad policy that prohibits or limits many types of company payments to physicians and requires disclosure of other payments, Massachusetts recently issued regulations that require disclosure by companies of payments to physicians for studies "that are designed or sponsored by marketing departments of manufacturers or that are undertaken to increase sales of a particular drug, biologic or medical device" (Lopes, 2009, p. 8). Payments for scientific research need not be disclosed.

Community Versus Academic Practice Environment

Chapter 5 reported on the extensive relationships between academic physicians and industry and discussed industry promotional activities undertaken in the context of graduate and undergraduate medical education. It reported on studies that suggest that industry relationships and promotional activities (e.g., detailing visits) in both academic and general practice settings may influence physician prescribing patterns and requests for additions to hospital formularies. It also reported on studies—conducted mostly in academic settings—that indicate that the provision of free drug samples to physicians may contribute to inappropriate prescribing practices, lower rates of use of generic and over-the-counter drugs, and increased drug costs.

Chapter 5 also noted that trainees in academic settings have ready access to the latest scientific information through faculty experts and advanced information technologies that they may use to search the medical literature; they do not require interactions with company sales representatives to obtain information on a new drug or its use. Faculty members—in addition to being in the forefront of knowledge development and evaluation in their own fields—also have ready access to the expertise of their colleagues. In contrast, community physicians have less access to such expertise, and that has been one argument in support of visits to community physicians by drug company sales representatives. Sales representatives are, however, tasked with promoting their company's products and not with providing a balanced assessment of the evidence for the use of different clinical options, including nonpharmacologic approaches.

One response to the informational needs of community physicians has been the development of accredited continuing medical education programs. Nevertheless, a recent historical review of pharmaceutical marketing and physician education suggested unintended consequences, that is, the provision of "novel sites of intersection between pharmaceutical marketing and physician education" (Podolsky and Greene, 2008, p. 833). Concern about such consequences has, in turn, produced new approaches, including the "academic detailing" programs described later in this chapter.

In research, the community practice environment is clearly different from the environment in academic medical centers and major teaching hospitals. Although the research may be reviewed in advance by an institutional review board, community physicians may receive no training in the standards of the ethical conduct of research, may have little contact with experienced clinical researchers, and may lack the knowledge needed to review contract or research descriptions provided by a company. In sum, the environment in which community physicians interact with industry may be quite different from the environment of academic physicians discussed in Chapter 5.

RESPONSES TO CONCERNS ABOUT INDUSTRY RELATIONSHIPS AND CONFLICTS OF INTEREST IN COMMUNITY PRACTICE

Responses to concerns about physician financial relationships with industry date back many years. For example, in 1972 the U.S. Congress acted to outlaw certain industry payments or other inducements to physicians. The discussion below focuses on the responses to those concerns made by professional societies, industry, and government. It does not examine responses by provider organizations, such as multispecialty group practices or hospitals. The committee found no systematic information on the responses by such organizations but identified examples of conflict of interest or other policies that restrict certain individual or organizational relationships with industry (see, e.g., Kaiser Permanente/TPMG [2004], Vesely [2005], and Henry Ford Health System [2007]). Consistent with the emphasis on professional values in this chapter, this section begins with a review of professional society policies.

Professional Societies

Several medical professional organizations have adopted guidelines, codes, or other statements that cover physician relationships with industry, but the committee found no comprehensive overview of statements (or the absence of statements) from professional societies. A selective review of society policies suggests that statements about gifts are fairly common, whereas statements about promotional speaking, ghostwriting, and consulting arrangements are not. A number of professional groups have endorsed a charter for medical professionalism that identifies "maintaining trust by managing conflicts of interest" as 1 of 10 key responsibilities of physicians (ABIM Foundation et al., 2002, p. 245).

Box 6-1 includes excerpts from general statements by AMA and ACP on gifts from industry to physicians. The AMA statement, which was first adopted in 1990, has been endorsed or used as a model by a number of other professional societies, including the American Academy of Pediatrics (Fallat and Glover, 2007), the American College of Obstetricians and Gynecologists (Morgan et al., 2006), and the American College of Rheumatology (ACR, 2007). AMA has also made specific recommendations regarding medical device representatives. It emphasizes that information from or training by such representatives should not be a substitute for the appropriate training of physicians and should be subject to facility policies that govern the presence of such representatives (e.g., informing patients, protecting privacy, and credentialing) (AMA, 2007).

Although ACP strongly discourages the acceptance of gifts and poses some pointed questions for physicians to consider before accepting them, it acknowledges that many physicians feel more comfortable with gifts than the tone of its position statement would imply (Coyle et al., 2002a). The statement observes that "[i]deally, physicians should not accept any promotional gifts or amenities, whatever their value or utility, if they have the potential to cloud professional judgment and compromise patient care" but "[a]s a practical matter, many physicians are comfortable" accepting gifts of modest value that may enhance medical practice or knowledge (p. 398).

BOX 6-1
Excerpts from Statements on Gifts by American Medical Association and American College of Physicians

American Medical Association

Ethical Opinion E-8.061: "Ultimately, it is the responsibility of individual physicians to minimize conflicts of interest that may be at odds with the best interest of patients and to access the necessary information to inform medical recommendations. . . . (1) Any gifts accepted by physicians individually should primarily entail a benefit to patients and should not be of substantial value. Accordingly, textbooks, modest meals, and other gifts are appropriate if they serve a genuine educational function. Cash payments should not be accepted. The use of drug samples for personal or family use is permissible as long as these practices do not interfere with patient access to drug samples. . . . (2) Individual gifts of minimal value are permissible as long as the gifts are related to the physician's work (e.g., pens and notepads). . . . (7) No gifts should be accepted if there are strings attached. For example, physicians should not accept gifts if they are given in relation to the physician's prescribing practices" (AMA, 2002 [updated]).

American College of Physicians

"The acceptance by a physician of gifts, hospitality, trips, and subsidies of all types from the health care industry that might diminish, or appear to others to diminish, the objectivity of professional judgment is strongly discouraged. As documented by some studies, the acceptance of even small gifts can affect clinical judgment and heighten the perception and/or reality of a conflict of interest. Accordingly, physicians need to gauge regularly whether any gift relationship is ethically appropriate and evaluate any potential for influence on clinical judgment. In making such evaluations, it is recommended that physicians consider such questions as 1) What would the public or my patients think of this arrangement? 2) What is the purpose of the industry offer? 3) What would my colleagues think about this arrangement? 4) What would I think if my own physician accepted this offer? In all instances, it is the individual responsibility of each physician to assess any potential relationship with industry to assure that it enhances patient care and medical knowledge and does not compromise clinical judgment" (Turton and Snyder, 2007, p. 469, revising Coyle et al., 2002a).

With respect to consulting, the ACP policy also advises physicians to "guard against conflicts of interest when invited to consult or speak for pay on behalf of a company" because "[i]t is likely that a company will retain only individuals who make statements or recommendations that are favorable to its products, thus compromising the physician's scientific objectivity" (Coyle et al., 2002a, p. 399). Furthermore,

> Physicians should also be circumspect if asked to deliver educational programming developed by a medical education and communication company. Such companies, which are largely financed through the pharmaceutical industry, are for-profit developers and vendors of continuing medical education. It is important that physicians retained as lecturers in such settings control the content of the educational modules they deliver rather than allow their presentations to be scripted by the company. Lecturers should screen industry-prepared presentation aids (such as slides and reference materials) to ensure their objectivity and should accept, modify, or refuse them on that basis. Presenters using such materials should disclose their source to audience members. Paid efforts to influence the profession or public opinion about specific medical products are particularly suspect. It is unethical, for example, for physicians to accept commissions for articles, editorials, or medical journal reviews that are actually ghostwritten by industry or public relations firms in an attempt to "manage the press" about certain products or services. (Coyle et al., 2002a, p. 399)

During the course of the committee's work, the Council of Medical Specialty Societies (CMSS) initiated a project to collect best practices on disclosure and limitation of conflict of interest and develop a statement on conflict of interest (The Associated Press, 2008). A CMSS task force recently recommended elements that specialty society policies should include, and it also proposed the development by CMSS of a template for such policies. The task force recommended that societies post their policies and provide information about the financial support that they receive from industry (CMSS, 2008). The CMSS earlier adopted a consensus statement on medical ethics that, among other provisions, states that:

- Physicians should resolve conflicts of interest in a way that gives primacy to the patient's interests.
- Physicians have an ethical obligation to preserve and protect the trust bestowed on them by society (CMSS, 1999, unpaged).

Although this chapter focuses on individual physicians, professional societies as organizations may also have financial relationships with industry. Such relationships include unrestricted educational grants, income from exhibitions and meetings, industry advertisements in the journals of professional societies, and funding for the development of practice guidelines. As discussed further in Chapter 8, such relationships can constitute institutional conflicts of interest, and the committee recommends the adoption of policies on such institution-level conflicts.

The committee found little information about the positions of state medical societies on individual or organizational relationships with medical product companies. The Wisconsin Medical Society announced in 2008 that its policy (which is not binding on physicians) is now that physicians should not accept gifts from companies whose products they prescribe to their patients. It noted that a "complete ban eases the burdens of compliance, biased decision making, and patient distrust" (WMS, 2008, unpaged).

Industry Codes and Company Actions

As mentioned above, the PhRMA *Code on Interactions with Healthcare Professionals* was revised in 2008 (and was effective in January 2009) and the AdvaMed code was also revised in 2008 (and was effective in July 2009). Some of the PhRMA code's provisions are summarized in Box 6-2. Overall, the revised code discourages noninformational physician-company relationships, such as speaker training programs at resorts and meals provided by sales representatives outside a physician's office or other medical setting. In addition, the revised code provides that the chief executive officers and compliance officers of companies certify yearly that they have a process in place to implement the code. Companies that do that will be identified on the association's website; AdvaMed has announced similar plans.

The 2008 revisions to the PhRMA code also include provisions about contracting arrangements. The document describes several factors as relevant to determining the legitimacy of such arrangement, including whether

- a written contract specifies the nature of the consulting services to be provided and the basis for payment of those services;
- a legitimate need for the consulting services has been identified in advance of requesting services and entering into arrangements with consultants;
- the criteria for selecting consultants are directly related to the identified purpose and the persons responsible for selecting the consultants have the expertise necessary to evaluate whether the particular health care professionals meet those criteria;
- the number of health care professionals retained is not greater than the number reasonably necessary to achieve the identified purpose;
- the retaining company maintains records concerning and makes appropriate use of the services provided by consultants; and
- the venue and circumstances of any meeting with consultants are conducive to the consulting services, and activities related to the services are the primary focus of the meeting; specifically, resorts are not appropriate venues (PhRMA, 2008, p. 8).

Partly in response to U.S. Department of Justice litigation and guidance from the Office of the Inspector General of the U.S. Department of Health

BOX 6-2
Summary of Selected Recent Revisions in the PhRMA *Code on Interactions with Healthcare Professionals*

Companies should not

- offer health care professionals any entertainment or recreational items or any gifts (e.g., notepads, mugs, and pens) that "do not advance disease or treatment education";
- create consulting arrangements as inducements or rewards for prescribing or recommending a particular medicine or course of treatment;
- create speaking engagements as inducements or rewards for prescribing a particular medicine or course of treatment or provide speaker payments above fair market value;
- fund continuing medical education programs as inducement to prescribe or recommend a particular medicine or course of treatment;
- directly subsidize the participation of a health care professional in such a program or in other conferences or professional meetings or create token consulting arrangements to do so indirectly; and
- directly provide meals at continuing medical education events.

Companies may, subject to certain standards,

- have sales representatives make informational visits to physicians and provide modest meals in connection with the visit;
- provide financial support to providers of continuing medical education so that they may reduce registration fees for programs;
- support professional and scientific meetings at appropriate locations in accord with the guidelines of the organizations supported;
- arrange for expert consultants on topics such as the marketplace, patient care, and products;
- sponsor speaker programs and provide training and reasonable compensation for speakers;
- provide scholarships for students and professionals to attend educational conferences; and
- provide educational and practice-related items of modest value to physicians.

and Human Services, some pharmaceutical companies have already revised their contracting practices. In addition, some individual pharmaceutical companies have announced that they will voluntarily post information about a range of payments to individual physicians. For example, Eli Lilly announced that it would create a publicly accessible registry of its payments to physicians beginning in 2009 (Lilly, 2008). Pfizer has released information about its grants and educational awards to medical, scientific, and patient organizations and has announced that it is eliminating grants to commercial providers of continuing medial education (Pfizer, 2008).

Government Responses

Chapters 1, 3, and 5 discussed various responses by federal and state governments to concerns about financial relationships involving physicians and industry. At the state level, these responses range from laws requiring company disclosure of certain payments to physicians to laws restricting or prohibiting certain relationships. As noted above, some federal agency policies require disclosure of certain physician ownership interests in health care facilities, and MedPAC has proposed a substantial expansion of disclosure of such interests.

As discussed in Chapter 2, conflicts of interest do not necessarily involve actual undue influence, but they may. In some cases, they may be illegal. Federal law prohibits "any remuneration (including any kickback, bribe, or rebate) directly or indirectly, overtly or covertly, in cash or in kind" in return for ordering, purchasing, or referring patients for services or items covered by a federal health care program (42 USC 1320a-7b(b)). Such remuneration has sometimes been disguised as payments to physicians for education, consulting, or research.

In 2003, the Office of the Inspector General of the U.S. Department of Health and Human Services issued guidance for pharmaceutical companies on complying with federal laws and regulations. The guidance included a discussion of how marketing and other relationships with physicians may be designed to reduce the risk of violations of the antikickback laws (OIG, 2003). It advised, for example, that payments for research, consulting, and advisory services be set at fair market value. The guidance also noted that certain practices that are common in other business areas may be illegal in the context of federal health care programs.

For the most part, prosecutions under the statute have been directed at the companies that offer inducements rather than at the individual physicians who accept them. Cases typically do not go to trial but end in financial settlements and compliance and monitoring arrangements (corporate integrity agreements) of some sort. Box 6-3 summarizes a few illustrative settlements of cases that involved various types of financial relationships between companies and physicians.[3]

[3] At the state level, state attorneys general have reached settlements with companies that are similar to those reached by the U.S. Department of Justice. For example, Oregon was the lead state in a $58 million settlement that involved 30 states and a 3-year investigation of deception in the marketing of rofecoxib (Vioxx), and the state was also involved in another multistate settlement involving charges of deceptive marketing of valdecoxib (Bextra) and celecoxib (Celebrex) (Oregon DOJ, 2008a,b).

BOX 6-3
Examples of Prosecutions Involving Kickbacks to Physicians

In 1997, a physician at the Tufts University health maintenance organization reported to federal investigators that a marketer for TAP Pharmaceuticals had offered him an educational grant if he would reverse a health plan decision to list a competing drug in the plan's formulary. Investigators taped company employees offering the physician $65,000 in "education" grants that he could use for any purpose. To settle these and other charges, the company agreed to pay the government $875,000 and enter into a corporate integrity agreement (DOJ, 2001; Studdert et al., 2004).

In 2006, Medtronic agreed to pay $40 million and enter into a corporate integrity agreement to settle charges of improper payments to physicians to promote the company's spinal devices. The improper payments included payments for physicians' attendance and expenses at medical education events and payments made under the guise of consulting, fellowship, royalty, and research activities (DOJ, 2006).

In 2007, the U.S. Department of Justice announced deferred prosecution agreements with four major orthopedic device manufacturers—Zimmer, Depuy, Biomet, and Smith & Nephew—that paid $311 million to settle allegations that they used consulting agreements and other payments as illegal inducements for physicians to use their products during the period from 2002 to 2006. The companies also entered into corporate integrity agreements that would involve extensive monitoring of their consulting needs and arrangements for an 18-month period (DOJ, 2007a).

In 2008, an Arkansas neurologist settled a U.S. Department of Justice civil suit for $1.5 million and also pled guilty to accepting kickbacks—gifts, funds for phony research studies, and sham consulting agreements—from Blackstone Medical, a medical device company (Demske, 2008).

In 2008, Merck reached an agreement with the U.S. Department of Justice to pay $650 million to settle charges that it overcharged Medicaid for three popular drugs and that its sales representatives had devised a variety of illegal arrangements (e.g., payments disguised as being for training, consultation, or market research) to induce physicians to use its products. The company also agreed to a 5-year corporate integrity agreement to prevent future improper conduct (DOJ, 2008).

For the orthopedic device companies mentioned in Box 6-3, the deferred prosecution agreements with the U.S. Department of Justice had some features that are similar to those in some of the conflict of interest policies and proposals discussed in this report. One was that the companies agreed to post on their websites the names of physician consultants and the payments made to them. In addition, new consulting agreements with physicians would require the physicians to agree to reveal the arrangement to their patients. For the 18-month period that they were in place, the deferred prosecution agreements provided that each company must undertake an assessment of its reasonable needs for educational consulting services and new product development consultants. They also provided for a federal monitor at each company to review compliance for all new and existing consulting relationships with the companies.

Academic Detailing and Other Prescriber Outreach Strategies

As one alternative to physician reliance on company sales representatives for information, "academic detailing" incorporates techniques that pharmaceutical company representatives use. Programs may use in-person visits to physicians by a clinical pharmacist or physician, provide educational materials and branded items, and offer individualized feedback on performance. The goal is to reduce inappropriate prescribing of targeted drugs, for example, inappropriate antibiotics and less effective vasodilators and analgesics. Randomized controlled trials have shown that such educational interventions are effective and have not found adverse clinical consequences (see, e.g., Soumerai and Avorn [1990], Solomon et al. [2001], van Eijk et al. [2001], and Simon et al. [2005]; but see also Lu et al. [2008]). These trials support other studies that suggest that the techniques that pharmaceutical company representatives commonly use are indeed effective in changing physician prescribing behavior.

Some states, including Pennsylvania, South Carolina, and Vermont, have initiated programs using such academic detailing. Pennsylvania's program has an operating budget of approximately $1 million per year, which funds about 1,000 detailing visits by a paid staff (Reck, 2008). Members of the U.S. Congress have proposed the creation of a federal program that would "provide grants or contracts for prescription drug education and outreach for healthcare providers and their patients" (HR 6752, July 31, 2008).

RECOMMENDATIONS

As described in this chapter, relationships between physicians in practice and drug and medical product companies are extensive and have prompted a range of responses from professional societies, government officials, and others. The environment of community medical practice presents challenges different from those posed in academic and research settings. In particular, physicians in community practice often have weaker ties with institutions than academic physicians and a greater degree of autonomy. In addition, although Chapters 3 and 5 cite questions about the implementation of conflict of interest policies by academic institutions, these institutions are generally in a stronger position to enforce employee adherence to conflict of interest policies than professional societies are to enforce member adherence to their policies and codes of ethics.

Voluntary Action by Individual Physicians

The committee's first recommendation on conflict of interest in medical practice generally parallels that made for academic medical centers, except that it is directed in the first instance at voluntary action by individual physicians. The recommendation also calls on professional societies and health care providers (including hospitals, nursing homes, and hospices) to adopt supportive policies; but the committee believed that it was appropriate to call on physicians directly to adopt practices that are consistent with high standards of professionalism.

RECOMMENDATION 6.1 Physicians, wherever their site of clinical practice, should

- **not accept items of material value from pharmaceutical, medical device, and biotechnology companies except when a transaction involves payment at fair market value for a legitimate service;**
- **not make educational presentations or publish scientific articles that are controlled by industry or contain substantial portions written by someone who is not identified as an author or who is not properly acknowledged;**
- **not enter into consulting arrangements unless they are based on written contracts for expert services to be paid for at fair market value;**
- **not meet with pharmaceutical and medical device sales representatives except by documented appointment and at the physician's express invitation; and**
- **not accept drug samples except in specified situations for patients who lack financial access to medications.**

Professional societies should amend their policies and codes of professional conduct to support these recommendations. Health care providers should establish policies for their employees and medical staff that are consistent with these recommendations.

The teaching mission of academic medical centers—which includes helping learners at all levels to think critically and appraise the evidence and providing appropriate role models and mentoring—provides strong arguments for the corresponding recommendations in Chapter 5. Furthermore, physicians in academic settings have ready access to objective, up-to-date information about new therapies, which is often not the case in community practice. The committee recognized the differences in academic and community environments but viewed critical thinking and the appraisal of evidence as key components of life-long learning and medical professionalism for all physicians, wherever their site of practice. The committee believes that entering into the relationships listed in Recommendation 6.1 creates unwarranted risks of compromising physician judgment and undermining public trust—risks that are not outweighed by prospective benefits for patients or society.

Evidence cited in earlier chapters and Appendix D suggests that gifts and drug samples can be influential even when their economic value is small. They primarily serve to create goodwill and a sense of reciprocity and partiality toward the marketing representatives who give them. (Gifts include meals provided to physicians and their employees as part of sales visits.) Moreover, some evidence suggests that they are associated with prescribing patterns that are inconsistent with evidence-based practice guidelines. Other evidence cited in Chapter 5 suggests that patients may have more negative attitudes toward such gifts and their potential impact on behavior than physicians do. The committee sees no convincing professional reasons to justify the acceptance of gifts or other items of material value from industry but does see the risk of bias and the loss of public trust.

To the extent that physicians outside academic institutions make educational presentations and prepare scientific publications, they should—like their counterparts who are faculty at academic institutions—refrain from participation in speakers bureaus and similar promotional activities and refuse authorship of ghostwritten articles. A physician should participate in consulting arrangements on the basis of a company's need for the physician's expertise. Such arrangements should be documented in contracts with specific tasks and deliverables and should be paid for at fair market value.

The recommendations about interactions with sales representatives are slightly different for academic and nonacademic physicians. The committee recognizes that physicians in academic settings have different responsibilities as educators and also have excellent access to information about the latest scientific and clinical developments. Physicians in busy community-based practices need objective information about new drugs and devices, as well as information that compares new drugs and devices with existing drugs and devices and that provides alternatives to drugs and devices. By making visits to physicians' offices, company representatives may provide this information in a convenient manner. In the future, however, with the continued growth of Internet resources and the development of prescriber outreach and other educational programs, alternative sources of timely, objective, up-to-date information should become more available and readily usable.

If a physician chooses to meet with pharmaceutical and device company representatives, certain conditions should apply. Meetings should be at the invitation of the physician and by appointment and should not involve gifts, including meals provided at the physician's office. In limited cases, it may be appropriate for meetings to take place in the presence of patients (with their informed consent), primarily when representatives are providing in-service education or assistance with devices or equipment.

A related issue is drug company access to physician prescribing information. Currently, drug companies can buy coded prescribing information from pharmacy benefits programs and pharmacy chains. Companies can also purchase data from the AMA Masterfile, which links physician license numbers with their names, addresses, and phone numbers. Some physicians and others have objected to this practice (Steinbrook, 2006). In response, AMA now allows physicians who do not want their identifying information to be provided to companies to fill out a form to request that their data not be made available to company sales representatives and their supervisors (O'Reilly, 2006). (Other company personnel could still have access to the information.) It would be preferable and a lesser burden on physicians for AMA to set the default option so that identifying information would not be provided unless a physician affirmatively agrees.

As discussed in Chapter 5, the committee recognizes that access to affordable medications is a serious problem for many Americans, but it believes that reliance on drug samples is an unsatisfactory response. Samples are typically available only for newer and heavily marketed drugs, which may have no proven clinical benefits over alternatives, including less expensive equivalent drugs or generics. Although a sample may be convenient for the patient, it may not be the most appropriate medication. Many samples are provided to patients with insurance coverage and to physicians and their families, groups that do not have impaired access to medications. In such situations, the convenience of samples is outweighed by their potential to undermine evidence-based, cost-effective prescribing. For patients with chronic illnesses who lack the ability to pay for medications, a sample should be a stopgap that is accompanied by referral of the patient to a public or pharmaceutical company assistance program that can provide continuity of treatment. If physicians decide to accept drug samples, they should be given to patients who lack financial access to medications in situations in which appropriate generic alternatives are not available and the medication can be continued at little or no cost to the patient for as long as the patient needs it. The committee recognizes that physicians in community practice may not have the option of using a centralized system of administration of drug samples, which is available in many academic medical centers. Some committee members were in favor of banning the acceptance of drug samples altogether and advocating for other mechanisms for providing access to drugs for indigent patients.

Recommendation 6.1 does not mention physician disclosure of financial relationships to patients. Patients could obtain that information, however, if the U.S. Congress were to require companies to disclose payments to physicians and to place that information on a searchable public database and also requires hospitals and other health care providers to report physician ownership interests. This option would avoid the interpersonal complexities involved with patients directly requesting or physicians directly providing such information. Patients and their families would need to be informed about the database, possibly through the use of brochures or notices in medical offices. Studies of patient use of the database would be a potential topic for the research agenda recommended in Chapter 9.

Continued Actions by Industry

The next recommendation promotes continued actions by pharmaceutical, medical device, and biotechnology companies to support the core values and missions of medicine. Some but not all of the recommended actions are covered by the revised codes issued by PhRMA (2008) and AdvaMed (2008) and by federal agency guidance to pharmaceutical companies (OIG, 2003).

RECOMMENDATION 6.2 Pharmaceutical, medical device, and biotechnology companies and their company foundations should have policies and practices against providing physicians with gifts, meals, drug samples (except for use by patients who lack financial access to medications), or other similar items of material value and against asking physicians to be authors of ghostwritten materials. Consulting arrangements should be for necessary services, documented in written contracts, and paid for at fair market value. Companies should not involve physicians and patients in marketing projects that are presented as clinical research.

The committee is encouraged that some companies have already taken steps to end company provision of certain gifts and meals and to develop new procedures for contracting with physicians for their consulting work. The revisions in the PhRMA and AdvaMed codes are also encouraging steps, especially if provisions to track and publicize adherence are meaningful. Public disclosure of commitment to the codes should put pressure on noncomplying companies and should also reduce any competitive disadvantage to those companies that do comply. The committee would, however, like to see the provisions on gifts extended, consistent with Recommendation 6.1. The adoption of Recommendation 3.4 (which proposes that the U.S. Congress establish a program that requires companies to report their payments to physicians, researchers, and institutions) should allow monitoring of some company practices.

If the levels of adherence to the policies and practices recommended here are low, governments may enact legislation to limit physician ties to companies, as the state of Massachusetts has. In general, committee members believed that voluntary limits should be given an opportunity to work and that legislation and regulation should be held as options if they do not. The reasoning was that this approach is more likely to reinforce professional values and allow more nuanced policies and standards that take into account the possibility of unintended consequences and that create fewer administrative burdens to be developed.

Other Recommendations in This Report

Other chapters of this report also offer some recommendations that could affect community physicians. To the extent they are involved in multiple activities that require the disclosure of financial interests (Recommendation 3.3), community physicians might face more specific disclosure requests but also more consistency in requests. If federal legislation requires pharmaceutical, device, and biotechnology companies to publicly report payments to physicians (Recommendation 3.4), some community physicians might choose to forgo certain relationships with industry that they find difficult to explain and justify. Community physicians who teach medical students or residents off-site would be affected by reforms in the policies of medical schools and teaching hospitals (Recommendation 5.1). A new system of funding continuing medical education (Recommendation 5.3) could lead to higher fees for attendees and reductions in the numbers, variety, and locations of course offerings. In addition, physicians who participate in professional society or other clinical practice guideline development activities might be limited in their involvement if they had conflicts of interest, especially conflicts involving promotional activities (Recommendation 7.1).

7

Conflicts of Interest and Development of Clinical Practice Guidelines

Clinical practice guidelines lie at the intersection of medical research, education, and practice. They build on medical research and serve an educational function. In clinical care, they may influence patient and physician decisions about health care interventions, health plan coverage for medical services, and assessments of the performance of individual physicians and institutions that provide health care.

Ideally, clinical practice guidelines are based on valid scientific evidence, critical assessment of that evidence, and objective clinical judgment that relates the evidence to the needs of practitioners and patients. Arguably, the most significant problem in the development of sound clinical practice guidelines is the lack of research that can be used to guide the development of comprehensive recommendations on clinical practice. Clinical trials often exclude children, older adults, and patients with multiple or uncommon diagnoses or complex personal situations. Given the lack of evidence on many clinical topics and patient populations and the frequent lack of consistent research findings, expert judgment based on clinical experience remains a significant element in the development of evidence-based practice guidelines. As the methods manual of the American College of Cardiology and the American Heart Association states, it is not often that there is "an abundance of evidence available that leads directly to an indisputable recommendation" (ACC/AHA, 2009, p. 27).

Financial relationships with pharmaceutical, medical device, and biotechnology companies may create conflicts of interest and a risk of undue influence on judgment both for entities that sponsor the development of clinical practice guidelines and for the individuals who participate in their development. In addition to financial relationships with industry, other potential sources of bias in the development of clinical practice guidelines include professional affiliations and practice specialization, reimbursement incentives, intellectual preconceptions and previously stated positions, and the desire for recognition and career advancement (see, e.g., Kahan et al. [1996], Ayanian et al. [1998], Murphy et al. [1998], Fitch et al. [1999], and Detsky [2006]).

This chapter begins with definitions and a brief historical overview and description of groups that develop clinical practice guidelines. It then reviews what the committee learned about the nature and the effects of sources of funding on the development of clinical practice guidelines, the financial interests of individual participants, and policies on financial relationships and conflicts of interest. A later section reviews other methods for promoting objectivity in the development of clinical practice guidelines and trust in those guidelines. The final section presents recommendations on how to reduce conflicts of interest in the development of clinical practice guidelines.

BACKGROUND AND CONTEXT

Definitions

As defined in an earlier Institute of Medicine (IOM) report, *clinical practice guidelines* are "systematically developed statements to assist practitioner and patient decisions about appropriate health care for specific clinical circumstances" (IOM, 1990, p. 8). The IOM report emphasized the role of formal evaluations of the evidence base for clinical practice guidelines and the linking of recommendations to those reviews. *Systematic reviews*, the common term used today for formal evaluations of the evidence, are highly structured assessments of the research literature that use explicit, previously defined methods and tools to identify, select, assess, and summarize research studies relevant to a technology, treatment of a clinical condition, or similar topic (see, e.g., OTA [1994] and Cochrane Collaboration [2005]). A *meta-analysis* is a quantitative summary of the data examined in a systematic review. As explained below, various groups have devised tools for assessing the extent to which a set of guidelines are based on systematic, evidence-based procedures.

Evolution of Clinical Practice Guidelines

The American College of Cardiology, the American College of Physicians, the National Institutes of Health (NIH) Consensus Development Program,[1] the U.S. Preventive Services Task Force, the Blue Cross and

[1] Since 1977, the Consensus Development Program at NIH has sponsored "an unbiased, independent, evidence-based assessment of complex medical issues" (NIH, undated). It orga-

Blue Shield Association, ECRI (now the ECRI Institute), and the RAND Corporation were, among others, leaders in devising systematic methods for assessing the evidence and developing clinical recommendations for practitioners, patients, payers, and others (see, e.g., IOM [1985, 1988] for contemporary descriptions of such activities). In 1989, the U.S. Congress created the Agency for Healthcare Policy and Research (AHCPR) and gave it responsibility for creating a public-private partnership to develop, disseminate, and evaluate clinical practice guidelines (P.L. 101-239). In 1995, the Congress came close to defunding the agency in response to lobbying by back surgeons who disagreed with the agency's guidelines for the treatment of low back pain developed by an AHCPR Patient Outcomes Research Team (Deyo et al., 1997; Gray et al., 2003; see also Clancy [2003], Gaus [2003], and Wennberg [2003]). Other government bodies charged with some aspect of technology assessment have also been defunded under circumstances that underscore the political sensitivity of this activity (for example, the National Center for Health Care Technology in 1982 and the congressional Office of Technology Assessment in 1995) (see, e.g., Bimber [1996], Rettig [1997], Eisenberg and Zarin [2002], and Keiper [2005]).

After its close call, AHCPR—rechristened the Agency for Healthcare Quality and Research (AHRQ)—withdrew from the work of developing clinical practice guidelines. Instead, the agency supports evidence-based practice centers that conduct systematic reviews that government agencies, professional societies, and other groups can request and use to develop guidelines and other recommendations. In 2008, AHRQ supported 14 such centers, 5 of which focused on assessments for the Centers for Medicare and Medicaid Services. One evidence review (performed under a grant from AHRQ) by the RAND Corporation's Evidence-Based Practice Center concluded that the quality of practice guidelines suffered as a result of the retreat of the agency from guideline development (Hasenfeld and Shekelle, 2003; see also Grilli et al. [2000]).

The U.S. Preventive Services Task Force, which was created several years before AHCPR/AHRQ but which is now part of the agency, continues to develop evidence-based guidelines for preventive services. It is currently supported by one evidence-based practice center. Other federal agencies, such as NIH and the Centers for Disease Control and Prevention, also develop practice guidelines.

To support the dissemination of the clinical practice guidelines developed and submitted by others, AHRQ sponsors the National Guideline

---

nizes conferences that are jointly sponsored and administered by one or more NIH institutes or centers and the Office of Medical Applications of Research, which is located in the Office of the Director of NIH. Other federal agencies may participate if their expertise is relevant to the topic. Currently, the Agency for Healthcare Research and Quality provides a systematic review of the conference topic from one of its Evidence-Based Practice Centers.

Clearinghouse. The guidelines posted by the clearinghouse are summarized in a common format that includes headings for information about the source(s) of funding and about financial disclosures or conflicts of interest.[2] Although the clearinghouse is the most comprehensive source of information on the funding of guideline development activities and on financial disclosures and conflicts of interest, its data have some significant limitations. The analysts who compile the guideline summaries primarily rely on source documents provided by the guideline sponsor, and those documents may be incomplete. For example, because the source documents are silent on the topic, "Not stated" entries for "financial relationships/conflict of interest" may be found in clearinghouse summaries of guidelines for groups such as the American College of Physicians and the U.S. Preventive Services Task Force. These two groups do, in fact, have a process of disclosing, evaluating, and managing conflicts of interest.[3] Given these and other limitations in the clearinghouse database, the committee used information from the database on funding sources and disclosures with caution.

The guideline initiatives described above and other initiatives have gradually but not fully replaced less rigorous guideline development efforts that lacked formal procedures, clear reporting of the authors involved with and the methods used for the systematic review of the evidence, and explicit links between the recommendations and the supporting evidence. Shortcomings in the processes for the development and reporting of clinical practice guidelines persist. These shortcomings include the incomplete disclosures of the financial relationships of the participants and the funding sources and informal procedures, which increase the opportunity for undue influence and bias (see, e.g., Shaneyfelt et al. [1999], Burgers et al. [2003], Harpole et al. [2003], Hasenfeld and Shekelle [2003], Shiffman et al. [2003], Boluyt et al. [2005], Guyatt et al. [2006], Poitras et al. [2007], Nix [2008], and Nuckols et al. [2008]).

---

[2] The criteria for the inclusion of a guideline in the clearinghouse relate to sponsorship, evidence of some kind of literature review, adoption of the guideline within the last 5 years, and print or online availability of the complete text of the guideline.

[3] To cite one example of how such omissions may occur, when U.S. Preventive Services Task Force guidelines are published in journals that require disclosures, they include a statement (compare, e.g., the guidelines on screening for lipid disorders in children as published in *Pediatrics* at USPSTF [2007a] and as published online at USPSTF [2007b]). In contrast, guidelines presented on the agency's website do not routinely include information about the group's conflict of interest policies and procedures or about the authors' financial relationships (see, e.g., guidelines on screening for sickle cell disease in newborns at USPSTF [2007c]). The processes for developing the guidelines were the same, but the information in the clearinghouse varies because the source documents varied in the information that they provided. A discussion of task force policies can be found online in the procedure manual, but the site does not highlight it (USPSTF, 2008).

Systematic Process for Developing Clinical Practice Guidelines

The adoption of explicit, systematic methods for reviewing evidence and developing and documenting practice guidelines is, as discussed further below, an important strategy for reducing the opportunities for bias, whether the source might be intellectual and professional preconceptions, financial interests, or something else. Table 7-1 depicts a generic process for developing evidence-based guidelines that is similar to that used by a number of government and professional societies. (Sponsor means the entity developing the guideline.)

At each step in this process, financial relationships may create conflicts of interest. Any of the responsible parties identified in Table 7-1 could have financial relationships with industry that could unduly influence recommendations—even when systematic reviews and other safeguards are employed. Thus, some groups have conflict of interest policies that apply not only to the expert panels that develop guidelines but also to some or all of the other responsible or involved parties. As described in Chapter 4, the evidence base itself can be biased to the extent that the publication of

TABLE 7-1 Basic Elements of Process for Developing Evidence-Based Practice Guidelines

Responsible Party	Activity
Sponsor	Select topic and provide financial and other resources
Sponsor	Appoint a panel to develop the guideline that balances relevant expertise and perspectives and that is subject to conflict of interest policies throughout the process
Panel	Develop a work plan and specify clinical questions and outcomes of interest
Panel or contractor	Conduct a systematic review of the relevant evidence by using standardized methods for selecting studies, analyzing and rating the evidence, identifying and evaluating benefits and harms, and presenting conclusions
Panel	Develop and agree on a draft guideline with recommendations explicitly linked to the evidence and expert judgment
Panel or sponsor	Distribute a draft for internal and external review
Reviewers	Review of guideline by external reviewers and internal reviewers (e.g., the governing board of a professional society)
Panel	Revise a draft and produce the final guideline
Sponsor or journal	Publish and disseminate the guideline
Sponsor	Monitor new research findings and determine whether a guideline should be updated

negative findings or findings unfavorable to a product have been delayed or suppressed.

Professional societies and other groups sometimes rely on evidence reviews conducted by AHRQ's Evidence-Based Practice Centers. (Professional societies and other groups can nominate topics for reviews. In late 2008, the agency's website listed 11 evidence reports on clinical topics as under development.) Others groups may use a combination of staff and expert panel members to conduct reviews. One reason for the latter course is the expense. Systematic reviews for a complex clinical topic may cost in the range of $300,000 to $350,000 or more (personal communication, Beth A. Collins Sharp, director, Evidence-Based Practice Centers Program, Agency for Healthcare Research and Quality, November 14, 2008). On the basis of the committee's review of descriptions of the systematic review process for several professional and patient advocacy groups, groups that rely on staff or volunteer experts vary considerably in the resources that they devote to such reviews, the rigor of their evidence review processes, and the products of these reviews.

Possible Benefits and Risks of Industry Involvement in Guideline Development

The committee found little systematic information about the funding of guidelines, the financial relationships of participants, or the effects of both. In developing this discussion and the recommendations in this chapter, it drew on testimony at its meeting and a convenience sample of information available on the Internet, as well as its experience and judgment.

Potential Benefits of Industry Relationships

Industry funding for the development of clinical practice guidelines may allow some groups to create guidelines on new topics when they otherwise would not. Groups that develop practice guidelines may also benefit from presentations by industry employees as part of the evidence consideration process, and industry employees may be asked to review evaluations of the evidence for their technical accuracy. Individual panel members who have financial relationships with industry often have expertise that is pertinent to the development of a guideline.

Risks of Industry Relationships

As observed above, relationships with industry and conflicts of interest in the development of clinical practice guidelines may exist at both the individual level (i.e., participants may have industry ties) and the institutional level (i.e., the sponsoring group may rely on industry funding for guidelines). These relationships raise the possibility of conflicts of interest and undue influence at each step in the guidelines development process.

Selection of topics Groups that require industry funding for the development of practice guidelines may propose topics that will attract industry funding (e.g., a guideline on how to use a product but not whether it should be used). Among the topics proposed to potential funders, companies may favor topics and questions for which the evidence is most likely to support conclusions favorable to a particular company.

Review of evidence Studies examining the association between industry ties and the outcomes of systematic reviews or meta-analyses raise concerns.[4] Although these studies do not deal explicitly with the entire process of developing clinical practice guidelines, they examine a key element. In one study, industry-sponsored meta-analyses of drug trials were less transparent about the methods that they used, were much more likely than Cochrane Collaboration reviews to recommend the experimental drug without reservation, and had fewer reservations about the methodological limitations of the trials included in the analysis (Jorgensen et al., 2006).[5] All of the industry-sponsored reviews but none of the Cochrane Collaboration reviews recommended the experimental drug without reservation.

Another study examined review articles on the health effects of secondhand smoke (Barnes and Bero, 1998). Ninety-four percent of the review articles written by individuals affiliated with the tobacco industry concluded that passive smoking is not harmful to health, whereas 13 percent of the reviews written by authors without such an affiliation made that conclusion. The association between the conclusion that secondhand smoke is not harmful and an affiliation with the tobacco industry persisted even after the analysts took into account the methodological quality of the review, the year of publication, the clinical topics examined, and whether the review was subject to peer review.

---

[4] As described in materials prepared for the Cochrane Collaboration (2002, unpaged), "meta-analysis is a two-stage process. The first stage is the extraction of data from each individual study and the calculation of a result for that study (the 'point estimate' or 'summary statistic'), with an estimate of the chance variation we would expect with studies like that (the 'confidence interval'). The second stage involves deciding whether it is appropriate to calculate a pooled average result across studies and, if so, calculating and presenting such a result. Part of this process is to give greater weight to the results from studies which give us more information, because these are likely to be closer to the truth we are trying to estimate."

[5] The authors identified 24 Cochrane Collaboration reviews for which another meta-analysis studied the same two drugs in the same disease and was published within 2 years of the Cochrane Collaboration review. (Eight of the 24 comparison guidelines were industry supported; 9 had no declared source of support; 7 reported nonprofit support or self-funding.)

As discussed in Chapter 4, which describes additional studies, a review of meta-analyses on hypertensive drugs found that financial ties to a single pharmaceutical company were not associated with findings that favored the company but were associated with favorable conclusions (Yank et al., 2007). The authors further noted that peer reviewers and journal editors did not prevent the publication of biased conclusions.

Expert panel deliberations The committee found no systematic studies of the relationship between participant financial relationships and the content of guidelines. One study did find, however, that only 7 percent of participants in guideline development surveyed believed that their own relationships with industry influenced their recommendations, but 19 percent believed that their coauthors' recommendations were influenced by such relationships (Choudhry et al., 2002). Because more than half of the participants reported no process for disclosing financial relationships, it is not clear how well informed the respondents were about their colleagues' relationships. (The extent of the relationships identified in the study is discussed below.)

Dissemination of guidelines Even if industry support is limited to the dissemination of guidelines, such support could influence the overall strategy for dissemination in ways that unduly favor a company's product. This is one interpretation of the controversy over guidelines related to sepsis summarized in Box 7-1 below.

GROUPS THAT DEVELOP CLINICAL PRACTICE GUIDELINES

A range of public and private groups develop or collaborate in the development of clinical practice guidelines (Table 7-2). On the basis of guidelines included in the National Guideline Clearinghouse, medical specialty societies are the most common developers of the guidelines; they accounted for almost 40 percent of the guidelines in the clearinghouse database in April 2008. Professional societies report that practice guidelines are among the most valued services that they provide (see, e.g., Bennett et al. [2003], Masur [2007], and Sagsveen [2008]). Evaluations of specialty society guidelines have sometimes been critical of their lack of systematic reviews of the evidence and other characteristics (see, e.g., Grilli et al. [2000]); but the committee's review indicates that many specialty societies have taken steps to make their procedures more systematic, transparent, and evidence based by hiring knowledgeable staff and developing methods, process manuals, and policies that include conflict of interest policies and procedures. The committee found less information about the clinical guideline development-related activities of disease-specific groups.

TABLE 7-2 Number of Clinical Practice Guidelines in the National Guideline Clearinghouse by Selected Types of Sponsors, as of March 16, 2009

Type of Sponsor	Number of Guidelines
Medical specialty society (U.S. and other)	959
Professional association (U.S. and other; mostly nonphysician or mixed groups)	408
Government agency (non-U.S.)	214
Federal/state/local government agency	165
Nonprofit organization	142
Independent expert panel	97
Academic institution (U.S. and other)	98
Disease-specific society (U.S. and other)	202
Hospital/medical center (U.S. and other)	26
For-profit organization	21
Managed care organization	11
Total, all guidelines, all sponsors	2,343

NOTE: Some guidelines are developed collaboratively by more than one type of sponsor. For example, a guideline may list as developers one or more professional societies and one or more disease-specific societies. The National Guideline Clearinghouse (NGC) search option does not generate unduplicated counts by category of sponsor. The unduplicated count presented here was provided by NGC staff. Nineteen of the 26 guidelines from a hospital or medical center were submitted by a single institution.
SOURCE: Personal communication, Mary Nix, Health Scientist Administrator, National Guideline Clearinghouse, March 22, 2009.

Public agencies also develop practice guidelines. U.S. federal and state agencies and public agencies from other countries accounted for more than 500 of the guidelines in the National Guideline Clearinghouse.

Some groups involved in guideline development have sought partners. For example, the American College of Cardiology and the American Heart Association have collaborated in their guideline development program since the 1980s (ACC/AHA, 2009). Several groups are investigating an international collaboration to develop guidelines for the care of respiratory diseases (personal communication, Holger Schunemann, M.D., Ph.D., chair, Department of Clinical Epidemiology and Biostatistics, McMaster University, February 19, 2009). Compared with the complexity of simply adding individuals with different professional and other backgrounds to a guideline development panel, the management of partnerships between and among agencies tends to be more complicated because each partner usually has, for example, its own policies and procedures. Nevertheless, the potential benefits of collaboration include the sharing of costs, broadening of the scope of the questions examined, and reductions in the number of dueling guidelines that may undermine the credibility and acceptance of recommendations.

FINANCIAL RELATIONSHIPS IN GUIDELINE DEVELOPMENT

Sources of Funding for Guidelines and Systematic Reviews

The committee found no systematic assessment of the public or private sources of funding for the development of clinical practice guidelines (see, e.g., Boyd [2008]) or systematic reviews of funding sources (Jorgensen et al., 2006). Nearly all (98 percent) of the summaries of more than 2,000 guidelines included in the National Guideline Clearinghouse as of April 21, 2008, contained a statement about the funding source, usually indicating that the group that developed the guideline had funded it (Nix, 2008). Some information is inconsistent. For example, in the summary statement for guidelines on bronchial intraepithelial neoplasia/early central airways lung cancer, the section on the source of funding states that a professional society funded it, whereas the section on financial disclosures/conflict of interest states that funding came from five pharmaceutical or biotechnology companies (NGC, 2009c; see also Kennedy et al. [2007]). Similarly, a guideline on the prevention and treatment of mucositis listed the two authoring groups as the source of funding, but the information on financial disclosures/conflicts of interest referred to unrestricted grants from unnamed companies (NGC, 2009h; see also Keefe et al. [2007]).

Some professional societies, such as the American College of Physicians, the American Academy of Neurology, the American Society of Hematology, and the American Society for Clinical Oncology, fund their guideline development programs from general revenues and, in some instances, grants from independent nonprofit organizations (ASCO, 2008; Sagsveen, 2008; personal communication, Martha Liggett, executive director, American Society of Hematology, February 24, 2008; personal communication, Vincenza Snow, director, Clinical Programs and Quality of Care, American College of Physicians, February 23, 2009). As discussed in Chapter 6, a society's general revenues may include a significant share from industry, for example, income generated by journal advertising or by pharmaceutical or device company exhibits at professional society meetings.

The committee is aware that some smaller professional societies that have sought to fund clinical guideline development and systematic reviews without industry support have found it difficult to do so (personal communication, Roger Chou, assistant professor of medicine and medical informatics and clinical epidemiology, Oregon Health Sciences University, April 2, 2008). Professional societies can, however, nominate topics for

AHRQ-supported systematic reviews, and if such a topic is selected, even a resource-limited society will have an evidence-based review with which to work.

Most, if not all, guidelines developed by government agencies in the United States (e.g., the U.S. Preventive Services Task Force) and elsewhere (e.g., the National Institute for Health and Clinical Excellence in the United Kingdom) are publicly funded. One controversial exception involving a Texas state agency is described in Box 7-1, which cites several controversies involving financial relationships in practice guidelines.

Practice guidelines are sometimes developed by ad hoc groups, which by their nature are not likely to have a well-developed infrastructure for the performance of evidence-based reviews and other activities, including procedures for identifying and managing conflicts of interest. Box 7-1 described one ad hoc initiative related to heart disease screening guidelines that provoked concerns about bias and conflict of interest.

The Cochrane Collaboration (an independent, nonprofit, international organization that produces systematic reviews, among other activities) does not allow industry funding for a review. It does, however, allow commercial contributions to a central pool of funds to be used for certain other activities, such as the translation of reviews into different languages (Cochrane Collaboration, 2006).

Although the committee found no systematic information, industry involvement in the dissemination of guidelines appears to be fairly common. For example, companies may buy copies of the journal issue in which a guideline is published. They may also develop derivative materials (e.g., summaries for lay audiences) based on the guideline. The committee was unable to systematically investigate whether dissemination activities resulted in materials that altered or elaborated on a guideline in ways that departed from the conclusions in the guideline itself.

Nature and Extent of Individual Relationships with Industry

The committee found little systematic study and documentation of financial relationships between industry and the individuals who author clinical practice guidelines. A 2002 study reported that the authors of practice guidelines had widespread financial relationships with the pharmaceutical industry (Choudhry et al., 2002).[6] Of 44 practice guidelines that Choudhry et al. initially reviewed, only 2 included disclosures of the authors' financial relationships with industry. A follow-up survey of 100 authors involved with 37 of the guidelines found that 87 percent of the authors had some

[6] The study covered guidelines that were published between 1991 and 1999, that had identifiable authors, and that had been endorsed by a "recognized" North American or European professional society.

BOX 7-1
Cases and Controversies Involving Conflicts of Interest in Guideline Development

In an investigation of pharmaceutical companies' use of educational grants (based on information provided by 23 companies), staff of the Finance Committee, U.S. Senate (2007) found that "several companies helped fund the Texas Medical Algorithm Program (TMAP) run by the Texas Department of State Health Services to develop psychiatric treatment algorithms" (p. 12). A whistleblower complaint led to the dismissal of the state employee who headed the effort and had served as a paid consultant to a company that benefited from the treatment guidelines (Waters, 2006, unpaged).

In 2006, the *Boston Globe* reported that an ad hoc group of physicians had solicited nearly $56,000 from several pharmaceutical companies to have their heart disease screening guidelines published in a supplement of a leading cardiology journal (Smith, 2006; see also, e.g., Naghavi et al. [2006]). The guidelines were subsequently criticized by an official of the National Heart, Lung, and Blood Institute, who pointed out that the supplement had been financed by a company that stood to profit from implementation of the recommendations, that the authors of the guidelines failed to reveal their relevant financial relationships with that company and others, and that the process for developing the guidelines was not evidence based or subject to rigorous review (Lauer, 2007).

Eichacker and colleagues (2006) alleged that industry funding was used to support a "three-pronged marketing strategy" to increase sales of drugs for the treatment of sepsis (p. 1640). They cited a marketing document, which is no longer available online, that described a strategy "to first raise awareness about rationing and then the disease state as a means of enhancing prospects of utilization" and then employ "highly-specific marketing initiatives to physicians and the medical trade media"; a grant would then be used to create a task force to study health care rationing in the intensive care unit; and lastly to "[r]aise awareness of severe sepsis and generate momentum towards development of treatment guidelines for the infection through establishment of the Surviving Sepsis Campaign" (AHRP, 2006, unpaged). The Infectious Diseases Society of America chose not to endorse the sepsis guidelines on the basis of concern about "the manner in which the guidelines were developed, the use of a suboptimal rating system, and their sponsorship by a drug company" (Eickhacker et al., 2006, p. 1642; see also Masur [2007]). A recent set of revisions to the guidelines reported no industry funding for guideline development meetings, and 7 of the 24 authors reported no "potential" conflicts of interest (Dellinger et al., 2008).

financial relationship or interaction with industry and that 59 percent had relationships with companies whose products were considered in the guideline. The most frequent relationship with companies involved honoraria for speaking (64 percent of the respondents, who reported an average of 7.3 companies as sources of the honoraria). Thirty-eight percent of the authors had an employee or consultant relationship with one or more companies. The majority of the authors surveyed reported no discussion of financial relationships during the guideline development process.[7]

Journal articles and other publications that contain practice guidelines vary greatly in the extent to which they include disclosures of the relevant financial relationships of the participants in the guideline development process. For the most part, disclosures emphasize financial relationships with pharmaceutical and device companies, although some describe ties to other kinds of organizations (e.g., federal research agencies and managed care organizations). Some guideline documents do not indicate whether the participants with no listed disclosures were explicitly asked to declare if they had no relevant relationships. The categorizations of the relationships are also not consistent across guideline disclosures. Some lump together relationships (e.g., research and consulting or honoraria and participation in speakers bureaus) that others report separately.

When guidelines include financial disclosure statements, the content is quite variable, as Box 7-2 illustrates. An analysis of the guideline summaries in the clearinghouse as of April 2008 found that almost half (47 percent) indicated "Not stated" under the summary heading for financial disclosure/conflict of interest (Nix, 2008). An earlier analysis found that the proportion of summaries that included some information on financial relationships or conflict of interest increased from just over 20 percent to approximately 50 percent from 1999 to 2006 (Tregear, 2007). (Most summaries in the clearinghouse are based on the source document cited for the guideline, but some reflect supplementary information provided by the groups submitting the guidelines.) In a later section, Box 7-3 provides additional examples of disclosures about conflict of interest policies.

---

[7] The committee also located an article reporting on a review by the Dutch Health Care Inspectorate of the influence of pharmaceutical companies in the development of practice guidelines in The Netherlands (Smulders and Thijs, 2007). As summarized in the English-language abstract, the agency concluded that "virtually all opinion leaders are financially supported by pharmaceutical companies, and therefore, potential conflicts of interest are unavoidable" (p. 2429). The agency recommended making potential conflicts more transparent by full disclosure of all relationships, especially financial relationships. It also suggested that allowing companies to review draft guidelines might reduce "undesirable initiatives" to influence guidelines, that individuals with certain kinds or levels of relationships might be precluded from participation in guidelines development, and that an independent review process might be instituted to assess guidelines for signs of interference by pharmaceutical companies.

BOX 7-2
Examples of Financial and Conflict of Interest Information Excerpted from Summaries in the National Guideline Clearinghouse

Example A
FINANCIAL DISCLOSURES/CONFLICTS OF INTEREST
Not stated. [This is the most common entry for the period from 1999 to 2006.]

Example B
FINANCIAL DISCLOSURES/CONFLICTS OF INTEREST
All participants involved in guideline development have disclosed potential conflicts of interest to their colleagues, and their potential conflicts have been documented for future reference. *They will not be published in any guideline, but kept on file for reference, if needed.* Participants have been asked to update their disclosures regularly throughout the guideline development process. [emphasis added; NGC, 2009e; see also NASS, 2008]

Example C
FINANCIAL DISCLOSURES/CONFLICTS OF INTEREST
All members of the Expert Panel complied with the Infectious Diseases Society of America (IDSA) policy on conflicts of interest, which requires disclosure of any financial or other interest that might be construed as constituting an actual, potential, or apparent conflict. Members of the Expert Panel were provided the IDSA's conflict of interest disclosure statement and were asked to identify ties to companies developing products that might be affected by promulgation of the guideline. Information was requested about employment, consultancies, stock ownership, honoraria, research funding, expert testimony, and membership on company advisory committees. The Panel made decisions on a case-by-case basis as to whether an individual's role should be limited as a result of a conflict. No limiting conflicts were identified.

Potential Conflicts of Interest: L.A.P. has served as a speaker and consultant to Schering-Plough and Pfizer. P.G.P. has received grant support from Schering-Plough, Pfizer, Merck, and Astellas; has been an ad hoc consultant for Pfizer; and has been a speaker for Pfizer and Astellas. C.A.K. has received research grants from Merck, Astellas, and Schering-Plough and serves on the speakers bureau for Merck, Astellas, Pfizer, and Schering-Plough. All other authors: no conflicts. [NGC, 2009d; see also Chapman et al. 2008]

Indirect evidence for widespread relationships with companies is presented in a study of participants involved with the development of the *Diagnostic and Statistical Manual of Mental Disorders* (Cosgrove et al., 2006). These diagnostic criteria, like practice guidelines, are based on expert reviews of the relevant evidence. (An AHRQ-funded study on conflicts of interest in commercial drug compendia should be published soon. Many health plans, including Medicare, use evidence summarized in compendia as a basis for payment and coverage decisions.)

The committee also found a few assessments of the adequacy of disclosures in studies that have applied the standardized evaluation tool AGREE (Appraisal of Guidelines Research and Evaluation), which is further described below. One of the evaluation criteria (Item 23) is whether a guideline document includes information about participant conflicts of interest. Another criterion (Item 22) is whether the guideline is editorially independent from the funding source. Studies have found shortcomings in reporting on conflicts of interest by participants and editorial independence in a wide array of clinical practice guidelines, including guidelines on stroke rehabilitation (Hurdowar et al., 2007), occupational medicine (Cates et al., 2006), pediatrics (Boluyt et al., 2005), lung cancer (Harpole et al., 2003), low back pain (Arnau et al., 2006), and nonsteroidal anti-inflammatory drug and acetaminophen treatment of osteoarthritis of the hip or knee (Wegman et al., 2004). It is not clear whether a lack of disclosure was related to the policies of the group developing the guidelines (e.g., no policy on disclosure or disclosures were not revealed) or the policies of particular journals (e.g., no request for disclosure). A study of 191 guidelines published in six leading journals in 1979, 1984, 1989, 1994, and 1999 found reporting of conflicts of interest only in the most recent year (1999) and then for only 7 of the 40 guidelines and 18 authors for that year (Papanikolaou et al., 2001). Although all the disclosures were in journals that had disclosure policies, only 4 percent of the articles in those journals included disclosures.

Consequences of Financial Relationships

The committee found no systematic studies that investigated the association between the funding source and the development process or the content of the clinical practice guidelines. As illustrated in Box 7-2, it did find cases that raised concerns about the influence of industry funding.

The committee also found no systematic studies of the relationship between participant financial relationships and the content of the guidelines.[8] As described above, a study by Choudhry and colleagues (2002) found that

[8] In a possibly relevant study of a different kind of panel, Lurie and colleagues (2006) examined the financial relationships and decisions reached in 221 meetings of 16 advisory committees of the Food and Drug Administration. They reported that in nearly three-quarters (73 percent) of the meetings at least one committee member had a financial link to the maker of a drug being considered by the committee or had a link to a competitor company. Overall, approximately one-quarter (28 percent) of the members reported conflicts. They concluded, "A weak relationship between certain types of conflicts and voting behaviors was detected, but excluding advisory committee members and voting consultants with conflicts would not have altered the overall vote outcome at any meeting studied" (p. 1921).

only 7 percent of participants in guideline development surveyed in their study believed that their own relationships with industry influenced their recommendations, but 19 percent felt that their coauthors' recommendations were influenced by such relationships. Also as described above, studies examining industry ties and the outcomes of systematic reviews raise concerns about undue influence.

A few case studies examine conflicts of interest for specific guidelines or guideline development programs. For example, in 2006, 14 of 16 members of a group that worked on the development of guidelines for the treatment of anemia in patients with chronic kidney disease received consultant fees, speaking fees, research funds, or some combination thereof from at least one company that could be affected by the guidelines (Coyne, 2007). The principal funder of the guidelines was a company that would be affected by the guidelines, and the chair and cochair of the work group had financial relationships with that company (KDOQI, 2007). The work group recommended that the dosage of a drug made by the company be raised, which could have substantially increased costs to the Medicare program. By coincidence, the guidelines were announced at the same time that research that showed adverse patient outcomes associated with the approach recommended by the guidelines was published. The lead investigator of the research allegedly informed the guideline development work group that the study in question had been terminated early, and he advised that they wait for the results before issuing the new guidelines. The group, however, chose not to wait. The entity that sponsored the work group recently described changes in its conflict of interest policies, which it described as providing "an even higher level of transparency" by providing that financial disclosures would be discussed at the meetings of guideline development groups, that those reviewing the evidence would be "empowered to assure that all guideline recommendations are supported by the evidence," that the organization's compliance officer would monitor guideline development activities and report to the organization's board on issues relating to conflict, and that no future guideline could be funded by a single industry sponsor (NKF, 2007).

POLICIES ON CONFLICTS OF INTEREST IN CLINICAL PRACTICE GUIDELINE DEVELOPMENT

Characteristics of Policies

The committee examined a convenience sample of conflict of interest policies identified through the National Guideline Clearinghouse, presentations at committee public meetings, organizational websites, documents describing guidelines, assessments of specific guidelines, other publications, and discussions with staff or members of organizations involved with guideline development. It found no systematic information on the conflict of interest policies of groups that develop clinical practice guidelines. Reviews by Boyd and Bero (2006) and Boyd (2008) likewise found no systematic descriptions or assessments of these policies.

The availability, representativeness, and quality of the available information are limited in several important ways. As noted above, even if the developers of guidelines have conflict of interest policies, they may not refer to them in individual guideline documents. This in turn means that the summaries in the National Guideline Clearinghouse are likely to have no information either. A number of groups have recently revised aspects of their policies, and the committee is aware of other groups that are considering changes. In some cases, these changes may not be reflected on websites or in publications.

From the policies examined, the committee identified several variations in organization conflict of interest policies and procedures. They vary in the

- information required for disclosure, including how detailed the information disclosed must be, how often disclosure is requested, and whether a panel member needs to explicitly state that he or she has no relationships to disclose;
- management of disclosed information, including who reviews it and whether other panel members are told of conflicts;
- procedures for managing the relationships disclosed, including limitations of participation by members with conflicts (such as serving as chair or cochair or voting);
- provisions for public disclosure of conflict of interest policies, funding sources, and individual financial relationships;
- procedures for managing relationships with companies that provide funding for guidelines development; and
- assignment of explicit responsibility for monitoring whether institutional policies are followed.

The frequent lack of transparency of conflict of interest policies limits the ability of guideline readers to consider financial relationships and conflicts of interest as part of their assessment of the credibility of a set of guidelines. To give a sense of what readers of guidelines may encounter, Box 7-3 includes additional examples of the range of summary statements in the National Guideline Clearinghouse. (See also Box 7-2.)

The committee found few descriptions of the policies used to manage the relationship between guideline developers and industry for groups that accept industry funding for guideline development. One exception is the

BOX 7-3
Examples of Conflict of Interest Policy Descriptions Excerpted from Summaries in the National Guideline Clearinghouse

Example A
FINANCIAL DISCLOSURES/CONFLICTS OF INTEREST
Not stated. [This is the most common entry for the period from 1999 to 2006.]

Example B
FINANCIAL DISCLOSURES/CONFLICTS OF INTEREST
To assure the integrity of the Advisory Committee on Immunization Practices (ACIP), the U.S. Department of Health and Human Services has taken steps to assure that there is technical compliance with ethics statutes and regulations regarding financial conflicts of interest. Concerns regarding the potential for the appearance of a conflict are addressed, or avoided altogether, through both pre- and postappointment considerations. Individuals with particular vaccine-related interests will not be considered for appointment to the committee. Potential nominees are screened for conflicts of interest, and if any are found, they are asked to divest or forgo certain vaccine-related activities. In addition, at the beginning of each ACIP meeting, each member is asked to declare his or her conflicts. Members with conflicts are not permitted to vote if a conflict involves the vaccine or biologic being voted upon. [NGC, 2009g; see also ACIP, 2007]

Example C
FINANCIAL DISCLOSURES/CONFLICTS OF INTEREST
The American Academy of Neurology (AAN) is committed to producing independent, critical and truthful clinical practice guidelines (CPGs). Significant efforts are made to minimize the potential for conflicts of interest to influence the recommendations of this CPG. To the extent possible, the AAN keeps separate those who have a financial stake in the success or failure of the products appraised in the CPGs and the developers of the guidelines. Conflict of interest forms were

American College of Chest Physicians, whose policies are summarized in Box 7-4.

Effectiveness of Policies

The committee identified no evaluations of the impact of conflict of interest policies on the content of guidelines or other outcomes. The review by Boyd and Bero (2006) also found no rigorous assessments of conflict of interest policies for guideline development and no evaluations of different strategies for implementing or enforcing them.

obtained from all authors and reviewed by an oversight committee prior to project initiation. AAN limits the participation of authors with substantial conflicts of interest. The AAN forbids commercial participation in, or funding of, guideline projects. Drafts of the guideline have been reviewed by at least three AAN committees, a network of neurologists, Neurology peer reviewers, and representatives from related fields. The AAN Guideline Author Conflict of Interest Policy can be viewed at www.aan.com. With regards to this specific report, all authors have stated that they have nothing to disclose. One of the authors performs epidural steroid injections. [NGC, 2009b; see also Armon et al., 2007]

Example D
FINANCIAL DISCLOSURES/CONFLICTS OF INTEREST
Standards and guidelines are to insure that individuals participating in professional activities are aware of author relationships with commercial companies that could potentially affect the information presented. The American Thyroid Association has endorsed the requirement that authors disclose any significant financial interest or affiliations they may have with the manufacturers of products or devices that may be discussed in the development of guidelines. In compliance with this policy, a superscript number placed by the name of an author denotes an author who has indicated an affiliation with organizations which have interests related to the content of these guidelines. The intent of this policy is to openly identify potential conflicts of interest so that physicians may form their own judgments about the guidelines with full disclosure of the facts; it remains for the audience to determine whether an author's outside interest may reflect a possible bias in either the exposition or the conclusions presented. [NGC, 2009f; see also Cooper et al., 2006a]

NOTE: As explained in the text of this chapter, the documents on which guideline summaries are based may not include references to organizational policies that have governed the development of the guideline. Thus, a "Not stated" response does not necessarily indicate that a group has no policy.

Other Strategies to Limit Bias in the Development of Clinical Practice Guidelines

Those committed to the development and implementation of sound, credible, and useful guidelines have devised a number of methods and tools that can be used to support the creation of such guidelines. Several are listed in Box 7-5, roughly according to the step in the process of guideline development described in Table 7-1. Arguably, the most important steps are the conduct of a systematic review of the evidence and the linking of recommendations to the evidence in an explicit fashion. The strategies—and continuing areas of debate and methodological refinement—are described in depth elsewhere (see, e.g., Higgins and Green [2008] and IOM [2008]).

BOX 7-4
Policies of American College of Chest Physicians on Industry Funding of Guideline Development

- Fund development activities are undertaken by the organization's executive office without the involvement or knowledge by the organizational unit responsible for guideline development, and each guideline ideally is either self-funded or funded by at least three to five outside sources.
- Names of sponsoring companies are not revealed to staff, society members, and other participants in guideline development until the information is disclosed in the final publication.
- Sponsors do not nominate topics, participate in meetings, or review drafts. They see the guideline only upon publication.
- The organization does not inform sponsors of the participants involved in developing a guideline, the specific questions investigated, the methodologists or evidence-based practice center involved in the evidence review, the reviewers, or meeting times or places.
- Guidelines refer to pharmaceuticals only by their generic names and not by their brand names.

SOURCE: Baumann et al., 2007; Lever and Lewis, 2008.

In general, they reinforce conflict of interest policies by limiting the opportunity for secondary financial interests to exert undue influence on the primary interest of developing sound guidelines.

Unfortunately, as Steinberg and Luce (2005) have observed, rigorous methods for clinical practice guideline development and reviews of the clinical evidence are not applied consistently, and the conclusions of evidence reviews are not always interpreted appropriately. Furthermore, given that the evidence base is weak in many areas, they advise, "physicians, policymakers, and others acting on the basis of judgments, recommendations, or measures . . . should not blindly assume that the label [evidence-based] truly applies" (p. 91).

As noted earlier, in addition to developing methods to limit bias, individuals and groups have been developing tools for standardizing the presentation of guidelines and assessing the quality of guidelines across several domains (see, e.g., IOM [1992], the AGREE Collaboration [2003], and Shiffman et al. [2003]). Methodologists have also developed tools that can be used to assess the quality of systematic reviews (Shea et al., 2007; see also Oxman et al. [2006a]). The 23-item AGREE instrument, which was developed by experts from 13 countries with funding from the European Union, includes two elements that relate to conflict of interest, specifically, that the "guideline is editorially independent from the funding

BOX 7-5
Other Strategies for Limiting Bias in Clinical Practice Guideline Development

Using an explicit process to select topics for clinical practice guideline development. Various groups and individuals have recommended a formal process and the use of explicit criteria for the selection of topics for guideline development (see, e.g., Battista and Hodge [1995], IOM [1995], and Oxman et al. [2006a]). Although the primary rationale is to use limited resources to evaluate areas that offer the greatest potential to improve the quality or effectiveness of health care, another potential benefit is a reduction in the opportunity for financial relationships and other sources of bias to influence the selection of topics.

Creating a diverse expert panel. The inclusion of individuals with a range of relevant professional and other backgrounds on guideline development panels can help check financial, professional, and other sources of bias; promote the fuller consideration of potential outcomes, relevant evidence, and aspects of implementation; and help win broader acceptance by professionals, consumers or patients, health care plans, and others who play roles in the successful implementation of guidelines (see, e.g., IOM [1990, 1992, 2008] and AGREE Collaboration [2003]).

Systematically reviewing relevant evidence. As summarized by Higgins and Green (2008, Section 1.2.2) for the Cochrane Collaboration, key elements of this critical step include

- "a clearly stated set of objectives with pre-defined eligibility criteria for studies;
- an explicit, reproducible methodology;
- a systematic search that attempts to identify all studies that would meet the eligibility criteria;
- an assessment of the validity of the findings of the included studies, for example, through the assessment of risk of bias; and
- a systematic presentation, and synthesis, of the characteristics and findings of the included studies."

Using systematic procedures to evaluate the evidence, employing expert judgment, and linking recommendations to the evidence. Methodologists have developed and tested formal processes for developing consensus and otherwise structuring the expert judgment process (see, e.g., Fink et al. [1984], Murphy et al. [1998], Verkerk et al. [2006], and Renfrew et al. [2008]). In addition, considerable effort has been invested in developing and testing explicit methods for reporting and rating the evidence relevant to guidelines and for rating the strength of the recommendations (see, e.g., Guyatt et al. [1995], Lohr [2004], and Schünemann et al. [2006], and Schünemann [2008]).

Obtaining expert reviews. An independent, expert review of the guidelines and related documents is an important tool that can be used to improve the identification, evaluation, and use of the evidence. The process used to select expert reviewers should explicitly identify and assess reviewer ties with potentially affected companies.

body" (Item 22) and that "[c]onflicts of interest of guideline development members have been recorded" (Item 23). In addition, the Conference on Guideline Standardization (COG) proposed a somewhat similar 18-item checklist for reporting (documenting) guidelines (Shiffman et al., 2003). The COG list includes the identification of the funding source or sponsor, its role in developing or reporting the guideline, and the disclosure of conflicts of interest.

These and other instruments are not intended to be used to assess the full substance of the guidelines. In and of themselves, they will not identify, for example, whether key evidence has been overlooked or incorrectly assessed, whether relevant benefits or harms have been ignored or improperly weighed, or whether critical barriers to implementation have been missed. Notwithstanding some shortcomings of guideline assessment tools, their development and application underscore that it is important for documents containing clinical practice guidelines to provide potential users of the guidelines with informative descriptions of the development process, the evidence base, the participants, and the applicable conflict of interest policies. When users of guidelines confront guidelines that lack such descriptions, they would be prudent to treat the guidelines with caution and search for other guidelines that provide appropriate documentation.

Even when the developers of clinical practice guidelines use sound methods, they are often limited by shortcomings in the evidence base. A review of the guidelines in the National Guideline Clearinghouse reveals recommendation after recommendation that is supported by weak, mixed, or no evidence. Both to support the development of practice guidelines and for other purposes, many groups in the United States and elsewhere have called for greatly increased public investments in comparative effectiveness research and analysis for at least two decades (for a small sampling, see IOM [1985, 2007, 2008], OTA [1994], CBO [2007], and MedPAC [2007]). At the end of the next section, the committee endorses the recommendations for such investments that another IOM committee made recently. Overall, the combination of a better evidence base for clinical practice guidelines and better tools for assessing that evidence not only strengthens the usefulness of practice guidelines but also reduces the potential for conflicts of interest to bias guidelines.

RECOMMENDATIONS

Given the important role that clinical practice guidelines play in many aspects of health care, it is important that these guidelines be free of industry influence and be viewed by clinicians, policy makers, patients, and others as objective and trustworthy. The committee found substantial variation in the extent to which different groups disclosed their conflict of interest policies and the financial ties to industry of the sponsoring group and the members of the guideline panel. It also found little systematic descriptions or assessments in the literature. On the basis of its judgment and experience (including experience with conflicting guidelines and guidelines not based on formal reviews of the evidence), the committee believes that the risk of undue industry influence on clinical practice guidelines is significant, and that risk justifies that strong steps be taken to strengthen conflict of interest policies governing the development of guidelines. Recommendation 7.1 proposes several such steps.

RECOMMENDATION 7.1 Groups that develop clinical practice guidelines should generally exclude as panel members individuals with conflicts of interest and should not accept direct funding for clinical practice guideline development from medical product companies or company foundations. Groups should publicly disclose with each guideline their conflict of interest policies and procedures and the sources and amounts of indirect or direct funding received for development of the guideline. In the exceptional situation in which avoidance of panel members with conflicts of interest is impossible because of the critical need for their expertise, then groups should

- **publicly document that they made a good-faith effort to find experts without conflicts of interest by issuing a public call for members and other recruitment measures;**
- **appoint a chair without a conflict of interest;**
- **limit members with conflicting interests to a distinct minority of the panel;**
- **exclude individuals who have a fiduciary or promotional relationship with a company that makes a product that may be affected by the guidelines;**
- **exclude panel members with conflicts from deliberating, drafting, or voting on specific recommendations; and**
- **publicly disclose the relevant conflicts of interest of panel members.**

Transparency is one key element of Recommendation 7.1. Groups should disclose their conflict of interest policies and their process for seeking members without conflicts of interest and its results. The disclosure of the relevant financial interests of members of guideline development panels should be sufficiently specific and comprehensive that it helps others judge the severity of the conflicts of interest, including allowing the identification of fiduciary interests (e.g., membership on company boards) and promotional relationships (e.g., participation in industry speakers bureaus).

Groups that develop guidelines should also disclose the sources and the amounts of funding provided for guideline development, including unrestricted company grants. Some committee members also wanted groups that develop guidelines to report publicly all their sources, amounts, and purposes of funding because industry contributions to general revenues (e.g., from journal advertising or unrestricted grants) could also create undue influence. The committee did not reach a consensus on this point. Other committee members were also concerned about the overall reliance of some professional and patient groups on industry funding, but they believed that this reporting of all sources and purposes of funding is not necessary, provided that groups developing guidelines adopt and implement rigorous evidence-based procedures, report indirect and direct funding sources for each guideline, and institute the conflict of interest policies and procedures recommended in this report. Another safeguard would be the continued development of processes for rating guidelines development processes, as described above. Moreover, if the U.S. Congress requires companies to report payments not only to individuals but also to a range of medical organizations, that information, in combination with the annual reports that many professional society and patient groups issue, should allow the calculation of industry funding as a share of total revenues.

Transparency also involves the inclusion of the specified information with each guideline that a group sponsors. Preferably, the information would accompany the written text, but it could—particularly if it is very lengthy—be provided by an Internet link that is maintained through the life of the guideline.

In addition to expanded disclosure about funding, the committee recommends an end to direct industry funding of clinical practice guidelines. It recognizes that this step might have the undesirable effect of reducing the involvement of professional societies in guideline development but believes that it is necessary to avoid the conflicts that come from industry financing. It is also likely that an increase in public support for systematic reviews of the evidence would buffer such effects because these reviews are an expensive part of the process of developing evidence-based guidelines. Professional societies and other groups with a shared interest in certain clinical problems could also collaborate on the development of guidelines and spread the costs. In addition, a pooling mechanism might be created—as has been suggested by some for continuing medical education—to support indirect industry funding of the development of clinical guidelines in certain broad categories.

Another important step is to exclude or substantially limit the participation of individuals with conflicts of interest on panels that develop clinical practice guidelines. As more academic institutions and other groups as well as individual professionals take the steps recommended in Chapters 5 and 6 of this report, it should be easier to find individuals who are free of conflicts of interest involving promotional relationships (e.g., participation in speakers bureaus). If groups conclude that participants with conflicts of interest are essential to provide the necessary expertise, they should demonstrate to the public that they have made a good faith but unsuccessful effort to find individuals with the required expertise and without conflicts of interest. They should also preclude individuals with conflicts of interest from chairing guideline development panels, restrict the number of individuals with conflicts of interest on panels to a distinct minority (e.g., to 25 to 30 percent of the membership), and prohibit members with conflicts of interest from drafting and deciding specific recommendations.

In addition to actions by the institutions directly involved in the development of guidelines, organizations with an interest in unbiased clinical practice guidelines can create incentives for groups that develop guidelines to adopt the recommendations presented in this report. The committee understands that the National Guideline Clearinghouse will be phasing in a requirement for the disclosure of conflicts of interest, but the committee recommends that it extend the requirement to include the disclosure of funding and policy information, consistent with Recommendation 7.1. It would also be desirable for the clearinghouse or some other entity to begin substantive assessments of the quality of clinical practice guidelines.

RECOMMENDATION 7.2 Accrediting and certification bodies, health insurers, public agencies, and other similar organizations should encourage institutions that develop clinical practice guidelines to adopt conflict of interest policies consistent with the recommendations in this report. Three desirable steps are for

- **journals to require that all clinical practice guidelines accepted for publication describe (or provide an Internet link to) the developer's conflict of interest policies, the sources and amounts of funding for the guideline, and the relevant financial interests of guideline panel members, if any;**
- **the National Guideline Clearinghouse to require that all clinical practice guidelines accepted for posting describe (or provide an Internet link to) the developer's conflict of interest policies, the sources and amounts of funding for development of the guideline, and the relevant financial interests of guideline panel members, if any; and**
- **accrediting and certification organizations, public and private health plans, and similar groups to avoid using clinical practice guidelines for performance measures, coverage decisions, and similar purposes if the guideline developers do not follow the practices recommended in this report.**

The committee expects that the adoption of the committee's recommendations will reduce the probability of undue influence from industry funding and may also reduce the number of conflicting and competing clinical practice guidelines. Some groups that have operated with undisclosed industry support or that have been unwilling to disclose the financial relationships of guideline development panel members may remove themselves from the guideline development process. Other groups may collaborate to share the costs of developing guidelines on topics of common interest.

Although the committee believes that an expanded role for public-sector sponsorship of the development of systematic reviews and clinical practice guidelines would be desirable, an examination of this issue is beyond its scope. The committee endorses the recommendation in a recent IOM report for expanded federal support for assessments of the effectiveness of clinical services (IOM, 2008). That report called for the U.S. Congress to direct the U.S. Department of Health and Human Services to designate a single entity with the responsibility and capacity to "to ensure production of credible, unbiased information about what is known and not known about clinical effectiveness" (p. 171). That entity would establish priorities for and manage the development of systematic reviews of clinical effectiveness, develop standards for such reviews and for clinical guidelines, and address conflicting guidelines. The report also recommended that accreditation organizations and other groups preferentially use guidelines developed by using the standards described in the report. In addition, it recommended that guideline development panels minimize bias by including a balance of competing interests, prohibit voting by participants with conflicts of interest, and publish conflicts that have been disclosed.

Other Relevant Recommendations in This Report

In addition to the two recommendations in this chapter, recommendations elsewhere in this report are relevant to institutions that develop clinical practice guidelines. Consensus standards on disclosure elements and procedures would make disclosures more informative as well as less burdensome for those making disclosures to multiple institutions (Recommendation 3.2). A national system for public reporting by companies of their payments to individuals and organizations would allow the easier verification of certain disclosures (Recommendation 3.4). Limitations on certain industry ties and practices (e.g., the receipt of gifts and participation in speakers bureaus) should reduce conflicts of interest among the pool of experts considered for participation in clinical practice guideline development (Recommendations 5.1, 6.1, and 6.2).

The adoption of explicit policies and procedures on institutional conflict of interest would challenge professional societies, patient advocacy groups, and other entities that develop clinical practice guidelines to confront the scope and appropriateness of their financial ties with industry, eliminate questionable ties, and prudently manage others (Recommendation 8.1). The next chapter discusses conflicts of interest at the level of institutions.

8

Institutional Conflicts of Interest

Financial relationships with industry exist at the institutional level as well as the individual level and may create conflicts of interest for academic medical centers, professional societies, and other institutions that carry out medical research, medical education, clinical care, or practice guideline development. Some of these relationships may generate significant benefits to an institution's primary missions. For example, gifts to endow named professorships or fund the construction of research facilities support the core teaching and research missions of academic medical centers. The committee heard testimony that new kinds of institutional relationships between academia and industry—beyond relationships involving individual faculty members—could promote the translation of basic discoveries into new therapies and thereby benefit society (Benz, 2008; Moses, 2008). The question for institutions as well as individuals is whether a relationship with industry can be maintained in a way that achieves the desired benefits but avoids the risks of undue influence on decision making and the loss of public trust.

Although several cases reported by the news media have called attention to institutional conflicts of interest in medicine, institutional conflicts of interest have generally received less attention than individual conflicts of interest. Institutional conflicts of interest often involve the financial interests of both the institution and its senior officials (Box 8-1).

The risks to core missions posed by institutional conflicts of interest can be as serious as those created by individual conflicts. Moreover, if institutions do not prudently manage relationships with industry and are exposed to public criticism for inadequately or improperly managing conflicts, the work of many individual researchers, educators, and clinicians associated

BOX 8-1
Cases and Controversies Involving Institutional Conflicts of Interest

After the 1999 death of Jesse Gelsinger during a clinical trial involving a gene transfer intervention conducted by a University of Pennsylvania research institute, various investigations raised questions about the university's oversight of the study and the research institute (Stolberg, 2000; Steinbrook, 2008c). The university and several past and present officials had financial interests in the biotechnology company that developed the intervention. The company contributed $25 million to the research institute's annual budget and had exclusive rights to develop products emerging from the trial and related research. In addition, the director of the institute, who was also the lead researcher, had founded the company and maintained a financial interest in it.

In 2005, reporters revealed that the Cleveland Clinic and its chief executive officer had undisclosed financial interests in a medical device firm (Armstrong, 2005). The firm's heart surgery device was used at the hospital and was promoted by its surgeons. Patients were not informed of the conflicts of interest. The board of the Cleveland Clinic subsequently adopted new policies on institutional conflict of interest.

Amgen, the manufacturer of epoetin, a drug that increases hemoglobin levels, was the founding and primary sponsor of the Kidney and Dialysis Outcomes Quality Initiative carried out by the National Kidney Foundation (Coyne, 2007; see also Chapter 7). This project issued practice guidelines recommending an increase in the target hemoglobin level for patients with chronic kidney disease, which would entail the use of higher doses of epoetin and increased sales of the sponsor's product.

In 2008, the chair of the Psychiatry Department at Emory University resigned that position after congressional investigators reported that he had failed to disclose the receipt of substantial consulting payments from pharmaceutical companies, in violation of university and federal government rules, and had also failed to comply with an agreement with the university that he limit such payments. One of the documents cited was a letter he sent to a university official pointing out that his multiple ties to pharmaceutical companies had benefited the university by attracting company funding for department career awards, an endowed chair, and other gifts (Harris, 2008).

with the institution may unfairly be called into question, even though they were not involved in the conduct that was criticized.

This chapter begins by defining institutional conflicts of interest and describing what has been documented about the extent of such conflicts. The discussion then reviews responses to institutional conflicts of interest and examines some of the challenges in managing such conflicts. The chapter concludes with recommendations, including a recommendation that the National Institutes of Health (NIH) require its grantees to adopt and apply policies on institutional conflicts of interest.

WHAT ARE INSTITUTIONAL CONFLICTS OF INTEREST?

Institutional conflicts of interest arise when an institution's own financial interests or those of its senior officials pose risks of undue influence on decisions involving the institution's primary interests. For academic institutions, such risks often involve the conduct of research within the institution that could affect the value of the institution's patents or its equity positions or options in biotechnology, pharmaceutical, or medical device companies. Conflicts of interest may also arise when institutions seek and receive gifts or grants from companies, for example, a gift of an endowed university chair or a grant for a professional society to develop a clinical practice guideline.

In addition, institutional conflicts of interest exist when senior officials who act on behalf of the institution have personal financial interests that may be affected by their administrative decisions. For instance, a department chair or dean who has a major equity holding in a medical device company could make decisions about faculty appointments and promotions or assignment of office or laboratory space in ways that favor the interests of the company but compromise the overall research, educational, or clinical mission of the institution. Similarly, a hospital official with such a holding would be at risk of undue influence in making decisions about the use of the company's products for patient care. In situations like these, an individual's financial relationship also implicates the institution's interests.

As emphasized in Chapter 2, conflicts of interest are defined in terms of the risk of undue influence and not actual bias or misconduct. Whether they are at the individual or the institutional level, conflict of interest policies seek to prevent compromised decision making rather than to try to remedy its consequences.

Institutional interests can be evaluated for the likelihood of undue influence and the seriousness of potential harms in ways analogous to those applicable to individual conflicts (see Chapter 2). Thus, assessments would consider the nature of the primary interest, the value and scope of the secondary interest, the extent of institutional accountability and discretion involving decisions about the primary interest at stake, and the seriousness of potential harms in relation to potential benefits (see also Emanuel and Steiner [1995]).

EXTENT OF INSTITUTIONAL RELATIONSHIPS WITH INDUSTRY

Because institutional conflicts of interest have not received as much attention as individual conflicts of interest, there is less evidence about their characteristics or impacts. The committee found little comprehensive information about the scope and nature of the ties of academic medical centers, professional societies, patient advocacy groups, and other institutions to pharmaceutical, medical device, and biotechnology companies. Such ties may involve various kinds of payments and gifts to an institution, institutional ownership interests in companies, patents, and the relationships of senior officials (for example, service on a company's board of directors). Most reports focus on prominent and usually egregious cases of misconduct, as illustrated in Box 8-1.

Chapter 4 reviewed the results of a survey of department chairs in medical schools and large independent teaching hospitals that found that 27 percent of preclinical departments and 16 percent of clinical departments received income from intellectual property licensing (Campbell et al., 2007b). (This income may be seen as a benefit of the provisions of the Bayh-Dole Act, which allow institutions to patent discoveries resulting from federally funded research and to grant exclusive licenses for others to develop those discoveries.) The survey also found that ties to industry were common among department chairs, who served as consultants (27 percent), members of a scientific advisory board (27 percent), paid speakers (14 percent), company officers (7 percent), and company board members (11 percent). The committee did not locate institution-level data on company funding of biomedical research, but Chapter 4 reported that the majority of such research in the United States is commercially funded.

For institutions as well as individuals who provide health care, conflicts of interest also arise from provider reimbursement methods, whether these involve fee for service, prospective payment per case, pay for performance, or other arrangements. In addition, conflicts may arise from provider ownership interests, for example, hospital ownership of subsidiary specialty centers to which the hospital's physicians refer patients. As noted in Chapter 6, however, consideration of payment methods and ownership interests in medical facilities are beyond the scope of this report.

Among universities, a Congressional Research Service report concluded that patents typically account for a small percentage of university research and development funding and that most significant income from patents has tended to come from single "blockbuster" patents (Schacht, 2008). The report did not look specifically at biomedical research institutions. The Association of University Technology Managers, which conducts an annual survey of technology transfer activities (including the licensing of patents and the launching of start-up companies), does not report information by scientific field.[1]

Most professional societies and disease-focused or patient advocacy groups do not make public the details of funding received from industry, but it appears that many groups depend on medical product companies for a significant share of their overall revenues and for specific activities (e.g., continuing medical education and the development of clinical practice guidelines). In connection with congressional inquiries about its relationships with pharmaceutical companies, the American Psychiatric Association (APA) reported that medical companies supplied about 28 percent of its annual income. An informal APA survey of other medical specialty societies indicated that this figure was about in the middle of the range of the income that companies provide these groups (from 2 to nearly 50 percent) (Stotland, 2008). An Associated Press story on pharmaceutical company spending to promote the awareness of fibromyalgia reported that companies contributed funds that amounted to 40 percent of the annual budget of the National Fibromyalgia Association (Perrone, 2009). Many groups list corporate donors but do not report how much of their income is derived from these donors. Groups that report sources of funding for activities such as clinical practice guideline development usually do not report the amount of company funding for an activity or what percentage of an activity's cost was accounted for by company funds. These data would assist with assessments of the risk of undue influence.

In a 2006 report for its board of directors, the American Academy of Family Physicians (AAFP) analyzed its resources and activities and concluded that it was not financially possible to forgo industry funding for any of its activities without imposing unacceptable cuts in services to members or increases in member costs. For its fiscal year 2006–2007 budget, AAFP projected that less than 38 percent of its income ($31 million of a total budget of $80 million) would come from dues and sales of products and services to members. Approximately 42 percent ($34 million) would come from the pharmaceutical industry, of which about 60 percent would come from advertising in the academy's journal and 13 percent would come from payments for exhibits at meetings (AAFP, 2006a). The report noted that the organization had sought to broaden its base of nondues funding beyond pharmaceutical companies by seeking grants from government and foundations for various activities and

[1] On the basis of its 2006 survey, the Association of University Technology Managers reported 12,672 actively managed licenses from patents as well as the introduction of 697 new products and 553 start-up companies (AUTM, 2007). It did not report the extent to which the institutions had financial stakes in the new products and companies. The survey covered 190 institutions, including 161 universities and 28 teaching hospitals and research institutions.

had also taken other steps to limit the influence of industry. If it stopped accepting all funding from industry, however, including journal advertising, the organization would have had to increase member dues by about $600 (to about $1,000 per year) to maintain the levels of service and the programs (e.g., existing educational activities at the same per program cost to members) that existed at that time (AAFP, 2006a).

The data presented in Chapter 6 showed that physician membership organizations obtained 49 percent of their income for accredited continuing medical education from a combination of commercial funding for activities, advertising, and exhibits at meetings. Medical school continuing medical education programs received about 62 percent of their income from these sources; for publishing and education companies, the figure was 73 percent.

RESPONSES TO INSTITUTIONAL CONFLICTS OF INTEREST

Federal regulations and laws have not consistently targeted institutional conflicts of interest. The U.S. Public Health Service (PHS) regulations on conflict of interest, which were issued in 1995 and which are included in Appendix B, cover only individual conflicts of interest and relationships with industry. Institutional conflicts of interest were deliberately not addressed (NIH, 1995). The guidance on financial relationships in research with human participants published by the U.S. Department of Health and Human Services discusses the identification and management of institutional as well as individual financial interests (HHS, 2004). The document suggests questions and procedures for institutional review boards (IRBs), investigators, and institutions to consider in evaluating institutional relationships. Federal antikickback rules apply to illegal payments to institutions as well as individuals. The recommendation by the Medicare Policy Advisory Commission (see Chapter 3) for industry reporting of consulting and other payments covers not only payments to physicians but also payments to medical schools, professional societies, and providers of continuing medical education (MedPAC, 2009). A bill introduced in the U.S. Congress in 2007 (S. 2029) and reintroduced in 2009 (Grassley, 2009) covers payments to individual physicians.

Several academic organizations have issued reports on institutional conflicts of interest, including the Association of American Medical Colleges (AAMC, 2002; AAMC-AAU, 2008), the Association of American Universities (AAMC-AAU, 2008), and the Council on Government Relations (COGR, 2003). The 2002 AAMC and 2008 AAMC-AAU reports dealt with institutional conflicts of interest in research with human participants.

The 2008 AAMC-AAU report was in part a response to evidence that academic medical centers had not implemented the recommendations set forth in the 2002 AAMC report. In an AAMC survey of its members, only 38 percent of the institutions that responded reported that they had a conflict of interest policy that applied to the institution's financial interest, although another 37 percent reported that they were developing such a policy (Ehringhaus et al., 2008). For institutions that had policies, the documents typically covered equity in nonpublicly held companies (90 percent) or publicly held companies (77 percent), royalties (80 percent), payments for reaching designated milestones in the course of a study (73 percent), and substantial gifts from a research sponsor (73 percent). The majority of institutions that had policies applied them to senior officials (71 percent), governing board members (66 percent), and members of the IRB (81 percent). In addition, the majority of respondents reported creating organizational arrangements to separate institutional responsibility for research from responsibility for investment management (94 percent) or technology transfer (61 percent). Although the most serious problem identified in the survey was the lack of policies at a majority of institutions, another concern was the incomplete coverage by policies of significant institutional interests.

In addition to reiterating the importance of such policies, the 2008 AAMC-AAU report set forth several guiding principles for institutional conflict of interest policies. They were

- "research and financial decision-making processes and agents must be separated";
- "decisions about whether or not to pursue a particular human subjects research project in the presence of an institutional conflict of interest should be governed by a 'rebuttable presumption' against doing the research at or under the auspices of the conflicted institution" unless a compelling case can be made to justify an exception; and
- institutional conflict of interests "will be addressed consistently throughout the institution, such that those subject to institutional financial conflict of interest policies, specifically officials of the institution and the institutions themselves, are subject to substantive reporting, disclosure, and management of their financial interests." (pp. 14–16)

The report also recommended the creation of a standing institutional conflict of interest committee and discussed procedures for the reporting of institutional financial interests and the managing of relationships that were determined to be conflicts of interest. Strategies could involve divesting the institution of an equity interest in a company, requiring senior officials to remove themselves from involvement with making decisions that might affect their conflicting interest, declining to perform research in which the institution has a financial stake (beyond the funding of the research itself), asking the IRB at another institution to review such research, or disclosing the institutional conflict of interest to research participants.

One university's policy lists several issues to be considered in evaluations of the circumstances that might justify institutional involvement in a human subjects research project despite a conflict of interest (University of Rochester, 2006). The case for the institution's participation in the project is stronger to the extent that

- the work is carried out at multiple sites (e.g., under the auspices of several institutions);
- the institution takes a relatively passive role in the conduct of the project (e.g., the gathering of data);
- the number of research subjects under the institution's supervision is small;
- an adverse effect on research subjects appears more likely if the institution is not used as a research site; and
- the investigators conducting the research or the university resources supporting the project are essential and are not readily available elsewhere.

In a position statement on organizational aspects of physician relationships with industry, the American College of Physicians (ACP) advised that "[m]edical professional societies that accept industry support or other external funding should be aware of potential bias and conflicts of interest" (Coyle et al., 2002b, p. 405). It recommended the adoption of explicit institutional policies on industry relationships, including policies that "avoid reliance on outside sources of support" and that guide the acceptance and disclosure of funding from industry and other outside sources. The ACP position on educational programs is that "it is unethical for academic institutions and educational organizations to accept any support that is explicitly or implicitly conditioned on industry's opportunity to influence the selection of instructors, speakers, invitees, topics, or content and materials of educational sessions" (Coyle et al., 2002b, p. 405).

In a 2006 statement, the Society for General Internal Medicine (SGIM) reported limits on the share of its annual operating budget that could come from external sources (SGIM, 2006). The limit on external sources of funding was 33 percent overall, with limits of 10 percent from health care-related for-profit entities in combination and 5 percent for any single such entity. (Thus, 67 percent of the operating budget must come from internal sources, such as member dues and fees.) Furthermore, the statement declared that the organization should not accept funds from

> for-profit companies (or not-for-profit entities funded largely by for-profit companies) for research or educational projects (including *individual* pre-courses, workshops or other presentations at the SGIM national or regional meetings) related to specific diseases, or to pharmaceuticals, medical devices, diagnostics, or other products or services purported to have direct health benefits to patients (regardless of whether the products are sold by that particular external funder). (p. 2)

The statement described such funds as "problematic" because their intent would seem to be "primarily promotional; that is, to directly or indirectly (through greater recognition of the disease in the population) encourage wider use of medical products, to the benefit of the sponsor" (p. 2). The statement stated that general meeting support may be solicited after program planners have determined the content of the meeting.

Chapter 6 discussed the actions that the Accreditation Council for Continuing Medical Education initiated to limit industry influence associated with providers' solicitation and acceptance of industry funding. Chapter 7 described the steps taken by some professional societies to insulate activities such as clinical practice guideline development from influence associated with industry funding. It also noted that some societies do not accept industry funding for guideline development.

SPECIAL CHALLENGES IN MANAGING INSTITUTIONAL CONFLICTS OF INTEREST

Although the committee found no systematic research on institutional conflicts of interest or the effects of institutional policies, it identified several challenges in managing such conflicts. One challenge is that identifying relevant institutional financial interests and conflicts may be difficult. Particularly in universities or other large institutions, no single individual or office may have knowledge of all such interests. Those responsible for identifying relationships may have to survey various parts of the institution to develop an inventory of relevant interests and relationship. In an academic medical center, for example, this inventory could cover the office responsible for technology transfer and intellectual property, the office or body that manages investments, the offices responsible for purchasing medical equipment, academic departments and other units that may receive gifts, and perhaps other offices or units as well. For senior officials, the usual process for disclosing individual financial interests will apply, although the review of disclosures will be at a higher level, for example, through a committee of the governing board, as recommended below.

Dealing with institutional conflicts of interest may be more difficult in some respects than dealing with individual conflicts of interest. In the case of individual conflicts in large institutions such as universities, medical schools, and major teaching hospitals, opportunities for review usually exist at multiple levels of the institution and involve authorities who are relatively independent and do not stand to gain personally from the secondary interests in question. In contrast, an independent review for institutional conflicts of interest may be difficult because the institutional officers themselves may stand to benefit indirectly from the conflict of interest and may be reluctant to question current or proposed relationships with companies that seem likely to improve the institution's financial welfare. For example, the reputation and tenure of chief executives and other high-level officials may depend on their success in strengthening the financial health of their institution. If senior officials who oversee technology transfer, intellectual property, and research grants are also charged with managing institutional conflicts of interest, they may find it difficult to resist pursuing a grant or may be reluctant to divest the institution of a property interest even if such actions are necessary to manage the conflict. The leaders of professional societies and patient advocacy groups that depend significantly on member dues or individual contributions may be reluctant to reject grants from industry, even though they create a risk of undue influence over activities such as the development of clinical practice guidelines or educational programs.

The potential for conflicts of interest among senior institutional officials is one reason for the committee's recommendation below that the key responsibility for oversight of institutional conflicts of interest be lodged with an institution's governing body. It is also a reason for the recommendation that independent members—individuals not affiliated with the institution—be included on board committees that review and manage institutional conflicts of interest.

Because the potential financial gain from a secondary institution-level interest may not be personal for institutional officials, their decisions may be more easily rationalized as serving the institution rather than themselves—even when officials also stand to gain in personal reputation. In fact, the gains often do serve the institution's primary mission, for example, when returns on investments or licenses are distributed to worthy research, educational, or patient care activities. Nonetheless, it is precisely because this argument for benefit is so plausible (and often valid) that serious institution-level conflicts of interest may be ignored or may not be reviewed carefully to assess whether they might, on balance, undermine rather than promote the primary missions of the institution.

For similar reasons, the public may—at least initially—be more tolerant of institutional conflicts of interest than individual conflicts of interest and may expect that institutions will pursue relationships to advance research, expand educational activities, or increase clinical resources. This tolerance may, in turn, reinforce the inclination of institutional leaders to downplay or ignore the resulting conflicts of interest. Because it is clear that universities and other health care institutions require resources to fulfill their missions and because society has encouraged institutions to pursue such resources, "[s]ociety may not view this as self-interested behavior and consequently may erroneously be more tolerant of circumstances in which an institution's financial interests may compromise the integrity of its missions than of similar situations involving individual conflict of interest" (Emanuel and Steiner, 1995, p. 263).

RECOMMENDATIONS

Because no decision maker in an institution is fully free of conflict in the case of institutional conflicts of interest, it is not possible to establish a fully independent process for assessing such conflicts. Although no perfect solution exists, the committee concluded that, on balance, the most suitable authority for making judgments about institutional conflicts is the board of trustees or an equivalent governing body.

In their fiduciary role, members of the board are responsible for giving priority to the longer-term interests of the institution. Because they stand at a greater distance from the daily pressures of decision making than an institution's senior officials, they should be able to assess more judiciously the positive or negative effects of financial interests on the institution's core mission. Board members also have access to comprehensive information about the finances of the institution, some of which may be confidential and not revealed to senior institutional officials. They may also be better positioned to help an institution's chief executive resolve disputes about conflicts of interest that involve different units within the institution. For example, in a university, faculty in the school of public health may be more concerned than faculty in the school of business about the potential for investments in certain products to create a risk to the missions of the whole institution.

In addition, the decisions made by a governing board are more salient within and beyond the institution than decisions made by staff. When the board takes up an issue, the concerned public is more likely to take notice.

RECOMMENDATION 8.1 The boards of trustees or the equivalent governing bodies of institutions engaged in medical research, medical education, patient care, or practice guideline development should establish their own standing committees on institutional conflicts of interest. These standing committees should

• have no members who themselves have conflicts of interest relevant to the activities of the institution;

• include at least one member who is not a member of the board or an employee or officer of the institution and who has some relevant expertise;

• create, as needed, administrative arrangements for the day-to-day oversight and management of institutional conflicts of interest, including those involving senior officials; and

• submit an annual report to the full board, which should be made public but in which the necessary modifications have been made to protect confidential information.

The standing board committee (or subcommittee) would regularly review the financial relationships of the institution itself to identify conflicts of interest with its primary mission or missions and would likewise review the financial relationships of senior officials. The board committee would also evaluate the adequacy of the policies and procedures established to deal with these relationships. This board committee would be different from the committee established to address individual conflicts of interests, as suggested in Recommendation 3.1.

Although the board should be accountable for institutional conflicts of interest, the committee recognizes that board members may not be well suited to carry out day-to-day oversight or conduct special investigations, especially in academic medical centers and other large institutions. The board may therefore decide to establish a mechanism for the day-to-day oversight of institutional conflicts of interest. This mechanism could take different forms at different institutions. For example, as AAMC and AAU have recommended, an academic institution might establish a faculty-staff committee that would oversee institutional conflicts of interest and that would be separate from any committee responsible for individual conflicts of interest. Such a committee (and any other support staff) could report to the board committee or to an officer of the institution who is not directly responsible for institutional investments, technology transfer, or research. Various options are reasonable; and the choices made may depend in part on the size, organization, and scope of an institution. In any case, the option selected should be consistent with the objectives of establishing and supporting governing board oversight of institutional conflicts of interest.

The recommended annual report from the board committee will provide an incentive for that committee to report on both what it has decided with respect to newly identified conflicts of interest and how its previous decisions (e.g., plans for eliminating or managing an institutional conflict of interest) have been implemented. Such reporting will also provide an incentive for rigorous review and accountability. The board committee is more likely to be diligent in its reviews if its members know that if they miss potential problems, their failure may be publicized for all to see, should these problems become the subject of official investigations or media reports. In certain cases, a tension may exist between the countervailing goals of public disclosure and keeping confidential certain personnel information and certain facts about current or pending intellectual property. Thus, the board's public reports may exclude some details because the information is confidential, but such exclusions should be rare.

To speed the adoption of institutional conflict of interest policies, NIH should extend the 1995 PHS regulations on conflict of interest to cover institutional as well as individual financial interests for institutions that receive PHS research grants. Such rules would also call attention to the issue and encourage institutions that do not receive research funds but that are engaged in medical education, clinical care, or the development of practice guidelines to voluntarily take action to avoid and oversee potential conflicts of interest. Ideally, the development of new PHS rules would be harmonized with corresponding revisions in the regulations of the National Science Foundation.

RECOMMENDATION 8.2 The National Institutes of Health should develop rules governing institutional conflicts of interest for research institutions covered by current U.S. Public Health Service regulations. The rules should require the reporting of identified institutional conflicts of interest and the steps that have been taken to eliminate or manage such conflicts.

Although the new PHS rules should be consistent with the recommendation in Recommendation 8.1 and other recommendations in this report, they need not be highly prescriptive or rigid, particularly given that experience with institutional conflict of interest policies appears to be more limited and is less well documented than policies governing individual conflicts. Provisions for monitoring and enforcement are, however, important both at the level of the NIH extramural program and within research institutions. Consistent with current PHS rules on individual conflicts of interest, Recommendation 8.2 calls for grantee reporting to NIH of identified institutional conflicts of interest.

NIH can encourage the appropriate and reasonably consistent implementation of the regulations by providing supplementary explanations and guidance, as it has recently done for its policies and regulations on individual conflicts of interest (see Chapter 3). It can also bring grantee representatives together to discuss their experiences and identify good practices in policy development and implementation. In addition, NIH can develop or commission case studies on common situations that raise concerns over conflicts of interest, such as institutional stakes in start-up companies that seek to sponsor research at the institution.

Although the 2008 AAMC-AAU report did not explicitly recommend governing board responsibility for policies on institutional conflicts of interest, their report can still provide useful guidance to NIH and to grantee institutions and a model for developing case studies to provide education on the evaluation of conflicts of interest. Because experience with and evaluations of institutional conflict of interest policies are limited, the investigation of such policies should be one focus of the research agenda recommended in Chapter 9. In addition, continued attention to this area—for example, further surveys of policy adoption—by AAMC would also be constructive.

The intent of the recommendations in this report is to promote a culture in which conflicts of interest are taken seriously by institutions and individuals engaged in medical research, education, and practice and practice guideline development. For this to happen, institutions must effectively manage their own conflicts and be seen to be doing so. The board and the senior officials set the tone for the institution. They should be accountable for making sure that their own institutional interests are in order.

9

Role of Supporting Organizations

Physicians, researchers, and the institutions that carry out medical research and education, provide patient care, and develop practice guidelines do not act in isolation but, rather, as part of complex intersecting systems. These systems can support or interfere with the adoption, implementation, and improvement of sound conflict of interest policies and can amplify or reduce the probability that financial relationships with industry may undermine primary professional or institutional obligations. Within these systems, a variety of organizations—public and private—can influence the policies and practices of institutions and uphold norms of professional integrity.

Chapter 1 distinguished between institutions that carry out medical research, education, clinical care, and practice guideline development and supporting organizations. Supporting organizations include accreditation and certification bodies, health insurance plans, membership groups such as the Association of American Medical Colleges (AAMC) and the World Association of Medical Journal Editors (WAME), and government agencies such as the National Institutes of Health (NIH). These entities may be seen as supporting organizations because they are in a position to influence the conflict of interest policies of the institutions that are the primary subject of this report. They can establish incentives for academic and other institutions to create more effective responses to conflicts of interest, including adopting and implementing the recommendations presented in this report. Some supporting organizations can also create incentives for individual physicians and researchers to follow conflict of interest policies and related codes of conduct. They can, more broadly, help create a culture of accountability that supports the integrity of professional judgment and sustains public confidence in that judgment.

The opportunities for supporting organizations to exert influence arise in different ways, depending on the roles and authority of the organization. Accrediting organizations set standards for medical schools, residency and fellowship programs, and institutions that provide health care. State agencies establish rules for the licensing and relicensing of individual physicians, and specialty boards design rules to certify and recertify physician specialists. The National Guidelines Clearinghouse sets conditions for the posting of clinical practice guidelines developed by professional societies and other groups. Public and private health insurers use a variety of financial and other incentives to influence the practices of institutions and individual physicians. The U.S. Department of Justice and the Office of Inspector General of the U.S. Department of Health and Human Services enforce antikickback and self-referral laws that prohibit or limit certain conflicts of interest. NIH promotes and oversees adherence to U.S. Public Health Service (PHS) regulations on conflict of interest for grantees. Professional societies and associations of health care and educational institutions articulate norms and ethical standards for their members. (Some professional societies are both organizations in this sense and also institutions that carry out research, education, and practice guideline development.) Although the Pharmaceutical Research and Manufacturers of America (PhRMA) and the Advanced Medical Technology Association (AdvaMed) represent companies, they establish codes of conduct for their members that may indirectly support medical professionals and institutions by discouraging member companies from interactions that create a risk of undue influence. (As described in Chapter 6, PhRMA and AdvaMed have indicated that they will publicly report on the companies that adopt their recently revised codes.)

Previous chapters have identified various shortcomings in the policies and practices of academic and other institutions. For example, as discussed in Chapter 3, some research institutions have been slow to adopt or adequately implement PHS requirements for conflict of interest policies, some academic medical centers have not adopted key AAMC policy recommendations, and some medical journals have not followed recommendations on conflict of interest from WAME and the International Committee of Medical Journal Editors (ICMJE). Furthermore, it may be difficult to determine a particular institution's policies. Postings on institutional websites may be incomplete or not up to date, and some institutions choose not to reveal their policies. Such a lack of transparency makes it difficult to assess whether an institution's policies are consistent with regulations or with recommendations of groups such as AAMC and WAME. As a result, opportunities to strengthen the institution's accountability for conflict of interest policies may be lost. Supporting organizations may promote consensus on the content of policies and also, in some situations, draw attention to the failure of institutions to adopt and implement the policies, which may then stimulate corrective action.

This chapter discusses ways in which these diverse supporting organizations can cooperate with and influence the academic and other institutions that have the primary responsibility for dealing with conflicts of interest in medical research, education, and practice. The chapter begins by considering some of the productive forms that support and cooperation can take. The discussion emphasizes the roles of collaboration, consensus building, and incentives in making conflict of interest policies more effective and compliance with them less burdensome. It also recognizes that policies need to be backed by enforcement and sanctions. The chapter concludes with two recommendations that supplement the mostly mission-specific recommendations of earlier chapters. The first calls on supporting organizations to develop incentives for medical institutions to become more accountable for preventing, identifying, and managing conflicts of interest. The second calls for more research to provide a stronger evidence base for evaluating and improving conflict of interest policies.

HOW SUPPORTING ORGANIZATIONS CAN INFLUENCE MEDICAL INSTITUTIONS

Consensus Building and Collaboration

Consensus building and collaboration can operate within the institutions that are the focus of this report. Such efforts seek to engage those affected by policies in the process of developing them to improve the policies (e.g., by identifying and understanding obstacles to the success of the policies) and to win acceptance or buy in by those affected. Supporting organizations may likewise be more successful if they engage research, educational, and other institutions in the process of designing incentives and setting standards and if they give those institutions some discretion on how to reach specific performance goals. The leaders of those institutions are often in the best position to identify barriers to accountability (including burdensome or confusing administrative procedures) and to suggest ways to overcome those barriers. They are also well situated to identify and reduce the unintended negative consequences of proposed policies or procedures.

Some lessons for collaborative efforts that can be made to improve conflict of interest policies and practices are suggested by quality improvement initiatives within health care organizations. The typical quality improvement program in health care actively engages frontline caregivers and managers in an interdisciplinary process of identifying and analyzing problems in the quality of care, devising preventive or corrective interventions, monitoring outcomes, and modifying interventions on the basis of the observed outcomes (Berwick, 1998). In this approach, the gathering and monitoring of outcomes data are crucial to identifying and reducing inappropriate variations in outcomes. In some cases, cross-institutional collaborations have helped institutions develop effective quality improvement programs. Some programs use transparency—the public reporting of organizational performance in relation to benchmarks—as a means of enhancing accountability and promoting competition to improve the quality of care. Accreditation agencies and voluntary groups have also encouraged this quality improvement process, and some universities have applied quality improvement models to university administration. The University of Wisconsin, for example, has an office of quality improvement that supports process improvement activities in administrative as well as academic areas, and its website showcases examples of activities that are potentially relevant for conflict of interest programs (University of Wisconsin, 2008).

There are, of course, significant differences between quality improvement procedures and conflict of interest policies. Nonetheless, the mechanisms of collaboration, consensus building, and outcome measurement can usefully guide the relationships between outside supporting organizations and institutions directly involved in medical research, education, and practice.

Some supporting organizations have been able to promote a consensus on important and often contentious aspects of conflict of interest policies. As described in earlier chapters, AAMC convened a broad group of affected parties that made recommendations about financial ties with industry in medical education (AAMC, 2008c). The parties included academic medical centers, teaching hospitals, industry, professional organizations, government agencies, and consumer groups. AAMC and the Association of American Universities convened another consensus development process to develop recommendations for improving the adoption and implementation of conflict of interest policies in human subjects research (AAMC-AAU, 2008). Over time, these and other initiatives have forged agreement on goals and recommendations regarding a number of controversial issues. Such collaborative consensus-building activities can address the practical concerns of individuals and institutions affected and make recommendations more credible and acceptable.

Incentives

Supporting organizations can devise incentives for institutions to adopt and implement conflict of interest policies. An example of an incentive for change in institutional policies and practices is the policy of the National Library of Medicine mentioned in Chapter 3. It will not cite or index articles from certain types of company-sponsored journal supplements unless they include specific disclosures about any financial relationships that guest editors and authors have with the company or with the commercial products discussed in the supplement.

Just as the Medicare program and private health insurers have turned to pay-for-performance programs to provide incentives for quality improvement, so could insurance organizations offer incentives to institutions to adopt and maintain effective conflict of interest policies and to individuals to refrain from engaging in undesirable relationships with pharmaceutical, medical device, and biotechnology companies. For example, if preferred provider organizations publicly identified those participating physicians who agreed to decline gifts and marketing payments from industry, many physicians might decide that the benefits of being so identified outweigh the benefits of accepting such gifts and payments.

Particular incentives can have both positive and negative aspects. For example, when it rated medical schools on aspects of their conflict of interest policies, the American Medical Student Association used the "sunshine" of publicity in ways that were positive for the schools that it viewed as having good policies and possibly embarrassing for the schools that it viewed as having deficient policies (AMSA, 2008b). Although public reporting should enhance transparency and motivate policy change, it is also possible that it could merely promote the documentation of policies rather than meaningful oversight or change. Furthermore, public reporting could discourage relationships with industry that appropriately promote institutional missions and professional goals.

Enforcement and Sanctions

On the basis of the literature reviewed for Chapters 3 and 6, the actual imposition of penalties does not seem to figure prominently in the enforcement of conflict of interest policies, except for cases that involve offenses such as violations of anti-kickback and self-referral laws. NIH surveys and site visits have uncovered shortcomings in the content and application of PHS conflict of interest regulations for research grantees, and it appears that federal officials have penalized institutions or required quality improvement or remedial programs only rarely and only in cases in which problems have been identified in other ways (e.g., congressional or media investigations) (see Kaiser [2008]). As described in Chapter 3, NIH opposed a recommendation from the Office of the Inspector General that it require additional information from grantees about identified conflicts of interest and the means for their resolution.

Although they should be applied thoughtfully, sanctions have important roles in limiting and managing conflicts of interest. For example, at the most basic level, a process needs to be in place for institutions to determine who has and who has not submitted the required financial disclosure forms. Usually, reminders should be sufficient for those who have not submitted forms, but penalties may also be needed, at least for blatant violations. Recent highly publicized incidents of significant underreporting of financial relationships to academic institutions call attention to the need for mechanisms to verify that the information disclosed is complete and accurate (e.g., through public reporting by industry of payments to physicians; see Recommendation 3.4). Again, sanctions may be appropriate for blatant cases of inaccurate disclosure. In addition, journal editors could take a stance more aggressive than they generally have thus far toward authors who violate their journals' disclosure and conflict of interest policies.

When noncompliance is egregious, penalties such as public censure or the suspension of individuals from certain positions (e.g., a principal investigator or department chair) may be necessary. Even accrediting agencies such as the Joint Commission (formerly the Joint Commission on the Accreditation of Healthcare Organizations) that have shifted from using more negative strategies to using more positive and cooperative strategies (e.g., acknowledging high performers and helping struggling performers improve) retain a range of sanctions for use against persistent or egregiously poor performers. Sanctions are, however, neither sufficient nor desirable as the sole instruments of accountability. They must be combined with a more ambitious and effective compliance strategy that employs collaboration, consensus building, and positive incentives.

RECOMMENDATIONS

Creating Incentives for Institutional Action

As this report has described, some institutions that carry out medical research, education, clinical care, and practice guideline development have no or inadequate conflict of interest policies. Some institutions may not even fully meet the requirements of current federal regulations, and others fail to undertake monitoring and enforcement activities. This report has also described shortcomings in adherence by individual physicians and researchers to academic medical center, journal, and other conflict of interest policies.

Ideally, physicians, scientists, and medical institutions should voluntarily adopt conflict of interest policies as a matter of professional responsibility and professional ethics. A commitment to patient well-being, valid scientific research, and evidence-based education would naturally lead professionals to voluntarily adopt strong measures to minimize the negative impact of conflicts of interest on objectivity and trust. No doubt many professionals have such an attitude and act on it. Realistically, however, the committee is aware that behaviors are shaped not only by personal commitments but also by cultural and social forces. The environment in which health care professionals carry out research, teach, provide clinical care, and develop practice guidelines should promote and reinforce a professional's internal tendency to avoid relationships that pose an unacceptable risk of improperly influencing his or her judgment. The same is true for institutions. Their commitment to improve the content and application of conflict of interest policies is more likely to be effective if strong and consistent support from multiple independent organizations exists alongside government regulations. Thus, Recommendation 9.1 calls for an array of public and private groups (that is, supporting organizations) to create incentives to promote the widespread acceptance of policies to limit and manage conflicts of interest.

RECOMMENDATION 9.1 **Accreditation and certification bodies, private health insurers, government agencies, and similar organizations should develop incentives to promote the adoption and effective implementation of conflict of interest policies by institutions engaged in medical research, medical education, clinical care, or practice guideline development. In developing the incentives, these organizations should involve the individuals and the institutions that would be affected.**

A number of specific suggestions about incentives were discussed above and in the earlier chapters on medical research, education, and practice and practice guideline development. Box 9-1 summarizes these and other

BOX 9-1
Examples of Methods That Supporting Organizations Can Use to Strengthen Conflict of Interest Policies

Oversight bodies that oversee or regulate medical education and practice

- Accreditation and specialty certification bodies could set standards for the adoption of conflict of interest policies by organizations that offer undergraduate, graduate, and continuing medical education. These bodies could also collect and make public information on the educational institutions that follow those standards.
- State licensing boards could require that the continuing medical education courses required for relicensure be provided only by institutions that have adopted conflict of interest policies and other relevant recommendations presented in this report.

BOX 9-1 Continued

Membership organizations

- AAMC, PhRMA, and AdvaMed could collect and make public information on which of their member organizations have adopted their recommended conflict of interest policies or codes of conduct. (Note that the last two organizations have announced that they will post the names of companies that have pledged to follow their recently revised codes.)
- WAME could collect and make public information on which medical journals have adopted the authorship, ghostwriting, and conflict of interest policies consistent with its policy statements and those of ICMJE.
- Professional societies and associations of professional organizations could set standards for conflict of interest provisions in professional codes and membership criteria, make their policies public, and establish awards for groups that have exemplary conflict of interest policies and procedures.

Private health insurance plans

- Private health insurance plans could establish incentives for hospitals and individual physicians to adopt conflict of interest policies, as recommended in this report. For example, the adoption of such policies could be a criterion for an institution to be a center of excellence or for a physician to be a member of a preferred provider program. Alternatively, the lists of physicians in a plan could include information on whether a physician has agreed to certain conflict of interest provisions. Health insurers could also establish similar incentives for other institutions that provide health care, such as skilled nursing facilities or dialysis units.
- Business coalitions, such as the Leapfrog Group, the National Business Group on Health, and the Pacific Business Group on Health, could encourage employers who purchase health insurance to provide financial incentives for health care plans and health care providers to adopt the relevant recommendations presented in this report.

Government agencies

- NIH could collect and make public information on research institutions that have policies that are not in full compliance with 1995 PHS regulations. It could expand its recent efforts to provide more guidance to grantee institutions covered by the PHS regulations, and it could also analyze a sample of grantee conflict of interest reports to understand and evaluate how grantees eliminate or manage those conflicts of interest that are identified.
- The National Library of Medicine could identify in its online databases those journals that have adopted the authorship guidelines of ICMJE or WAME. For example, a symbol could be placed near the name of the journal when it appears in the listing of an article.
- The National Guidelines Clearinghouse could include only clinical practice guidelines that follow the recommendations presented in this report, including the provision of information about the sponsoring group's conflict of interest policies, the sources and amounts of industry funding for the guideline, the steps taken to identify participants without conflicts of interest, and the limits placed on participation in decision making by members with conflicts of interest.

examples of what supporting organizations can do. Many involve collecting and making public information about which institutions have adopted and applied the recommended policies. The committee expects that the prospect of such reporting would motivate institutions to close the gaps and loopholes in their conflict of interest policies or to provide a vigorous justification of why their policies depart from the recommendations.

If voluntary measures to deal with conflicts of interest are perceived to be weak or ineffectual, then calls for additional legislation or regulation or the more intrusive or punitive enforcement of existing laws will likely grow. The opportunity to preempt sweeping and potentially burdensome legal requirements should give a sense of urgency to voluntary efforts to establish and implement conflict of interest policies that reassure the public and those who make public policy. Government directives and prohibitions can be blunt instruments for dealing with conflict of interest problems, which often call for subtle judgments of risks and benefits and which involve many uncertainties. They also may not be as sensitive as voluntarily adopted measures to the administrative burdens of compliance or the possibility of unintended adverse consequences. This caution should not be interpreted as an endorsement of lax agency oversight or the lax application of existing conflict of interest rules.

Building the Evidence Base for Policy Improvement

As has been observed throughout this report, little systematic information about conflict of interest policies is available. This lack of information extends from basic descriptive information about policies to evaluations of the effects of different kinds of policies and implementation strategies.

> **RECOMMENDATION 9.2 To strengthen the evidence base for the design and application of conflict of interest policies, the U.S. Department of Health and Human Services should coordinate the development and funding of a research agenda to study the impact of conflicts of interest on the quality of medical research, education, and practice and on practice guideline development and to examine the positive and negative effects of conflict of interest policies on these outcomes.**

Within the U.S. Department of Health and Human Services, NIH, the Agency for Healthcare Quality and Research, and the Food and Drug Administration should be involved in defining a research agenda that addresses questions and concerns about implementing, enforcing, and possibly refining conflict of interest policies. The research agenda not only should investigate government policies, however, but also should investigate the policies that academic medical centers, professional societies, and other private groups have adopted.

Research on the characteristics and outcomes of conflict of interest policies would be desirable for several reasons. First, research could clarify which relationships are associated with higher or lower risks of undue influence or loss of trust, as well as the magnitudes of such associations. Second, such research may identify which conflict of interest policies and procedures are effective in achieving the desired outcomes and under what circumstances various policies are likely to be more effective. These data could then guide modifications in policies and procedures. Third, research on conflict of interest policies may identify unintended adverse consequences of well-intentioned policies and, in turn, inform corrective policy changes. Unintended negative consequences might include disproportionate administrative burdens and the inhibition of constructive collaborations between academia and industry. Strengthening the evidence base should allow institutions to improve their conflict of interest policies to better protect the integrity of their missions and to maintain the trust of the public.

References

AAFP (American Academy of Family Physicians). 2006a. *Board of Directors Report V to the 2006 Congress of Delegates*. Leawood, KS: AAFP. http://www.aafp.org/online/etc/medialib/aafp_org/documents/about/congress/2006/bd-rpts/brdrptv.Par.0001.File.tmp/Board%20Report%20V%20on%20AAFP%20and%20Nondues%20Revenue.pdf (accessed April 8, 2009).

AAFP. 2006b. *Full Disclosure for CME Activities: American Family Physician authors*. Leawood, KS: AAFP. http://www.aafp.org/online/etc/medialib/aafp_org/documents/news_pubs/afp/afpconflictofinterestform.Par.0001.File.tmp/COI-form-2008.pdf (accessed August 12, 2008).

AAMC (Association of American Medical Colleges). 1998. *Guidelines for Dealing with Faculty Conflicts of Commitment and Conflicts of Interest in Research*. Adopted by AAMC Executive Council, February 1990; revised, January 1998. Washington, DC: AAMC.

AAMC. 2001. *Protecting Subjects, Preserving Trust, Promoting Progress: Policy and Guidelines for the Oversight of Individual Financial Interests in Human Subjects Research*. Washington, DC: AAMC. http://www.aamc.org/research/coi/firstreport.pdf (accessed June 23, 2008).

AAMC. 2002. *Protecting Subjects, Preserving Trust, Promoting Progress II: Principles and Recommendations for Oversight of an Institution's Financial Interests in Human Subjects Research*. Washington, DC: AAMC. http://www.aamc.org/research/coi/2002coireport.pdf (accessed September 19, 2008).

AAMC. 2004. *Clinical Trial Contracts: A Discussion of Four Selected Provisions*. Washington, DC: AAMC. https://services.aamc.org/Publications/showfile.cfm?file=version6.pdf&prd_id=76&prv_id=75&pdf_id=6 (accessed February 21, 2009).

AAMC. 2008a. Table 3: applicants to U.S. medical schools by state of legal residence, 1997-2008. In *AAMC Facts*. Washington, DC: AAMC. http://www.aamc.org/data/facts/2008/2008slr.htm (accessed March 22, 2009).

AAMC. 2008b. *Compact Between Biomedical Graduate Students and Their Research Advisors*. Washington, DC: AAMC. https://services.aamc.org/Publications/showfile.cfm?file=version127.pdf (accessed February 18, 2009).

AAMC. 2008c. *Industry Funding of Medical Education*. Washington, DC: AAMC. https://services.aamc.org/Publications/showfile.cfm?file=version114.pdf&prd_id=232 (accessed October 10, 2008).

AAMC. 2008d. *Medical Schools*. Washington, DC: AAMC. http://www.aamc.org/medicalschools.htm (accessed November 17, 2008).

AAMC. 2008e. Table 26: total active enrollment by U.S. medical school and sex, 2003-2008. In *AAMC Facts*. Washington, DC: AAMC. http://www.aamc.org/data/facts/2008/school-enrll0308.htm (accessed March 4, 2009).

AAMC-AAU (Association of American Universities). 2008. *Protecting Patients, Preserving Integrity, Advancing Health: Accelerating the Implementation of COI Policies in Human Subjects Research*. Report of the AAMC-AAU Advisory Committee on Financial Conflicts of Interest in Human Subjects Research. Washington, DC: AAMC. https://services.aamc.org/Publications/showfile.cfm?file=version107.pdf&prd_id=220&prv_id=268&pdf_id=107 (accessed September 19, 2008).

AAU. 2001. *Report on Individual and Institutional Financial Conflict of Interest*. Report of the AAU Task Force on Research Accountability. Washington, DC: AAU. http://www.aau.edu/research/COI.01.pdf (accessed August 1, 2008).

AAUP (American Association of University Professors). 2004. *Statement on Corporate Funding of Academic Research*. Washington, DC: AAUP. http://www.aaup.org/NR/rdonlyres/7B12F7B9-FA00-44DD-999F-FFA21AAE1F39/0/CorporateFundingonAcaResearch.pdf (accessed April 17, 2009).

AAUP/ACE (American Council on Education). 1965. On preventing conflicts of interest in government-sponsored research at universities; a joint statement of the Council of the American Association of University Professors and The American Council on Education. *AAUP Bulletin* 51:42-43.

ABIM (American Board of Internal Medicine) Foundation, ACP-ASIM (American College of Physicians-American Society of Internal Medicine) Foundation, and European Federation of Internal Medicine. 2002. Medical professionalism in the new millennium: a physician charter. *Annals of Internal Medicine* 136(3):243-246.

ABMS (American Board of Medical Specialties). 2007. *American Board of Medical Specialties Board Certification Editorial Background*. Evanston, IL: ABMS. http://www.abms.org/news_and_events/media_newsroom/pdf/abms_editorialbackground.pdf (accessed September 25, 2008).

ACC/AHA (American College of Cardiology/American Heart Association). 2009. *Methodology Manual for ACC/AHA Guideline Writing Committees*. Report of the ACC/AHA Task Force on Practice Guidelines. Washington, DC: ACC/AHA. http://www.acc.org/qualityandscience/clinical/manual/pdfs/methodology.pdf (accessed April 8, 2009).

ACCME (Accreditation Council for Continuing Medical Education). 2005. *ACCME's Glossary of Terms and Abbreviations*. Chicago, IL: ACCME. http://cores33webs.mede.uic.edu/capp/public/public_docs/accme_glossary_of_terms.pdf (accessed October 22, 2008).

ACCME. 2008a. *ACCME Annual Report Data 2007*. Chicago, IL: ACCME. http://www.accme.org/dir_docs/doc_upload/207fa8e2-bdbe-47f8-9b65-52477f9faade_uploaddocument.pdf (accessed October 22, 2008).

ACCME. 2008b. *Accredited CME Is Education That Matters to Patient Care*. Chicago, IL: ACCME. http://www.accme.org/dir_docs/doc_upload/d6b96a50-084c-485b-b71a-6b405b9c07d8_uploaddocument.pdf (accessed December 30, 2008).

ACCME. 2008c. *Executive Summary of the November 2008 Meetings of the ACCME Board of Directors*. Chicago, IL: ACCME. http://www.accme.org/dir_docs/whats_new/607a2906-dda2-4e9d-b6cf-7922723b46a1_uploadfile.pdf (accessed February 22, 2009).

ACCME. 2008d. *For Comment: ACCME Proposes Additional Features of Independence in Accredited Continuing Medical Education*. Chicago, IL: ACCME. http://www.accme.org/dir_docs/doc_upload/d64b68f6-9525-43af-9074-719f92ad7c97_uploaddocument.pdf (accessed October 7, 2008).

ACCME. 2009. *List of Accredited Providers.* Chicago, IL: ACCME. http://www.accme.org/index.cfm/fa/home.popular/popular_id/66be063a-8081-40f2-9615-042a733485d8.cfm (accessed March 23, 2009).

ACE (American Council on Education). 2007. *Working Paper on Conflict of Interest.* Washington, DC: ACE. http://www.acenet.edu/AM/Template.cfm?Section=Home&TEMPLATE=/CM/ContentDisplay.cfm&CONTENTID=26137 (accessed April 17, 2009).

ACGME (Accreditation Council for Graduate Medical Education). 2002. *Principles to Guide the Relationship Between Graduate Medical Education and Industry.* Chicago, IL: ACGME. http://www.acgme.org/acWebsite/positionPapers/pp_GMEGuide.pdf (accessed August 12, 2008).

ACGME. 2007a. *ACGME Institutional Requirements.* Chicago, IL: ACGME. http://www.acgme.org/acWebsite/irc/irc_IRCpr07012007.pdf (accessed September 3, 2008).

ACGME. 2007b. *The ACGME at a Glance.* Chicago, IL: ACGME. http://www.acgme.org/acWebsite/newsRoom/newsRm_acGlance.asp (accessed September 3, 2008).

ACGME. 2008. *Glossary of Terms.* Chicago, IL: ACGME. http://www.acgme.org/acwebsite/about/ab_acgmeglossary.pdf (accessed August 12, 2008).

ACIP (Advisory Committee on Immunization Practices). 2007. Recommended adult immunization schedule: United States, October 2007-September 2008. *Annals of Internal Medicine* 147(10):725-729.

ACN (American College of Neuropsychopharmacology). 2004. Executive summary. In *Preliminary Report of the Task Force on SSRIs and Suicidal Behavior in Youth.* Nashville, TN: ACN. http://www.acnp.org/asset.axd?id=aad01592-01b2-4672-ad28-119537460ffa (accessed December 15, 2008).

ACR (American College of Radiology). 2007a. *ACR Practice Guideline for the Performance of Total Body Irradiation.* Reston, VA: ACR.

ACR (American College of Rheumatology). 2007b. *Code of Ethics of the American College of Rheumatology, Inc.* http://www.rheumatology.org/about/codeofethics/index.pdf (accessed September 2, 2008).

Adair, R. F., and L. R. Holmgren. 2005. Do drug samples influence resident prescribing behavior? A randomized trial. *American Journal of Medicine* 118(8):881-884.

AdvaMed (Advanced Medical Technology Association). 2008. *Code of Ethics on Interactions with Health Care Professionals.* Effective July 1, 2009. Washington, DC: AdvaMed. http://www.advamed.org/NR/rdonlyres/61D30455-F7E9-4081-B219-12D6CE347585/0/AdvaMedCodeofEthicsRevisedandRestatedEffective20090701.pdf (accessed February 9, 2009).

AFMI (*Annals of Family Medicine,* Inc.). 2008. *Annals of Family Medicine Manuscript Agreement.* Leawood, KS: AFMI. http://www.annfammed.org/misc/pdfsanddocs/ManuscriptAgreement08.doc (accessed December 30, 2008).

AGREE (Appraisal of Guidelines Research and Evaluation) Collaboration. 2003. *AGREE Instrument Training Manual.* http://www.agreecollaboration.org/pdf/aitraining.pdf (accessed February 23, 2009).

AHRP (Alliance for Human Research Protection). 2006. *Vioxx Redux: FDA on the Sidelines as Marketing Subsumes Evidence: Surviving Sepsis-NEJM.* New York, NY: AHRP. http://www.ahrp.org/cms/index2.php?option=com_content&do_pdf=1&id=366 (accessed April 25, 2008).

AJN (*American Journal of Nephrology*). 2008. *Guidelines for Authors.* http://content.karger.com/ProdukteDB/produkte.asp?Aktion=JournalGuidelines&ProduktNr=223979 (accessed September 15, 2008).

Alpert, J. S., S. Furman, and L. Smaha. 2002. Conflicts of interest: science, money, and health. *Archives of Internal Medicine* 162(6):635-637.

AMA (American Medical Association). 2002. *Opinion E-8.061: Clarifying Addendum [to Opinion 8.061, "Gifts to physicians from industry"]*. Chicago, IL: AMA. http://www.ama-assn.org/ama/pub/category/4263.html (accessed September 2, 2008).

AMA. 2006. *The Physician's Recognition Award and Credit System: Information for Accredited Providers and Physicians*. Chicago, IL: AMA. http://www.ama-assn.org/ama1/pub/upload/mm/455/pra2006.pdf (accessed September 15, 2008).

AMA. 2007. Opinion 8.047: industry representatives in clinical settings. *Code of Medical Ethics*. http://www.ama-assn.org/ama1/pub/upload/mm/Code_of_Med_Eth/opinion/opinion8047.html (accessed April 8, 2009).

AMA. 2008a. Continuing medical education for licensure reregistration. In *State Medical Licensure Requirements and Statistics 2009*. Chicago, IL: AMA. http://www.ama-assn.org/ama1/pub/upload/mm/40/table16-2009.pdf (accessed February 10, 2009)

AMA. 2008b. *Guidance on New Procedures for CME*. Chicago, IL: AMA. http://www.ama-assn.org/ama/pub/education-careers/continuing-medical-education/physicians-recognition-award-credit-system/cme-help/guidance-new-procedure-cme.shtml (accessed February 16, 2009).

AMA. 2008c. *Reference Committee Highlights: 2008 Annual Meeting for the AMA House of Delegates*. Chicago, IL: AMA. http://www.ama-assn.org/ama1/pub/upload/mm/471/refcomhighlights.pdf (accessed January 29, 2009).

AMSA (American Medical Student Association). 2008a. *Focus on Pharm Free*. Reston, VA: AMSA. http://www.amsa.org/prof/focus.cfm (accessed August 1, 2008).

AMSA. 2008b. *PharmFree Scorecard 2008*. Reston, VA: AMSA. http://amsascorecard.org/ (accessed September 19, 2008).

Ancker, J. S., and A. Flanagin. 2007. A comparison of conflict of interest policies at peer-reviewed journals in different scientific disciplines. *Science and Engineering Ethics* 13(2):147-157.

Andersen, M., J. Kragstrup, and J. Sondergaard. 2006. How conducting a clinical trial affects physicians' guideline adherence and drug preferences. *Journal of the American Medical Association* 295(23):2759-2764.

Angel, J. E. 2003. Industry sponsorship of continuing medical education. *Journal of the American Medical Association* 290(9):1149-1150; author reply 1150.

APA (American Psychiatric Association). 2008. *Minutes*. APA Board of Trustees meeting, Arlington, VA, March 9-10. Arlington, VA: APA.

Arenberg, D. 2007. Bronchioloalveolar lung cancer: ACCP evidence-based clinical practice guidelines (2nd edition). *Chest* 132(3 Suppl.):306S-313S.

Armon, C., C. E. Argoff, J. Samuels, and M. M. Backonja. 2007. Assessment: use of epidural steroid injections to treat radicular lumbosacral pain: report of the Therapeutics and Technology Assessment Subcommittee of the American Academy of Neurology. *Neurology* 68(10):723-729.

Armstrong, D. 2005. Surgery journal threatens ban for authors' hidden conflicts. *Wall Street Journal*, December 28, B1.

Armstrong, D. 2006. Medical reviews face criticism over lapses. *Wall Street Journal*, July 19, B1, B2.

Arnau, J. M., A. Vallano, A. Lopez, F. Pellise, M. J. Delgado, and N. Prat. 2006. A critical review of guidelines for low back pain treatment. *European Spine Journal* 15(5):543-553.

ASCO (American Society of Clinical Oncology). 2007. *Journal of Clinical Oncology Author Disclosure Declaration*. Alexandria, VA: ASCO. http://jco.ascopubs.org/misc/jco_disclosure_contribution.pdf (accessed November 11, 2008).

ASCO. 2008. *American Society of Clinical Oncology Guideline Procedures Manual*. Alexandria, VA: ASCO. http://www.asco.org/ASCO/Quality+Care+%26+Guidelines/Practice+Guidelines/development+process (accessed February 27, 2009).

ASH (American Society of Hematology). 2008. Principles, policies, and procedures related to conflict-of-interest. Written statement given to the Institute of Medicine Committee on Conflict of Interest in Medical Research, Education, and Practice, Washington, DC.

The Associated Press. 2008. *Medical Experts Fight Drug Industry Influence.* http://www.ctv.ca/servlet/ArticleNews/story/CTVNews/20080911/medical_schools_080911/20080911?hub=Health (accessed December 15, 2008).

ATS (American Thoracic Society). 2008. *Policy on Management of Conflict of Interest in Official ATS Documents, Projects, and Conferences.* New York, NY: ATS. http://www.thoracic.org/sections/about-ats/coi-management/resources/coi-policy.pdf (accessed August 19, 2008).

AUTM (Association of University Technology Managers). 2007. *AUTM U.S. Licensing Activity Survey: FY2006.* Deerfield, IL: AUTM. http://www.autm.net/Content/NavigationMenu/Surveys/LicensingSurveysAUTM/FY2006LicensingActivitySurvey/AUTM_06_US_LSS_FNL.pdf (accessed January 10, 2009).

Avorn, J. 2006. Dangerous deception—hiding the evidence of adverse drug effects. *New England Journal of Medicine* 355(21):2169-2171.

Avorn, J., and S. B. Soumerai. 1983. Improving drug-therapy decisions through educational outreach. A randomized controlled trial of academically based "detailing." *New England Journal of Medicine* 308(24):1457-1463.

Ayanian, J. Z., M. B. Landrum, S. L. Normand, E. Guadagnoli, and B. J. McNeil. 1998. Rating the appropriateness of coronary angiography—do practicing physicians agree with an expert panel and with each other? *New England Journal of Medicine* 338(26):1896-1904.

Ayres, C. G., and H. M. Griffith. 2007. Perceived barriers to and facilitators of the implementation of priority clinical preventive services guidelines. *American Journal of Managed Care* 13(3):150-155.

Bahtsevani, C., G. Uden, and A. Willman. 2004. Outcomes of evidence-based clinical practice guidelines: a systematic review. *International Journal of Technology Assessment in Health Care* 20(4):427-433.

Bailey, R. 2008. *Scrutinizing Industry-Funded Science: The Crusade Against Conflicts of Interest.* New York: American Council on Science and Health. http://www.acsh.org/docLib/20080401_scrutinizing.pdf (accessed October 10, 2008).

Barnes, B. E., J. G. Cole, C. T. King, R. Zukowski, T. Allgier-Baker, D. M. Rubio, and L. E. Thorndyke. 2007. A risk stratification tool to assess commercial influences on continuing medical education. *Journal of Continuing Education in the Health Professions* 27(4):234-240.

Barnes, D. E., and L. A. Bero. 1998. Why review articles on the health effects of passive smoking reach different conclusions. *Journal of the American Medical Association* 279(19):1566-1570.

Baru, J. S., D. A. Bloom, K. Muraszko, and C. E. Koop. 2001. John Holter's shunt. *Journal of the American College of Surgeons* 192(1):79-85.

Battista, R. N., and M. J. Hodge. 1995. Setting priorities and selecting topics for clinical practice guidelines. *Canadian Medical Association Journal* 153(9):1233-1237.

Baumann, M. H., S. Z. Lewis, and D. Gutterman. 2007. ACCP evidence-based guideline development: a successful and transparent approach addressing conflict of interest, funding, and patient-centered recommendations. *Chest* 132(3):1015-1024.

Baxter, P. 2006. Medicine and the pharmaceutical industry. *Developmental Medicine and Child Neurology* 48(8):627.

Beauchamp, T. L., and J. F. Childress. 2009. *Principles of Biomedical Ethics*, 6th ed. New York: Oxford University Press.

Bekelman, J. E., Y. Li, and C. P. Gross. 2003. Scope and impact of financial conflicts of interest in biomedical research: a systematic review. *Journal of the American Medical Association* 289(4):454-465.

Bellin, M., S. McCarthy, L. Drevlow, and C. Pierach. 2004. Medical students' exposure to pharmaceutical industry marketing: a survey at one U.S. medical school. *Academic Medicine* 79(11):1041-1045.

Benet, L. Z. 2008. Perspectives on financial relationships and conflicts of interest in basic and early stage translational research: reflections on 28 years of organized COI experience at UCSF. Presentation to the Institute of Medicine Committee on Conflict of Interest in Medical Research, Education, and Practice, Washington, DC, May 22.

Bennett, C. L., M. R. Somerfield, D. G. Pfister, C. Tomori, S. Yakren, and P. B. Bach. 2003. Perspectives on the value of American Society of Clinical Oncology clinical guidelines as reported by oncologists and health maintenance organizations. *Journal of Clinical Oncology* 21(5):937-941.

Bennett, K. J., D. L. Sackett, R. B. Haynes, V. R. Neufeld, P. Tugwell, and R. Roberts. 1987. A controlled trial of teaching critical appraisal of the clinical literature to medical students. *Journal of the American Medical Association* 257(18):2451-2454.

Benz, E. 2008. Untitled. Presentation to the Institute of Medicine Committee on Conflict of Interest in Medical Research, Education, and Practice, Washington, DC, May 22.

Bero, L. 2008. "Experimental" institutional models for corporate funding of academic research: unknown effects on the research enterprise. *Journal of Clinical Epidemiology* 61(7):629-633.

Bero, L., and D. Rennie. 1996. Influences on the quality of published drug studies. *International Journal of Technology Assessment in Health Care* 12(2):209-237.

Bero, L., A. Galbraith, and D. Rennie. 1992. The publication of sponsored symposiums in medical journals. *New England Journal of Medicine* 327(16):1135-1140.

Bero, L., S. Glantz, and M. K. Hong. 2005. The limits of competing interest disclosures. *Tobacco Control* 14(2):118-126.

Bero, L., F. Oostvogel, P. Bacchetti, and K. Lee. 2007. Factors associated with findings of published trials of drug-drug comparisons: why some statins appear more efficacious than others. *PLoS Medicine* 4(6):e184.

Berwick, D. M. 1998. Developing and testing changes in delivery of care. *Annals of Internal Medicine* 128(8):651-656.

Bhargava, N., J. Qureshi, and N. Vakil. 2007. Funding source and conflict of interest disclosures by authors and editors in gastroenterology specialty journals. *American Journal of Gastroenterology* 102(6):1146-1150.

Bimber, B. 1996. *The Politics of Expertise in Congress: The Rise and Fall of the Office of Technology Assessment.* Albany, NY: State University of New York Press.

Bird, S. J., and R. E. Spier. 2005. The complexity of competing and conflicting interests. *Science and Engineering Ethics* 11(4):515-517.

Blake, R. L., Jr., and E. K. Early. 1995. Patients' attitudes about gifts to physicians from pharmaceutical companies. *Journal of the American Board of Family Practice* 8(6):457-464.

Blumenthal, D. 2004. Doctors and drug companies. *New England Journal of Medicine* 351(18):1885-1890.

Blumenthal, D., E. G. Campbell, N. Causino, and K. S. Louis. 1996a. Participation of life-science faculty in research relationships with industry. *New England Journal of Medicine* 335(23):1734-1739.

Blumenthal, D., N. Causino, E. Campbell, and K. S. Louis. 1996b. Relationships between academic institutions and industry in the life sciences—an industry survey. *New England Journal of Medicine* 334(6):368-373.

Blumenthal, D., E. G. Campbell, M. S. Anderson, N. Causino, and K. S. Louis. 1997. Withholding research results in academic life science. Evidence from a national survey of faculty. *Journal of the American Medical Association* 277(15):1224-1228.

Bodenheimer, T. 2000. Uneasy alliance—clinical investigators and the pharmaceutical industry. *New England Journal of Medicine* 342(20):1539-1544.

Bodenheimer, T., R. A. Berenson, and P. Rudolf. 2007. The primary care-specialty income gap: why it matters. *Annals of Internal Medicine* 146(4):301-306.

Bok, D. 2003. *Universities in the Marketplace*. Princeton, NJ: Princeton University Press.

Boltri, J. M., E. R. Gordon, and R. L. Vogel. 2002. Effect of antihypertensive samples on physician prescribing patterns. *Family Medicine* 34(10):729-731.

Boluyt, N., C. R. Lincke, and M. Offringa. 2005. Quality of evidence-based pediatric guidelines. *Pediatrics* 115(5):1378-1391.

Bombardier, C., L. Laine, A. Reicin, D. Shapiro, R. Burgos-Vargas, B. Davis, R. Day, et al. 2000. Comparison of upper gastrointestinal toxicity of rofecoxib and naproxen in patients with rheumatoid arthritis. VIGOR Study Group. *New England Journal of Medicine* 343(21):1520-1528, 2 p following 1528.

Bond, E. C., and S. Glynn. 1995. Recent trends in support for biomedical research and development. In *Sources of Medical Technology: Universities and Industry*. Washington, DC: National Academy Press.

Borgert, C. J. 2007. Conflict of interest or contravention of science? *Regulatory Toxicology and Pharmacology* 48(1):4-5.

Borie, D. C., J. J. O'Shea, and P. S. Changelian. 2004. JAK3 inhibition, a viable new modality of immunosuppression for solid organ transplants. *Trends in Molecular Medicine* 10(11):532-541.

Bossuyt, P. M., J. B. Reitsma, D. E. Bruns, C. A. Gatsonis, P. P. Glasziou, L. M. Irwig, J. G. Lijmer, et al. 2003. Towards complete and accurate reporting of studies of diagnostic accuracy: the STARD initiative. Standards for Reporting of Diagnostic Accuracy. *Clinical Chemistry* 49(1):1-6.

Boston University. 2007. *Policies for Interactions Among Clinicians at Boston Medical Center and Boston University School of Medicine and Representatives of the Healthcare Industry.* Boston, MA: Boston University, http://www.bu.edu/cms/www.bumc.bu.edu/busm-od/files/Images/Policies/BMC-BUSM%20Industry%20Interactions%20_July%2026_.pdf (accessed September 25, 2008).

Bowman, M. A. 1986. The impact of drug company funding on the content of continuing medical education. *Journal of Continuing Education in the Health Professions* 6(1):66-69.

Bowman, M. A., and D. L. Pearle. 1988. Changes in drug prescribing patterns related to commercial company funding of continuing medical education. *Journal of Continuing Education in the Health Professions* 8(1):13-20.

Boyd, E. A. 2008. Individual and organizational financial relationships with industry: what do we know? Presentation to the Institute of Medicine Committee on Conflict of Interest in Medical Research, Education, and Practice, Washington, DC, May 22.

Boyd, E. A., and L. A. Bero. 2000. Assessing faculty financial relationships with industry: a case study. *Journal of the American Medical Association* 284(17):2209-2214.

Boyd, E. A., and L. A. Bero. 2006. Improving the use of research evidence in guideline development. 4. Managing conflicts of interests. *Health Research Policy and Systems* 4:16.

Boyd, E. A., and L. A. Bero. 2007. Defining financial conflicts and managing research relationships: an analysis of university conflict of interest committee decisions. *Science and Engineering Ethics* 13(4):415-435.

Boyd, E. A., M. K. Cho, and L. A. Bero. 2003. Financial conflict-of-interest policies in clinical research: issues for clinical investigators. *Academic Medicine* 78(8):769-774.

Boyd, E. A., S. Lipton, and L. A. Bero. 2004. Implementation of financial disclosure policies to manage conflicts of interest. *Health Affairs* 23(2):206-214.

Brandeis, L. D. 1914. What publicity can do. In *Other People's Money and How the Bankers Use It*. New York: Frederick A Stokes Company.

Braunwald, E., A. S. Fauci, D. Kasper, S. Hauser, D. Longo, and J. L. Jameson. 2001. *Harrison's Principles of Internal Medicine*, vol. 2. New York: McGraw-Hill Professional.

Bravo, N. R. 2008. *Director's Column: Managing Financial Conflicts of Interests*. Bethesda, MD: Office of Extramural News, National Institutes of Health. http://nexus.od.nih.gov/nexus/nexus.aspx?ID=81&Month=6&Year=2008 (accessed December 2, 2008).

Brennan, T. A., and M. M. Mello. 2007. Sunshine laws and the pharmaceutical industry. *Journal of the American Medical Association* 297(11):1255-1257.

Brennan, T. A., D. J. Rothman, L. Blank, D. Blumenthal, S. C. Chimonas, J. J. Cohen, J. Goldman, et al. 2006. Health industry practices that create conflicts of interest: a policy proposal for academic medical centers. *Journal of the American Medical Association* 295(4):429-433.

Brewer, D. 1998. The effect of drug sampling policies on residents' prescribing. *Family Medicine* 30(7):482-486.

Brody, B. 2006a. Intellectual property and biotechnology: the U.S. internal experience—Part I. *Kennedy Institute of Ethics Journal* 16(1):1-37.

Brody, B. 2006b. Intellectual property and biotechnology: the U.S. internal experience—Part II. *Kennedy Institute of Ethics Journal* 16(2):105-128.

Brody, H. 2007. *Hooked: Ethics, the Medical Profession, and the Pharmaceutical Industry*. Lanham, MD: Rowman & Littlefield Publishers, Inc.

Brotzman, G. L., and D. H. Mark. 1993. The effect on resident attitudes of regulatory policies regarding pharmaceutical representative activities. *Journal of General Internal Medicine* 8(3):130-134.

Budiansky, S. 1983. Academic interest conflicts: laxity of Californian practice. *Nature* 301(5896):102.

Burgers, J. S., R. Grol, N. S. Klazinga, M. Makela, and J. Zaat. 2003. Towards evidence-based clinical practice: an international survey of 18 clinical guideline programs. *International Journal for Quality in Health Care* 15(1):31-45.

Burton, T. M. 2006. Amid alarm bells, a blood substitute keeps pumping; ten in trial have heart attacks, but data aren't published; FDA allows a new study; doctors' pleas are ignored. *Wall Street Journal*, February 22, A1, A12.

Business Wire. 2008. National study by PeopleMetrics Rx confirms importance of emotional connection between pharmaceutical sales reps and physicians. *Business Wire*, August 11. http://www.reuters.com/article/pressRelease/idUS168653+11-Aug-2008+BW20080811 (accessed September 25, 2008).

Cain, D., G. Loewenstein, and D. Moore. 2005. The dirt on coming clean: the perverse effects of disclosing conflicts of interest. *Journal of Legal Studies* 34:1-25.

Camilleri, M., G. L. Gamble, S. L. Kopecky, M. B. Wood, and M. L. Hockema. 2005. Principles and process in the development of the Mayo Clinic's individual and institutional conflict of interest policy. *Mayo Clinic Proceedings* 80(10):1340-1346.

Campbell, E. G., and D. Blumenthal. 2000. Academic industry relationships in biotechnology: a primer on policy and practice. *Cloning* 2(3):129-136.

Campbell, E. G., K. S. Louis, and D. Blumenthal. 1998. Looking a gift horse in the mouth: corporate gifts supporting life sciences research. *Journal of the American Medical Association* 279(13):995-999.

Campbell, E. G., B. R. Clarridge, M. Gokhale, L. Birenbaum, S. Hilgartner, N. A. Holtzman, and D. Blumenthal. 2002. Data withholding in academic genetics: evidence from a national survey. *Journal of the American Medical Association* 287(4):473-480.

Campbell, E. G., J. B. Powers, D. Blumenthal, and B. Biles. 2004. Inside the triple helix: technology transfer and commercialization in the life sciences. *Health Affairs* 23(1):64-76.

Campbell, E. G., J. S. Weissman, C. Vogeli, B. R. Clarridge, M. Abraham, J. E. Marder, and G. Koski. 2006. Financial relationships between institutional review board members and industry. *New England Journal of Medicine* 355(22):2321-2329.

Campbell, E. G., R. L. Gruen, J. Mountford, L. G. Miller, P. D. Cleary, and D. Blumenthal. 2007a. A national survey of physician-industry relationships. *New England Journal of Medicine* 356(17):1742-1750.

Campbell, E. G., J. S. Weissman, S. Ehringhaus, S. R. Rao, B. Moy, S. Feibelmann, and Susan Dorr Goold. 2007b. Institutional academic-industry relationships. *Journal of the American Medical Association* 298(15):1779-1786.

Campbell, S. M., M. Hann, M. O. Roland, J. A. Quayle, and P. G. Shekelle. 1999. The effect of panel membership and feedback on ratings in a two-round Delphi survey: results of a randomized controlled trial. *Medical Care* 37(9):964-968.

Campbell, W. A. 2007. The high cost of free lunch. *Obstetrics and Gynecology* 110(4):931-932; author reply 932-933.

Caplan, R. M. 1996. History of the Society of Medical College Directors of Continuing Medical Education (SMCDCME): the first twelve years, 1976-1988. *The Journal of Continuing Education in the Health Professions* 16:14-24.

Carlat, D. 2007. Dr. Drug Rep. *The New York Times*, November 25, Sec. 6, p. 64.

Carlson, G. A., P. S. Jensen, R. L. Findling, R. E. Meyer, J. Calabrese, M. P. DelBello, G. Emslie, et al. 2003. Methodological issues and controversies in clinical trials with child and adolescent patients with bipolar disorder: report of a consensus conference. *Journal of Child and Adolescent Psychopharmacology* 13(1):13-27.

Carpenter, D. In press. The ambiguous emergence of an organizational identity: pharmaceutical regulation at the FDA, 1947-1961. In *Reputation and Power: Organizational Image and Pharmaceutical Regulation at the FDA*, edited by D. Carpenter. Princeton, NJ: Princeton University Press. http://www.fas.harvard.edu/~polecon/EmergenceofAmerican PharmceuticalRegulation.pdf (accessed February 10, 2009).

Carroll, A. E., R. C. Vreeman, J. Buddenbaum, and T. S. Inui. 2007. To what extent do educational interventions impact medical trainees' attitudes and behaviors regarding industry-trainee and industry-physician relationships? *Pediatrics* 120(6):e1528-e1535.

Cassell, G. 2008. Untitled. Presentation for Eli Lilly and Company to the Institute of Medicine Committee on Conflict of Interest in Medical Research, Education, and Practice, Washington, DC, May 22.

Cates, J. R., D. N. Young, D. S. Bowerman, and R. C. Porter. 2006. An independent AGREE evaluation of the Occupational Medicine Practice Guidelines. *The Spine Journal* 6(1):72-77.

CBO (Congressional Budget Office). 1986. *Physician Reimbursement Under Medicare: Options for Change*. Washington, DC: CBO. http://www.cbo.gov/ftpdocs/59xx/doc5967/doc13b-Entire.pdf (accessed September 25, 2008).

CBO. 2007. *Research on the Comparative Effectiveness of Medical Treatments: Options for an Expanded Federal Role*. Testimony by Director Peter R. Orszag before the House Ways and Means Subcommittee on Health, June 12. http://www.cbo.gov/ftpdocs/82xx/doc8209/Comparative_Testimony.pdf.

Cech, T. R., and J. S. Leonard. 2001. Conflicts of interest—moving beyond disclosure. *Science* 291(5506):989.

CEJA (Council on Ethical and Judicial Affairs, American Medical Association). 2008. *Industry Support of Professional Education in Medicine*. CEJA Report 1-A-08. Chicago, IL: CEJA. http://www.acme-assn.org/advocacy_pg/ceja1.doc (accessed September 15, 2008).

Chabner, B. A. 2008. Conflict of interest: in the eye of the beholder? *The Oncologist* 13(3): 212-213.

Chaillet, N., E. Dube, M. Dugas, F. Audibert, C. Tourigny, W. D. Fraser, and A. Dumont. 2006. Evidence-based strategies for implementing guidelines in obstetrics: a systematic review. *Obstetrics and Gynecology* 108(5):1234-1245.

Chan, A. W., A. Hrobjartsson, M. T. Haahr, P. C. Gotzsche, and D. G. Altman. 2004a. Empirical evidence for selective reporting of outcomes in randomized trials: comparison of protocols to published articles. *Journal of the American Medical Association* 291(20):2457-2465.

Chan, A. W., K. Krleza-Jeric, I. Schmid, and D. G. Altman. 2004b. Outcome reporting bias in randomized trials funded by the Canadian Institutes of Health Research. *Canadian Medical Association Journal* 171(7):735-740.

Changelian, P. S., D. Moshinsky, C. F. Kuhn, M. E. Flanagan, M. J. Munchhof, T. M. Harris, J. L. Doty, J. Sun, C. R. Kent, K. S. Magnuson, D. G. Perregaux, P. S. Sawyer, and E. M. Kudlacz. 2008. The specificity of JAK3 kinase inhibitors. *Blood* 111(4):2155-2157.

Chapman, S. W., W. E. Dismukes, L. A. Proia, R. W. Bradsher, P. G. Pappas, M. G. Threlkeld, and C. A. Kauffman. 2008. Clinical practice guidelines for the management of blastomycosis: 2008 update by the Infectious Diseases Society of America. *Clinical Infectious Diseases* 46(12):1801-1812.

Chaudhry, S., S. Schroter, R. Smith, and J. Morris. 2002. Does declaration of competing interests affect readers' perceptions? A randomised trial. *British Medical Journal* 325(7377):1391-1392.

Chew, L. D., T. S. O'Young, T. K. Hazlet, K. A. Bradley, C. Maynard, and D. S. Lessler. 2000. A physician survey of the effect of drug sample availability on physicians' behavior. *Journal of General Internal Medicine* 15(7):478-483.

Chimonas, S., T. A. Brennan, and D. J. Rothman. 2007. Physicians and drug representatives: exploring the dynamics of the relationship. *Journal of General Internal Medicine* 22(2):184-190.

Chiong, W. 2003. Industry-to-physician marketing and the cost of prescription drugs. *American Journal of Bioethics* 3(3):W28-W29.

Cho, M. K., R. Shohara, A. Schissel, and D. Rennie. 2000. Policies on faculty conflicts of interest at US universities. *Journal of the American Medical Association* 284(17):2203-2208.

Choudhry, N. K., H. T. Stelfox, and A. S. Detsky. 2002. Relationships between authors of clinical practice guidelines and the pharmaceutical industry. *Journal of the American Medical Association* 287(5):612-617.

Chren, M. M., and C. S. Landefeld. 1994. Physicians' behavior and their interactions with drug companies. A controlled study of physicians who requested additions to a hospital drug formulary. *Journal of the American Medical Association* 271(9):684-689.

Christie, J. D., I. M. Rosen, L. M. Bellini, T. V. Inglesby, J. Lindsay, A. Alper, and D. A. Asch. 1998. Prescription drug use and self-prescription among resident physicians. *Journal of the American Medical Association* 280(14):1253-1255.

Citron, P. 2008. Medical device considerations. Presentation to the Institute of Medicine Committee on Conflict of Interest in Medical Research, Education, and Practice, Washington, DC, January 21.

Clamon, J. B. 2003. The search for a cure: combating the problem of conflicts of interest that currently plagues biomedical research. *Iowa Law Review* 89(1):235-271.

Clancy, C. M. 2003. Back to the future. *Health Affairs* Suppl Web Exclusives: W3-314–W3-316.

CMS (Centers for Medicare and Medicaid Services). 2006. *National Coverage Determinations with Data Collection as a Condition of Coverage: Coverage with Evidence Development.* Baltimore, MD: CMS. http://www.cms.hhs.gov/mcd/ncpc_view_document.asp?id=8 (accessed October 7, 2008).

CMS. 2008. *Factsheet: Physician Self-Referral and Hospital Ownership Disclosure Provisions in the IPPS FY 2009 Final Rule.* Baltimore, MD: CMS. http://www.Cms.Hhs.Gov/Apps/Media/Press/Factsheet.Asp?Counter=3226&Intnumperpage=10&Checkdate=&Checkkey=&Srchtype=1&Numdays=3500&Srchopt=0&Srchdata=&Keywordtype=All&Chknewstype=6&Intpage=&Showall=&Pyear=&Year=&Desc=False&Cboorder=Date (accessed March 21, 2009).

CMSS (Council of Medical Specialty Societies). 1999. *Ethics Statement.* Chicago, IL: CMSS. http://www.cmss.org/print.cfm?itemid=1100 (accessed November 20, 2008).

CMSS. 2008. *CMSS Task Force on Professionalism and Conflict of Interest in Medicine: Recommendations.* Chicago, IL: CMSS. http://www.cmss.org/index.cfm?p=readmore&itemID=1358&detail=News%20Items (accessed February 26, 2009).

Cochrane Collaboration. 2002. *An Introduction to Meta-Analysis.* Baltimore, MD: Cochrane Collaboration. http://www.cochrane-net.org/openlearning/html/mod3-2.htm (accessed March 23, 2009).

Cochrane Collaboration. 2005. *Glossary of Terms in the Cochrane Collaboration.* Baltimore, MD: Cochrane Collaboration. http://www.cochrane.org/resources/handbook/glossary.pdf (accessed July 17, 2008).

Cochrane Collaboration. 2006. *Commercial Sponsorship and the Cochrane Collaboration.* Baltimore, MD: Cochrane Collaboration. http://www.cochrane.org/docs/commercial-sponsorship.htm (accessed March 21, 2009).

COGR (Council on Governmental Relations). 2002. *Recognizing and Managing Personal Financial Conflicts of Interest.* Washington, DC: COGR. http://www.cogr.edu/docs/COIFinal.pdf (accessed September 19, 2008).

COGR. 2003. *Approaches to Developing an Institutional Conflict of Interest Policy.* Washington, DC: COGR. http://www.cogr.edu/files/publications_Conflicts.cfm (accessed November 11, 2008).

Columbia College of Physicians and Surgeons. 2008. *New Conflict of Interest Policy Regarding Education and Clinical Care for P&S Faculty.* New York: Columbia College of Physicians and Surgeons. http://www.columbia.edu/cu/administration/policylibrary/policies/00bb9c661ce31c31011eda93ef3c0008/PS_COI_policy_2008_FINAL_1232028040523.pdf (accessed March 23, 2009).

Columbia University. 2009. *Columbia University Policy on Financial Conflicts of Interest and Research.* New York: Columbia University. http://evpr.columbia.edu/files_sponsored projectprocedures/imce_shared/COI_Policy_4_3_09_new.pdf (accessed April 10, 2009).

Columbia University. Undated. *Responsible Conduct of Research: Conflicts of Interest.* New York, NY: Columbia University. http://www.columbia.edu/ccnmtl/projects/rcr/rcr_conflicts/ (accessed March 21, 2009).

CONSORT Group. 2001. The revised CONSORT statement for reporting randomized trials: explanation and elaboration. *Annals of Internal Medicine* 134(8):663-694.

CONSORT Group. 2007. *About CONSORT.* http://www.consort-statement.org/?o=1014 (accessed September 26, 2008).

Cook, D. M., E. A. Boyd, C. Grossmann, and L. A. Bero. 2007. Reporting science and conflicts of interest in the lay press. *PLoS ONE* 2(12):e1266.

Cooper, D. S., G. M. Doherty, B. R. Haugen, R. T. Kloos, S. L. Lee, S. J. Mandel, E. L. Mazzaferri, et al. 2006a. Management guidelines for patients with thyroid nodules and differentiated thyroid cancer. *Thyroid* 16(2):109-142.

Cooper, R. J., M. Gupta, M. S. Wilkes, and J. R. Hoffman. 2006b. Conflict of interest disclosure policies and practices in peer-reviewed biomedical journals. *Journal of General Internal Medicine* 21(12):1248-1252.

Cosgrove, L., S. Krimsky, M. Vijayaraghavan, and L. Schneider. 2006. Financial ties between DSM-IV panel members and the pharmaceutical industry. *Psychotherapy and Psychosomatics* 75(3):154-160.

Cottingham, A. H., A. L. Suchman, D. K. Litzelman, R. M. Frankel, D. L. Mossbarger, P. R. Williamson, D. C. Baldwin, Jr., and T. S. Inui. 2008. Enhancing the informal curriculum of a medical school: a case study in organizational culture change. *Journal of General Internal Medicine* 23(6):715-722.

Council on Scientific Affairs and Council on Ethical and Judicial Affairs. 1990. Conflicts of interest in medical center/industry research relationships. *Journal of the American Medical Association* 263(20):2790-2793.

Coyle, S. L., Ethics and Human Rights Committee, and American College of Physicians-American Society of Internal Medicine. 2002a. Physician-industry relations. Part 1. Individual physicians. *Annals of Internal Medicine* 136(5):396-402.

Coyle, S. L., Ethics and Human Rights Committee, and American College of Physicians-American Society of Internal Medicine. 2002b. Physician-industry relations. Part 2. Organizational issues. *Annals of Internal Medicine* 136(5):403-406.

Coyne, D. W. 2007. Influence of industry on renal guideline development. *Clinical Journal of the American Society of Nephrology* 2(1):3-7; discussion 13-14.

CTSA (Clinical and Translational Science Awards). 2009. *About CTSA*. http://www.ctsaweb.org/index.cfm?fuseaction=home.aboutHome (accessed March 19, 2009).

Culliton, B. J. 1982. The academic-industrial complex. *Science* 216(4549):960-962.

Curfman, G. D., S. Morrissey, and J. M. Drazen. 2005. Expression of concern: Bombardier et al., "Comparison of upper gastrointestinal toxicity of rofecoxib and naproxen in patients with rheumatoid arthritis," N Engl J Med 2000;343:1520-8. *New England Journal of Medicine* 353(26):2813-2814.

Cutrona, S. L., S. Woolhandler, K. E. Lasser, D. H. Bor, D. McCormick, and D. U. Himmelstein. 2008. Characteristics of recipients of free prescription drug samples: a nationally representative analysis. *American Journal of Public Health* 98(2):284-289.

Dana, J., and G. Loewenstein. 2003. A social science perspective on gifts to physicians from industry. *Journal of the American Medical Association* 290(2):252-255.

Darves, B. 2007. *Physician Employment and Compensation Outlook for '07*. http://www.nejmjobs.org/career-resources/physician-compensation-trends.aspx (accessed September 17, 2008).

Daugherty, K. K. 2005. Samples: to use or not to use? *Journal of Clinical Pharmacy and Therapeutics* 30(6):505-510.

Davidoff, F. 2002. Between the lines: navigating the uncharted territory of industry-sponsored research. *Health Affairs* 21(2):235-242.

Davidoff, F., C. D. DeAngelis, J. M. Drazen, M. G. Nicholls, J. Hoey, L. Hojgaard, R. Horton, et al. 2001. Sponsorship, authorship and accountability. *Canadian Medical Association Journal* 165(6):786-788.

Davidson, J. M., A. M. Aquino, S. C. Woodward, and W. W. Wilfinger. 1999. Sustained microgravity reduces intrinsic wound healing and growth factor responses in the rat. *FASEB Journal* 13(2):325-329.

Davis, M. 1998. Conflict of interest. In *Encyclopedia of Applied Ethics*, edited by R. Chadwick. London: Academic Press.

Davis, M., and A. Stark. 2001. *Conflict of Interest in the Professions*. New York: Oxford University Press.

Dawson, D. L. 2006. Training in carotid artery stenting: do carotid simulation systems really help? *Vascular* 14(5):256-263.

de Haas, E. R., H. C. de Vijlder, W. S. van Reesema, J. J. van Everdingen, and H. A. Neumann. 2007. Quality of clinical practice guidelines in dermatological oncology. *Journal of the European Academy of Dermatology and Venereology* 21(9):1193-1198.

DeAngelis, C. D. 2006. The influence of money on medical science. *Journal of the American Medical Association* 296(8):996-998.

DeAngelis, C. D., and P. B. Fontanarosa. 2008. Impugning the integrity of medical science: the adverse effects of industry influence. *Journal of the American Medical Association* 299(15):1833-1835.

DeAngelis, C. D., P. B. Fontanarosa, and A. Flanagin. 2001. Reporting financial conflicts of interest and relationships between investigators and research sponsors. *Journal of the American Medical Association* 286(1):89-91.

Decker, R. S., L. Wimsatt, A. G. Trice, and J. A. Konstan. 2007. *A Profile of Federal-Grant Administrative Burden Among Federal Demonstration Partnership Faculty.* Report of the Faculty Standing Committee of the Federal Demonstration Partnership. Washington, DC: Federal Demonstration Partnership. http://www.thefdp.org/Faculty%20burden%20survey%20report%20-%20complete.pdf (accessed July 2, 2008).

Dellinger, R. P., M. M. Levy, J. M. Carlet, J. Bion, M. M. Parker, R. Jaeschke, K. Reinhart, et al. 2008. Surviving Sepsis Campaign: international guidelines for management of severe sepsis and septic shock: 2008. *Intensive Care Medicine* 34(1):17-60.

DeMaria, A. N. 2004. Authors, industry, and review articles. *Journal of the American College of Cardiology* 43(6):1130-1131.

Demske, G. E. 2008. *Examining the Relationship Between the Medical Device Industry and Physicians.* Testimony before the Special Committee on Aging, U.S. Senate, February 27. http://aging.senate.gov/events/hr188gd2.pdf (accessed August 11, 2008).

DeRenzo, E. G. 2005. Conflict-of-interest policy at the National Institutes of Health: the pendulum swings wildly. *Kennedy Institute of Ethics Journal* 15(2):199-210.

Detsky, A. S. 2006. Sources of bias for authors of clinical practice guidelines. *Canadian Medical Association Journal* 175(9):1033, 1035.

Deyo, R. A., B. M. Psaty, G. Simon, E. H. Wagner, and G. S. Omenn. 1997. The messenger under attack—intimidation of researchers by special-interest groups. *New England Journal of Medicine* 336(16):1176-1180.

Dicken, P., L. J. Grant, and S. Jones. 2000. An evaluation of the characteristics and performance of neonatal phototherapy equipment. *Physiological Measurement* 21(4):493-503.

Dickersin, K. 1990. The existence of publication bias and risk factors for its occurrence. *Journal of the American Medical Association* 263(10):1385-1389.

Dickersin, K., S. Chan, T. C. Chalmers, H. S. Sacks, and H. Smith, Jr. 1987. Publication bias and clinical trials. *Controlled Clinical Trials* 8(4):343-353.

Dickersin, K., Y. I. Min, and C. L. Meinert. 1992. Factors influencing publication of research results. Follow-up of applications submitted to two institutional review boards. *Journal of the American Medical Association* 267(3):374-378.

Dickler, R. M. 2007. Untitled. Letter on behalf of the Association of American Medical Colleges to Glenn Hackbarth, Chair of Medicare Payment Advisory Commission, January 4. http://www.aamc.org/advocacy/teachhosp/medpac/hackbarth_final.pdf (accessed September 3, 2008).

DiMasi, J. A., R. W. Hansen, and H. G. Grabowski. 2003. The price of innovation: new estimates of drug development costs. *Journal of Health Economics* 22(2):151-185.

DiMasi, J. A., R. W. Hansen, and H. G. Grabowski. 2004. *Assessing Claims About the Cost of New Drug Development: A Critique of the Public Citizen and TB Alliance Reports.* http://csdd.tufts.edu/_documents/www/Doc_231_45_735.pdf (accessed October 10, 2008).

Dinan, M. A., K. P. Weinfurt, J. Y. Friedman, J. S. Allsbrook, J. Gottlieb, K. A. Schulman, M. A. Hall, J. K. Dhillon, and J. Sugarman. 2006. Comparison of conflict of interest policies and reported practices in academic medical centers in the United States. *Accountability in Research* 13(4):325-342.

DOJ (U.S. Department of Justice). 2001. *Tap Pharmaceutical Products Inc. and Seven Others Charged with Health Care Crimes; Company Agrees to Pay $875 Million to Settle Charges.* Press release, October 3. Washington, DC: DOJ. http://www.usdoj.gov/opa/pr/2001/October/513civ.htm (accessed September 17, 2008).

DOJ. 2004. *Warner-Lambert to Pay $430 Million to Resolve Criminal & Civil Health Care Liability Relating to Off-Label Promotion.* Press release, May 13. Washington, DC: DOJ. http://www.usdoj.gov/opa/pr/2004/May/04_civ_322.htm (accessed September 25, 2008).

DOJ. 2006. *Medtronic to Pay United States $40 Million to Settle Kickback Allegations.* Press release, July 18. Washington, DC: DOJ. http://www.usdoj.gov/opa/pr/2006/July/06_civ_445.html (accessed September 25, 2008).

DOJ. 2007a. *Five Companies in Hip and Knee Replacement Industry Avoid Prosecution by Agreeing to Compliance Rules and Monitoring.* Press release, September 27. Washington, DC: DOJ. http://www.usdoj.gov/usao/nj/press/files/pdffiles/hips0927.rel.pdf (accessed July 28, 2008).

DOJ. 2007b. *Jazz Pharmaceuticals, Inc. Agrees to Pay $20 Million to Resolve Criminal and Civil Allegations in "Off-Label" Marketing Investigation.* Press release, July 13. Washington, DC: DOJ. http://www.usdoj.gov/usao/nye/pr/2007/2007jul13a.html (accessed September 25, 2008).

DOJ. 2008. *Merck to Pay More Than $650 Million to Resolve Claims of Fraudulent Price Reporting and Kickbacks.* Press release, February 7. Washington, DC: DOJ. http://www.usdoj.gov/opa/pr/2008/February/08_civ_094.html (accessed September 17, 2008).

Drazen, J. M., and G. D. Curfman. 2002. Financial associations of authors. *New England Journal of Medicine* 346(24):1901-1902.

Druker, B. J., F. Guilhot, S. G. O'Brien, I. Gathmann, H. Kantarjian, N. Gattermann, M. W. Deininger, et al. 2006. Five-year follow-up of patients receiving imatinib for chronic myeloid leukemia. *New England Journal of Medicine* 355(23):2408-2417.

Duderstadt, J. J. 2000. *A University for the 21st Century.* Ann Arbor: University of Michigan Press.

Duffy, S. P. 2003. Pharmaceutical companies to pay $1.2B in Medicare fraud. *The Legal Intelligencer*, June 24. http://www.law.com/jsp/article.jsp?id=1056139882090 (accessed August 11, 2008).

Duvall, D. G. 2006. Conflict of interest or ideological divide: the need for ongoing collaboration between physicians and industry. *Current Medical Research and Opinion* 22(9):1807-1812.

Easterbrook, P. J., J. A. Berlin, R. Gopalan, and D. R. Matthews. 1991. Publication bias in clinical research. *Lancet* 337(8746):867-872.

Eaton, L. 2005. Medical editors issue guidance on ghost writing. *British Medical Journal* 330(7498):988.

EBM Working Group. 1992. Evidence-based medicine. A new approach to teaching the practice of medicine. *Journal of the American Medical Association* 268(17):2420-2425.

ECRI Institute. 2007. Sales representatives and other outsiders in the OR. *Operating Room Risk Management*, November, vol. 2. Plymouth Meeting, PA: ECRI Institute. https://www.ecri.org/Documents/Sample_ORRM_Outsiders_in_the_OR_Report.pdf (accessed December 30, 2008).

Editors. 2007. Probing STROBE. *Epidemiology* 18(6):789-790.

Edwards, J. C., L. Szczepanski, J. Szechinski, A. Filipowicz-Sosnowska, P. Emery, D. R. Close, R. M. Stevens, et al. 2004. Efficacy of B-cell-targeted therapy with rituximab in patients with rheumatoid arthritis. *New England Journal of Medicine* 350(25):2572-2581.

EHP (Environmental Health Perspectives). 2009. Instructions to authors. *Environmental Health Perspectives* 115(7):366-371. http://www.ehponline.org/docs/admin/instructions.pdf (accessed August 12, 2008).

Ehringhaus, S., and D. Korn. 2004. *U.S. Medical School Policies on Individual Financial Conflicts of Interest: Results of an AAMC Survey.* Washington, DC: Association of American Medical Colleges. http://www.aamc.org/research/coi/coiresults2003.pdf (accessed October 21, 2008).

Ehringhaus, S., and D. Korn. 2006. *Principles for Protecting Integrity in the Conduct and Reporting of Clinical Trials.* Washington, DC: Association of American Medical Colleges. http://www.aamc.org/research/clinicaltrialsreporting/clinicaltrialsreporting.pdf (accessed October 22, 2008).

Ehringhaus, S., J. S. Weissman, J. L. Sears, S. D. Goold, S. Feibelmann, and E. G. Campbell. 2008. Responses of medical schools to institutional conflicts of interest. *Journal of the American Medical Association* 299(6):665-671.

Eichacker, P. Q., C. Natanson, and R. L. Danner. 2006. Surviving sepsis—practice guidelines, marketing campaigns, and Eli Lilly. *New England Journal of Medicine* 355(16): 1640-1642.

Eichacker, P. Q., C. Natanson, and R. L. Danner. 2007. Separating practice guidelines from pharmaceutical marketing. *Critical Care Medicine* 35(12):2877-2878; author reply 2878-2880.

Eisenberg, J. M., and D. Zarin. 2002. Health technology assessment in the United States. Past, present, and future. *International Journal of Technology Assessment in Health Care* 18(2):192-198.

Elliott, C. 2004. Pharma goes to the laundry: public relations and the business of medical education. *Hastings Center Report* 34(5):18-23.

Elliott, C. 2006. The drug pushers. *Atlantic Magazine*, April. http://www.theatlantic.com/doc/200604/drug-reps/3 (accessed November 21, 2008).

Emanuel, E., and D. Steiner. 1995. Institutional conflict of interest. *New England Journal of Medicine* 332(4):262-267.

Emanuel, E., and D. F. Thompson. 2008. The concept of conflicts of interest. In *The Oxford Textbook of Clinical Research Ethics*, edited by E. Emanuel, C. Grady, R. Crouch, R. Lie, F. Miller, and D. Wendler. New York: Oxford University Press.

EPIC Investigators. 1994. Use of a monoclonal antibody directed against the platelet glycoprotein IIb/IIIa receptor in high-risk coronary angioplasty. The EPIC Investigation. *New England Journal of Medicine* 330(14):956-961.

Epstein, A. M. 2007a. Pay for performance at the tipping point. *New England Journal of Medicine* 356(5):515-517.

Epstein, A. M., T. H. Lee, and M. B. Hamel. 2004. Paying physicians for high-quality care. *New England Journal of Medicine* 350(4):406-410.

Epstein, R. A. 2005. Pharma furor: why two high-profile attacks on big drug companies flunk the test of basic economics. *Legal Affairs Magazine*, January/February. http://www.legalaffairs.org/issues/January-February-2005/review_epstein_janfeb05.msp (accessed September 15, 2008).

Epstein, R. A. 2007b. Conflicts of interest in health care: who guards the guardians? *Perspectives in Biology and Medicine* 50(1):72-88.

Erde, E. L. 1996. Conflicts of interests in medicine: a philosophical and ethical morphology. In *Conflicts of Interest in Clinical Practice and Research*, edited by R. G. Spece, D. S. Shimm, and A. E. Buchanan. New York: Oxford University Press

Ethics, Law, and Humanities Committee of the American Academy of Neurology. 2001. Practice advisory: participation of neurologists in direct-to-consumer advertising. *Neurology* 56(8):995-996.

Fahrenthold, D. A. 2006. U.S. criminal charges filed against scientist; undisclosed consulting deals at issue. *The Washington Post*, December 5, B06.

Fallat, M. E., and J. Glover. 2007. Professionalism in pediatrics. *Pediatrics* 120(4): e1123-e1133.

Farrell, R. J., Y. Ang, P. Kileen, D. S. O'Briain, D. Kelleher, P. W. Keeling, and D. G. Weir. 2000. Increased incidence of non-Hodgkin's lymphoma in inflammatory bowel disease patients on immunosuppressive therapy but overall risk is low. *Gut* 47(4):514-519.

FASEB (Federation of American Societies for Experimental Biology). 2008. *COI Toolkit: Recommendations, Tools, and Resources for the Conduct and Management of Financial Relationships Between Academia and Industry in Biomedical Research.* Bethesda, MD: FASEB. http://opa.faseb.org/pages/Advocacy/coi/Toolkit.htm (accessed March 21, 2009).

FDA (U.S. Food and Drug Administration). 1995. *Confidential Financial Disclosure Report for Special Government Employees.* Silver Spring, MD: FDA. http://www.fda.gov/oc/advisory/conflictofinterest/disclosure.pdf (accessed July 3, 2008).

FDA. 1997. Guidance for industry: industry-supported scientific and educational activities. *Federal Register* 62(232):64093-64100.

FDA. 2000. *FDA Guidance on Conflict of Interest for Advisory Committee Members, Consultants and Experts—Table of Contents.* Silver Spring, MD: FDA. http://www.fda.gov/oc/advisory/conflictofinterest/guidance.html (accessed July 3, 2008).

FDA. 2001. *Guidance: Financial Disclosure by Clinical Investigators.* Silver Spring, MD: FDA. http://www.fda.gov/oc/guidance/financialdis.html (accessed February 2, 2009).

FDA. 2004a. *Innovation or Stagnation: Challenge and Opportunity on the Critical Path to New Medical Products.* Washington, DC: U.S. Department of Health and Human Services. http://www.fda.gov/oc/initiatives/criticalpath/whitepaper.html (accessed February 18, 2009).

FDA. 2004b. *RE: P040012 ACCULINK Carotid Stent System and RX ACCULINK Carotid Stent System.* Letter from Dr. Tillman, Center for Devices and Radiological Health, to Ms. Anastas, Guidant Corporation, August 30. http://www.fda.gov/cdrh/pdf4/P040012a.pdf (accessed October 7, 2008).

FDA. 2008a. *Guidance for the Public, FDA Advisory Committee Members, and FDA Staff: Public Availability of Advisory Committee Members' Financial Interest Information and Waivers.* Silver Spring, MD: FDA. http://www.fda.gov/oc/advisory/GuidancePolicyRegs/ACDisclosureFINALGuidance080408.pdf (accessed August 18, 2008).

FDA. 2008b. *Guidance for the Public, FDA Advisory Committee Members, and FDA Staff on Procedures for Determining Conflict of Interest and Eligibility for Participation in FDA Advisory Committees.* Silver Spring, MD: FDA. http://www.fda.gov/oc/advisory/GuidancePolicyRegs/ACWaiverCriteriaFINALGuidance080408.pdf (accessed August 12, 2008).

Finance Committee, U.S. Senate. 2007. *Use of Educational Grants by Pharmaceutical Manufacturers.* Washington, DC: U.S. Government Printing Office. http://www.acme-assn.org/home/prb042507a.pdf (accessed November 21, 2008).

Finance Committee, U.S. Senate. 2008. *Support for S.2029, the Grassley-Kohl Physician Payments Sunshine Act.* Washington, DC: U.S. Government Printing Office. http://finance.senate.gov/press/Gpress/2008/prg071608a.pdf (accessed August 12, 2008).

Fink, A., J. Kosecoff, M. Chassin, and R. H. Brook. 1984. Consensus methods: characteristics and guidelines for use. *American Journal of Public Health* 74(9):979-983.

Finkelstein, S. N., K. A. Isaacson, and J. J. Frishkopf. 1984. The process of evaluating medical technologies for third-party coverage. *Journal of Health Care Technology* 1(2):89-102.

Finn, P. B. 2006. The negotiation and development of a clinical trial agreement. *Journal of Biolaw & Business* 9(2):21-27.

Fitch, K., P. Lazaro, M. D. Aguilar, Y. Martin, and S. J. Bernstein. 1999. Physician recommendations for coronary revascularization: variations by clinical specialty. *The European Journal of Public Health* 9(3):181-187.

Fitz, M. M., D. Homan, S. Reddy, C. H. Griffith III, E. Baker, and K. P. Simpson. 2007. The hidden curriculum: medical students' changing opinions toward the pharmaceutical industry. *Academic Medicine* 82(10 Suppl.):S1-S3.

Flanagin, A., L. A. Carey, P. B. Fontanarosa, S. G. Phillips, B. P. Pace, G. D. Lundberg, and D. Rennie. 1998. Prevalence of articles with honorary authors and ghost authors in peer-reviewed medical journals. *Journal of the American Medical Association* 280(3):222-224.

Flanagin, A., P. B. Fontanarosa, and C. D. DeAngelis. 2006. Update on JAMA's conflict of interest policy. *Journal of the American Medical Association* 296(2):220-221.

Fletcher, S. W. 2008. Chairman's summary of the conference. In *Continuing Education in the Health Professions: Improving Healthcare Through Lifelong Learning*, edited by M. Hager. New York: Josiah Macy, Jr., Foundation.

Flewell, M. N. 2007. A look ahead . . . oncology sales force effectiveness in an era of unprecedented competition. *Oncology Business Review*, June. http://www.oncbiz.com/documents/OBRjune07_ImpactRX.pdf (accessed August 27, 2007).

Fontanarosa, P. B., and C. D. DeAngelis. 2008. Publication of clinical trials in JAMA. *Journal of the American Medical Association* 299(1):95-96.

Fontanarosa, P. B., A. Flanagin, and C. D. DeAngelis. 2005. Reporting conflicts of interest, financial aspects of research, and role of sponsors in funded studies. *Journal of the American Medical Association* 294(1):110-111.

Frankel, M. S. 1996. Perception, reality, and the political context of conflict of interest in university-industry relationships. *Academic Medicine* 71(12):1297-1304.

Friedman, P. J. 1992. The troublesome semantics of conflict of interest. *Ethics & Behavior* 2(4):245-251.

Frohlich, E. P. 2007. The high cost of free lunch. *Obstetrics and Gynecology* 110(4):931; author reply 932-933.

Fugh-Berman, A. 2005. The corporate coauthor. *Journal of General Internal Medicine* 20(6):546-548.

Fugh-Berman, A., and S. Ahari. 2007. Following the script: how drug reps make friends and influence doctors. *PLoS Medicine* 4(4):e150.

Fugh-Berman, A., and S. Batt. 2006. This may sting a bit. *Virtual Mentor* 8(6):412-415. http://virtualmentor.ama-assn.org/2006/06/oped1-0606.html (accessed October 10, 2008).

Fung, A., M. Graham, and D. Weil. 2007. *Full Disclosure: The Perils and Promise of Transparency.* New York, NY: Cambridge University Press.

Gagnon, M. A., and J. Lexchin. 2008. The cost of pushing pills: a new estimate of pharmaceutical promotion expenditures in the United States. *PLoS Medicine* 5(1):e1.

GAO (U.S. General Accounting Office [Now the U.S. Government Accountability Office]). 1995. *Increased HMO Oversight Could Improve Quality and Access to Care.* Report to the Special Committee on Aging, U.S. Senate. Washington, DC: GAO. http://www.gao.gov/archive/1995/he95155.pdf (accessed February 10, 2009).

GAO. 2001. *HHS Direction Needed to Address Financial Conflicts of Interest.* Report to the Ranking Minority Member, Subcommittee on Public Health, Committee on Health, Education, Labor, and Pensions, U.S. Senate. Washington, DC: GAO. http://www.gao.gov/new.items/d0289.pdf (accessed February 10, 2009).

GAO. 2003. *Most Federal Agencies Need to Better Protect Against Financial Conflicts of Interest.* Report to the Honorable Richard C. Shelby, U.S. Senate. Washington, DC: GAO. http://www.gao.gov/new.items/d0431.pdf (accessed August 1, 2008).

Garb, S. 1960. Teaching medical students to evaluate drug advertising. *Journal of Medical Education* 35:729-739.

Garber, A. M. 2001. Evidence-based coverage policy. *Health Affairs* 20(5):62-82.

Gaus, C. R. 2003. An insider's perspective on the near-death experience of AHCPR. *Health Affairs* Suppl Web Exclusives:W3-311–W3-313.

Gelijns, A. C., and S. O. Thier. 2002. Medical innovation and institutional interdependence: rethinking university-industry connections. *Journal of the American Medical Association* 287(1):72-77.

Geppert, C. M. 2007. Medical education and the pharmaceutical industry: a review of ethical guidelines and their implications for psychiatric training. *Academic Psychiatry* 31(1):32-39.

Gibbons, R. V., F. J. Landry, D. L. Blouch, D. L. Jones, F. K. Williams, C. R. Lucey, and K. Kroenke. 1998. A comparison of physicians' and patients' attitudes toward pharmaceutical industry gifts. *Journal of General Internal Medicine* 13(3):151-154.

Gibson, L. 2004. GlaxoSmithKline to publish clinical trials after US lawsuit. *British Medical Journal* 328(7455):1513.

Gilbert, S. 2008. The invisible hand in medical education. *Bioethics Forum*, March 14. http://www.thehastingscenter.org/bioethicsforum/post.aspx?id=736&terms=the+invisible+hand+and+%23filename+*.html (accessed October 10, 2008).

Ginsburg, P. B., and J. M. Grossman. 2005. When the price isn't right: how inadvertent payment incentives drive medical care. *Health Affairs* Suppl Web Exclusives:W5-376–W5-384.

Ginzberg, E., and A. Dutka. 1989. *The Financing of Biomedical Research.* Baltimore, MD: The Johns Hopkins University Press.

Glaser, B. E., and L. A. Bero. 2005. Attitudes of academic and clinical researchers toward financial ties in research: a systematic review. *Science and Engineering Ethics* 11(4):553-573.

Goldblum, O. M., and M. J. Franzblau. 2006. Academic medical centers and conflicts of interest. *Journal of the American Medical Association* 295(24):2845-2846; author reply 2848-2849.

Golden, G. A., J. N. Parochka, and K. M. Overstreet. 2002. Medical education and communication companies: an updated in-depth profile. *Journal of Continuing Education in the Health Professions* 22(1):55-62.

Golder, S., and Y. K. Loke. 2008. Is there evidence for biased reporting of published adverse effects data in pharmaceutical industry-funded studies? *British Journal of Clinical Pharmacology* 66(6):767-773.

Goldner, J. A. 2000. Dealing with conflicts of interest in biomedical research: IRB oversight as the next best solution to the abolitionist approach. *Journal of Law, Medicine and Ethics* 28(4):379-404.

Goldsmith, L. A. 2006. Conflict of interest and the JID. *Journal of Investigative Dermatology* 126:2147-2148.

Goldstein, J. 2008. Implant firms pay doctors millions; as joint replacements have increased, so have payments to surgeons. *The Philadelphia Inquirer*, June 29, A01.

Goldstein, N. 2006. Financial conflicts of interest in biomedical human subject research. *Journal of Biolaw & Business* 9(1):26-37.

Goozner, M. 2004. *Unrevealed: Non-Disclosure of Conflicts of Interest in Four Leading Medical and Scientific Journals.* Washington, DC: Center for Science in the Public Interest. http://cspinet.org/new/pdf/unrevealed_final.pdf (accessed November 11, 2008).

Goroll, A. H., R. A. Berenson, S. C. Schoenbaum, and L. B. Gardner. 2007. Fundamental reform of payment for adult primary care: comprehensive payment for comprehensive care. *Journal of General Internal Medicine* 22(3):410-415.

Gott, V. L., D. E. Alejo, and D. E. Cameron. 2003. Mechanical heart valves: 50 years of evolution. *Annals of Thoracic Surgery* 76(6):S2230-S2239.

Gotzsche, P. C., A. Hrobjartsson, H. K. Johansen, M. T. Haahr, D. G. Altman, and A. W. Chan. 2006. Constraints on publication rights in industry-initiated clinical trials. *Journal of the American Medical Association* 295(14):1645-1646.

Gotzsche, P. C., A. Hrobjartsson, H. K. Johansen, M. T. Haahr, D. G. Altman, and A. W. Chan. 2007. Ghost authorship in industry-initiated randomised trials. *PLoS Medicine* 4(1):e19.

Gourley, R. H. 1966. Teaching the evaluation of drug advertising to medical students. *Virginia Medical Monthly (1918)* 93(8):459-461.

GRADE Working Group. 2004. Grading quality of evidence and strength of recommendations. *British Medical Journal* 328(7454):1490.

Grassley, C. 2008a. *Grassley Works to Protect Medicare Dollars, Empower Patients with Information.* Press release, July 25. http://www.senate.gov/~finance/press/Gpress/2008/prg072508.pdf (accessed September 17, 2008).

Grassley, C. 2008b. Payment to physicians. *Congressional Record—Senate*, p. S5030. http://frwebgate.access.gpo.gov/cgi-bin/getpage.cgi?dbname=2008_record&page=S5030&position=all (accessed July 17, 2008).

Grassley, C. 2009. *Grassley Works to Disclose Financial Ties Between Drug Companies and Doctors.* Press release, January 22. http://grassley.senate.gov/news/Article.cfm?customel_dataPageID_1502=18901 (accessed February 26, 2009).

Gray, B. H., M. K. Gusmano, and S. R. Collins. 2003. AHCPR and the changing politics of health services research. *Health Affairs* Suppl Web Exclusives:W3-283–W3-307.

Gray, S. W., F. J. Hlubocky, M. J. Ratain, and C. K. Daugherty. 2007. Attitudes toward research participation and investigator conflicts of interest among advanced cancer patients participating in early phase clinical trials. *Journal of Clinical Oncology* 25(23):3488-3494.

Greene, J. A. 2007. Pharmaceutical marketing research and the prescribing physician. *Annals of Internal Medicine* 146(10):742-748.

Grilli, R., N. Magrini, A. Penna, G. Mura, and A. Liberati. 2000. Practice guidelines developed by specialty societies: the need for a critical appraisal. *Lancet* 355(9198):103-106.

Grimshaw, J. M., and I. T. Russell. 1993. Effect of clinical guidelines on medical practice: a systematic review of rigorous evaluations. *Lancet* 342(8883):1317-1322.

Grimshaw, J. M., L. Shirran, R. Thomas, G. Mowatt, C. Fraser, L. Bero, R. Grilli, et al. 2001. Changing provider behavior: an overview of systematic reviews of interventions. *Medical Care* 39(8 Suppl. 2):II2-II45.

Grimshaw, J. M., M. Eccles, R. Thomas, G. MacLennan, C. Ramsay, C. Fraser, and L. Vale. 2006. Toward evidence-based quality improvement. Evidence (and its limitations) of the effectiveness of guideline dissemination and implementation strategies 1966-1998. *Journal of General Internal Medicine* 21(Suppl. 2):S14-S20.

Gross, C. P. 2007. Conflict of interest and clinical research. Presentation to the Institute of Medicine Committee on Conflict of Interest in Medical Research, Education, and Practice, Washington, DC, November 6.

Gross, C. P., A. R. Gupta, and H. M. Krumholz. 2003. Disclosure of financial competing interests in randomised controlled trials: cross sectional review. *British Medical Journal* 326(7388):526-527.

Groves, K. E., I. Sketris, and S. E. Tett. 2003. Prescription drug samples—does this marketing strategy counteract policies for quality use of medicines? *Journal of Clinical Pharmacy and Therapeutics* 28(4):259-271.

Guirguis-Blake, J., N. Calonge, T. Miller, A. Siu, S. Teutsch, and E. Whitlock. 2007. Current processes of the U.S. Preventive Services Task Force: refining evidence-based recommendation development. *Annals of Internal Medicine* 147(2):117-122.

Guyatt, G. H., and D. Rennie. 2002. *Users' Guides to the Medical Literature: A Manual for Evidence-Based Clinical Practice.* Chicago, IL: American Medical Association.

Guyatt, G. H., D. L. Sackett, J. C. Sinclair, R. Hayward, D. J. Cook, and R. J. Cook. 1995. Users' guides to the medical literature. IX. A method for grading health care recommendations. Evidence-Based Medicine Working Group. *Journal of the American Medical Association* 274(22):1800-1804.

Guyatt, G. H., G. Vist, Y. Falck-Ytter, R. Kunz, N. Magrini, and H. Schunemann. 2006. An emerging consensus on grading recommendations? *ACP Journal Club* 144(1):A8-A9.

Guyatt, G. H., A. D. Oxman, R. Kunz, G. E. Vist, Y. Falck-Ytter, and H. J. Schunemann. 2008. What is "quality of evidence" and why is it important to clinicians? *British Medical Journal* 336(7651):995-998.

Hafferty, F. W. 1998. Beyond curriculum reform: confronting medicine's hidden curriculum. *Academic Medicine* 73(4):403-407.

Haidet, P. 2008. Where we're headed: a new wave of scholarship on educating medical professionalism. *Journal of General Internal Medicine* 23(7):1118-1119.

Haivas, I., S. Schroter, F. Waechter, and R. Smith. 2004. Editors' declaration of their own conflicts of interest. *Canadian Medical Association Journal* 171(5):475-476.

Hall, M. A., E. Dugan, R. Balkrishnan, and D. Bradley. 2002. How disclosing HMO physician incentives affects trust. *Health Affairs* 21(2):197-206.

Halperin, E. C., P. Hutchison, and R. C. Barrier, Jr. 2004. A population-based study of the prevalence and influence of gifts to radiation oncologists from pharmaceutical companies and medical equipment manufacturers. *International Journal of Radiation Oncology, Biology, Physics* 59(5):1477-1483.

Hampson, L. A., M. Agrawal, S. Joffe, C. P. Gross, J. Verter, and E. J. Emanuel. 2006. Patients' views on financial conflicts of interest in cancer research trials. *New England Journal of Medicine* 355(22):2330-2337.

Hampson, L. A., J. E. Bekelman, and C. Gross. 2008. Empirical data on conflicts of interest. In *The Oxford Textbook of Clinical Research Ethics*, edited by E. Emanuel, C. Grady, R. A. Crouch, R. K. Lie, F. G. Miller, and D. Wendler. New York: Oxford University Press.

Hardell, L., M. J. Walker, B. Walhjalt, L. S. Friedman, and E. D. Richter. 2007. Secret ties to industry and conflicting interests in cancer research. *American Journal of Industrial Medicine* 50(3):227-233.

Harpole, L. H., M. J. Kelley, G. Schreiber, E. M. Toloza, J. Kolimaga, and D. C. McCrory. 2003. Assessment of the scope and quality of clinical practice guidelines in lung cancer. *Chest* 123(1 Suppl.):7S-20S.

Harris, G. 2005. Ban on federal scientists' consulting nears. *The New York Times*, February 1, A15.

Harris, G. 2008. Top psychiatrist didn't report drug makers' pay. *The New York Times*, October 4, A1.

Harris, G., and B. Carey. 2008. Researchers fail to reveal full drug pay. *The New York Times*, June 8, A1.

The Harvard Crimson. 1988. Interesting conflicts: medical school. http://www.thecrimson.com/article.aspx?ref=144875 (accessed July 28, 2008).

Hasenfeld, R., and P. G. Shekelle. 2003. Is the methodological quality of guidelines declining in the US? Comparison of the quality of US Agency for Health Care Policy and Research (AHCPR) guidelines with those published subsequently. *Quality and Safety in Health Care* 12(6):428-434.

Hauser, R. G., and B. J. Maron. 2005. Lessons from the failure and recall of an implantable cardioverter-defibrillator. *Circulation* 112(13):2040-2042.

Hauser, S. L., E. Waubant, D. L. Arnold, T. Vollmer, J. Antel, R. J. Fox, A. Bar-Or, et al. 2008. B-cell depletion with rituximab in relapsing-remitting multiple sclerosis. *New England Journal of Medicine* 358(7):676-688.

Healy, D. 2006. Did regulators fail over selective serotonin reuptake inhibitors? *British Medical Journal* 333(7558):92-95.

Healy, D., and D. Cattell. 2003. Interface between authorship, industry and science in the domain of therapeutics. *British Journal of Psychiatry* 183:22-27.

Hemminki, E. 1980. Study of information submitted by drug companies to licensing authorities. *British Medical Journal* 280(6217):833-836.

Henderson, J. A., and J. J. Smith. 2003. Financial conflict of interest in medical research: overview and analysis of institutional controls. *Food and Drug Law Journal* 58(2):251-267.

Henry Ford Health System. 2007. *Vendor Policy and Procedures*. Detroit, MI: Henry Ford Health System. http://www.henryford.com/documents/Purchasing/Vendor%20Visitation%20Policyfinal0108.pdf (accessed February 10, 2009).

Henschke, C. I., and D. F. Yankelevitz. 2008. Unreported financial disclosures. *Journal of the American Medical Association* 299(15):1770; discussion 1771.

Hensley, S. 2005. To sell their drugs, companies increasingly rely on doctors. *Wall Street Journal*, July 15, A5.

Hensley, S., and B. Martinez. 2005. To sell their drugs, companies increasingly rely on doctors. *Wall Street Journal*, July 15, A1, A2.

Heres, S., J. Davis, K. Maino, E. Jetzinger, W. Kissling, and S. Leucht. 2006. Why olanzapine beats risperidone, risperidone beats quetiapine, and quetiapine beats olanzapine: an exploratory analysis of head-to-head comparison studies of second-generation antipsychotics. *American Journal of Psychiatry* 163(2):185-194.

Herrin, J., J. A. Etchason, J. P. Kahan, R. H. Brook, and D. J. Ballard. 1997. Effect of panel composition on physician ratings of appropriateness of abdominal aortic aneurysm surgery: elucidating differences between multispecialty panel results and specialty society recommendations. *Health Policy* 42(1):67-81.

HHS (U.S. Department of Health and Human Services). 2004. *Financial Relationships and Interests in Research Involving Human Subjects: Guidance for Human Subject Protection*. Washington, DC: DHHS. http://www.hhs.gov/ohrp/humansubjects/finreltn/fguid.pdf (accessed July 16, 2008).

HHS. 2005. Supplemental standards of ethical conduct and financial disclosure requirements for employees of the Department of Health and Human Services. *Federal Register* 70(168):51559-51574. http://www.nih.gov/about/ethics/08252005supplementalfinancialdisclosure.pdf (accessed February 2, 2009).

HHS. 2008. *Physician Self-Referral and Hospital Ownership Disclosure Provisions in the IPPS FY 2009 Final Rule*. Press release, August 4. Washington, DC: DHHS. http://www.cms.hhs.gov/apps/media/fact_sheets.asp (accessed September 16, 2008).

Higgins, J. P., and S. Green, eds. 2008. *Cochrane Handbook for Systematic Reviews of Interventions*, Version 5.0.1. Baltimore, MD: The Cochrane Collaboration. http://www.cochrane-handbook.org/ (accessed February 23, 2009)

Hill, K. P., J. S. Ross, D. S. Egilman, and H. M. Krumholz. 2008. The ADVANTAGE seeding trial: a review of internal documents. *Annals of Internal Medicine* 149(4):251-258.

Hillman, A. L. 1987. Financial incentives for physicians in HMOs. Is there a conflict of interest? *New England Journal of Medicine* 317(27):1743-1748.

Hillman, B. J., C. A. Joseph, M. R. Mabry, J. H. Sunshine, S. D. Kennedy, and M. Noether. 1990. Frequency and costs of diagnostic imaging in office practice—a comparison of self-referring and radiologist-referring physicians. *New England Journal of Medicine* 323(23):1604-1608.

The House of Commons Health Committee (United Kingdom). 2005. *The Influence of the Pharmaceutical Industry.* Fourth Report of Session 2004–05. London: House of Commons. http://www.parliament.the-stationery-office.co.uk/pa/cm200405/cmselect/cmhealth/42/42.pdf (accessed October 9, 2008).

Hrachovec, J. B., and M. Mora. 2001. Reporting of 6-month vs 12-month data in a clinical trial of celecoxib. *Journal of the American Medical Association* 286(19):2398; author reply 2399-2400.

Hsiao, W. C., D. L. Dunn, and D. K. Verrilli. 1993. Assessing the implementation of physician-payment reform. *New England Journal of Medicine* 328(13):928-933.

Huddle, T. S. 2008. Drug reps and the academic medical center: a case for management rather than prohibition. *Perspectives in Biology and Medicine* 51(2):251-260.

Hurdowar, A., I. D. Graham, M. Bayley, M. Harrison, S. Wood-Dauphinee, and S. Bhogal. 2007. Quality of stroke rehabilitation clinical practice guidelines. *Journal of Evaluation in Clinical Practice* 13(4):657-664.

Huth, E. J., and K. Case. 2004. The URM: twenty-five years old. *Science Editor* 27:17-21.

Hyman, P. L., M. E. Hochman, J. G. Shaw, and M. A. Steinman. 2007. Attitudes of preclinical and clinical medical students toward interactions with the pharmaceutical industry. *Academic Medicine* 82(1):94-99.

ICMJE (International Committee of Medical Journal Editors). 2008. *Uniform Requirements for Manuscripts Submitted to Biomedical Journals: Writing and Editing for Biomedical Publication.* http://www.icmje.org/icmje.pdf (accessed December 31, 2008).

Ingelfinger, J. R. 2007. Through the looking glass: anemia guidelines, vested interests, and distortions. *Clinical Journal of the American Society of Nephrology* 2(3):415-417.

IOM (Institute of Medicine). 1985. *Assessing Medical Technologies.* Washington, DC: National Academy Press.

IOM. 1988. *Medical Technology Assessment Directory: A Pilot Reference to Organizations, Assessments, and Information Resources.* Washington, DC: National Academy Press.

IOM. 1990. *Clinical Practice Guidelines: Directions for a New Program.* Washington, DC: National Academy Press.

IOM. 1991. *Patient Outcomes Research Teams: Managing Conflict of Interest.* Washington, DC: National Academy Press.

IOM. 1992. *Guidelines for Clinical Practice: From Development to Use.* Washington, DC: National Academy Press.

IOM. 1995. *Setting Priorities for Clinical Practice Guidelines.* Washington, DC: National Academy Press.

IOM. 2001. *Preserving Public Trust: Accreditation and Human Research Participant Protection Programs.* Washington, DC: National Academy Press.

IOM. 2003. *Responsible Research: A Systems Approach to Protecting Research Participants.* Washington, DC: The National Academies Press.

IOM. 2004. *The Ethical Conduct of Clinical Research Involving Children*. Washington, DC: The National Academies Press.

IOM. 2006. *Rewarding Provider Performance: Aligning Incentives in Medicare*. Washington, DC: The National Academies Press.

IOM. 2007. *Learning What Works Best: The Nation's Need for Evidence on Comparative Effectiveness in Health Care*. Washington, DC: The National Academies Press.

IOM. 2008. *Knowing What Works in Health Care: A Roadmap for the Nation*. Washington, DC: The National Academies Press.

IOM. 2009. *Projects: Committee on Planning a Continuing Health Care Professional Education Institute*. http://www.iom.edu/CMS/3809/59584.aspx (accessed February 18, 2009).

IOM/NRC (National Research Council). 2002. *Integrity in Scientific Research: Creating an Environment That Promotes Responsible Conduct*. Washington, DC: The National Academies Press.

Ivanis, A., D. Hren, D. Sambunjak, M. Marusič, and A. Marusič. 2008. Quantification of authors' contributions and eligibility for authorship: randomized study in a general medical journal. *Journal of General Internal Medicine* 23(9):1303-1310.

Jacobs, J. J., J. O. Galante, S. K. Mirza, and T. Zdeblick. 2006. Relationships with industry: critical for new technology or an unnecessary evil? *Journal of Bone and Joint Surgery* 88(7):1650-1663.

Jansen, L. A., and D. P. Sulmasy. 2003. Bioethics, conflicts of interest, & the limits of transparency. *Hastings Center Report* 33(4):40-43.

Jeffrey, K. 2001. *Machines in Our Hearts: The Cardiac Pacemaker, the Implantable Defibrillator, and American Health Care*. Baltimore, MD: The Johns Hopkins University Press.

Johns, M. M., M. Barnes, and P. S. Florencio. 2003. Restoring balance to industry-academia relationships in an era of institutional financial conflicts of interest: promoting research while maintaining trust. *Journal of the American Medical Association* 289(6):741-746.

Johns Hopkins University School of Medicine. 2009. *Johns Hopkins Medicine Policy on Interaction with Industry*. http://www.hopkinsmedicine.org/Research/OPC/JHM industryinteractionpolicyFINAL.pdf (accessed April 10, 2009).

Johnson, J. A. 1982. *Biotechnology: Commercialization of Academic Research*. Congressional Research Service Report, Issue IB81160. Washington, DC: Congressional Research Service. http://digital.library.unt.edu/govdocs/crs/permalink/meta-crs-8589:1 (accessed August 1, 2008).

Jolly, P. 2007. *Medical School Tuition and Young Physician Indebtedness: An Update to the 2004 Report*. Washington, DC: Association of American Medical Colleges. http://www.brynmawr.edu/healthpro/documents/AAMC_2004Med_Debt_Report.pdf (accessed August 12, 2008).

Jordan, K. A. 2003. Financial conflicts of interest in human subjects research: proposals for a more effective regulatory scheme. *Washington and Lee Law Review* 60(1):15-109.

Jorgensen, A. W., J. Hilden, and P. C. Gotzsche. 2006. Cochrane reviews compared with industry supported meta-analyses and other meta-analyses of the same drugs: systematic review. *British Medical Journal* 333(7572):782-785.

Jost, T. S. 2009. Oversight of marketing relationships between physicians and the drug and device industry: a comparative study. In *Medizin und Haftung, Festschrift für Erwin Deutsch zum 80*, edited by H. Ahrens, C. vonBar, G. Fischer, A. Spickhoff, and J. Taupitz. Berlin: Springer-Verlag.

Kahan, J. P., R. E. Park, L. L. Leape, S. J. Bernstein, L. H. Hilborne, L. Parker, C. J. Kamberg, et al. 1996. Variations by specialty in physician ratings of the appropriateness and necessity of indications for procedures. *Medical Care* 34(6):512-523.

Kahn, J. O., D. W. Cherng, K. Mayer, H. Murray, and S. Lagakos. 2000. Evaluation of HIV-1 immunogen, an immunologic modifier, administered to patients infected with HIV having 300 to 549 × 10^6/L CD4 cell counts: a randomized controlled trial. *Journal of the American Medical Association* 284(17):2193-2202.

Kaiser, J. 2008. NIH suspends grant to Emory University. *ScienceNOW Daily News*, October 14. http://sciencenow.sciencemag.org/cgi/content/full/2008/1014/1 (accessed February 19, 2009).

Kaiser Permanente/TPMG (The Permanente Medical Group). 2004. *TPMG Policy Manual: Conflict of Interest Policy.* http://www.sccgov.org/SCC/docs/SCC%20Public%20Portal/keyboard%20agenda/Committee%20Agenda/2007/April%2011,%202007/TMP Keyboard201889142.pdf (accessed February 10, 2009).

Kane, G. M. 2008. *Conference Proceedings.* Mayo CME Consensus Conference, Rochester, MN, September 25-26. Rochester, MN: Mayo Clinic. http://www.sacme.org/site/sacme/assets/pdf/Mayo_CME_Consensus_Conf_Proceedings_1-20-09.pdf (accessed February 27, 2009).

Kao, A. C., A. M. Zaslavsky, D. C. Green, J. P. Koplan, and P. D. Cleary. 2001. Physician incentives and disclosure of payment methods to patients. *Journal of General Internal Medicine* 16(3):181-188.

Kassirer, J. P. 2001. Financial conflict of interest: an unresolved ethical frontier. *American Journal of Law and Medicine* 27(2-3):149-162.

Kassirer, J. P. 2004. *On the Take: How Medicine's Complicity with Big Business Can Endanger Your Health.* New York, NY: Oxford University Press.

Kastelein, J. J., F. Akdim, E. S. Stroes, A. H. Zwinderman, M. L. Bots, A. F. Stalenhoef, F. L. Visseren, et al. 2008. Simvastatin with or without ezetimibe in familial hypercholesterolemia. *New England Journal of Medicine* 358(14):1431-1443.

Katz, H. P., S. E. Goldfinger, and S. W. Fletcher. 2002. Academia-industry collaboration in continuing medical education: description of two approaches. *Journal of Continuing Education in the Health Professions* 22(1):43-54.

Kaushansky, K. 2008. Untitled. Presentation for the American Society of Hematology to the Institute of Medicine Committee on Conflicts of Interest in Medical Research, Education, and Practice, Washington, DC, May 22.

KDOQI (Kidney Disease Outcomes Quality Initiative). 2007. KDOQI Clinical Practice Guideline and Clinical Practice Recommendations for anemia in chronic kidney disease: 2007 update of hemoglobin target. *American Journal of Kidney Diseases* 50(3):471-530.

Keefe, D. M., M. M. Schubert, L. S. Elting, S. T. Sonis, J. B. Epstein, J. E. Raber-Durlacher, C. A. Migliorati, D. B. McGuire, R. D. Hutchins, and D. E. Peterson. 2007. Updated clinical practice guidelines for the prevention and treatment of mucositis. *Cancer* 109(5):820-831.

Keim, S. M., M. Z. Mays, and D. Grant. 2004. Interactions between emergency medicine programs and the pharmaceutical industry. *Academic Emergency Medicine* 11(1):19-26.

Keiper, A. 2005. Science and Congress. *The New Atlantis* Fall 2004/Winter 2005(7):19-50.

Kennedy, T. C., A. McWilliams, E. Edell, T. Sutedja, G. Downie, R. Yung, A. Gazdar, et al. 2007. Bronchial intraepithelial neoplasia/early central airways lung cancer: ACCP evidence-based clinical practice guidelines (2nd edition). *Chest* 132(3 Suppl.):221S-233S.

Keszler, M., and D. J. Durand. 2001. Neonatal high-frequency ventilation. Past, present, and future. *Clinics in Perinatology* 28(3):579-607.

KFF (Kaiser Family Foundation). 2002. *National Survey of Physicians part II: Doctors and Prescription Drugs.* Menlo Park, CA: KFF. http://www.kff.org/rxdrugs/loader.cfm?url=/commonspot/security/getfile.cfm&PageID=13965 (accessed August 12, 2008).

Kim, S. Y., R. W. Millard, P. Nisbet, C. Cox, and E. D. Caine. 2004. Potential research participants' views regarding researcher and institutional financial conflicts of interest. *Journal of Medical Ethics* 30(1):73-79.

King-Casas, B., D. Tomlin, C. Anen, C. F. Camerer, S. R. Quartz, and P. R. Montague. 2005. Getting to know you: reputation and trust in a two-person economic exchange. *Science* 308(5718):78-83.

Klanica, K. 2005. Conflicts of interest in medical research: how much conflict should exceed legal boundaries? *Journal of Biolaw & Business* 8(3):37-45.

Klein, J. E., and A. R. Fleischman. 2002. The private practicing physician-investigator: ethical implications of clinical research in the office setting. *Hastings Center Report* 32(4):22-26.

Kodish, E., T. Murray, and P. Whitehouse. 1996. Conflict of interest in university-industry research relationships: realities, politics, and values. *Academic Medicine* 71(12): 1287-1290.

Kopelow, M. 2008. Untitled. Presentation to the Institute of Medicine Committee on Conflicts of Interest in Medical Research, Education, and Practice, Washington, DC, January 21.

Kovaleski, D. 2008. *No Pharma Funding.* http://meetingsnet.com/cmepharma/cme/no_pharma_funding_012808/index.html (accessed January 29, 2009).

Krimsky, S. 2003. *Science in the Private Interest: Has the Lure of Profits Corrupted Biomedical Research?* Lanham, MD: Rowman & Littlefield Publishers.

Krimsky, S., and L. S. Rothenberg. 2001. Conflict of interest policies in science and medical journals: editorial practices and author disclosures. *Science and Engineering Ethics* 7(2):205-218.

Krimsky, S., L. S. Rothenberg, P. Stott, and G. Kyle. 1996. Financial interests of authors in scientific journals: a pilot study of 14 publications. *Science and Engineering Ethics* 2(4):395-410.

Kuehn, B. M. 2005. Pharmaceutical industry funding for residencies sparks controversy. *Journal of the American Medical Association* 293(13):1572-1580.

Kulynych, J. J. 2007. Some thoughts about the evaluation of non-clinical functional magnetic resonance imaging. *American Journal of Bioethics* 7(9):57-58.

Kurth, T., J. M. Gaziano, N. R. Cook, G. Logroscino, H. C. Diener, and J. E. Buring. 2006. Migraine and risk of cardiovascular disease in women. *Journal of the American Medical Association* 296(3):283-291.

Lagnado, M. 2002. Haunted papers. *Lancet* 359(9309):902.

Lahiri, S., C. Levenstein, D. I. Nelson, and B. J. Rosenberg. 2005. The cost effectiveness of occupational health interventions: prevention of silicosis. *American Journal of Industrial Medicine* 48(6):503-514.

Landefeld, C. S., and M. A. Steinman. 2009. The Neurontin legacy—marketing through misinformation and manipulation. *New England Journal of Medicine* 360(2):103-106.

Landrum, M. B., B. J. McNeil, L. Silva, and S. L. Normand. 1999. Understanding variability in physician ratings of the appropriateness of coronary angiography after acute myocardial infarction. *Journal of Clinical Epidemiology* 52(4):309-319.

Lane, K., and R. Berkow. 1999. The Merck Manual: a century of medical publishing and practice. *CBE Views* 22(4):112-113.

Langwell, K. M., and L. M. Nelson. 1986. Physician payment systems: a review of history, alternatives and evidence. *Medical Care Review* 43(1):5-58.

Larson, R. J., L. M. Schwartz, S. Woloshin, and H. G. Welch. 2005. Advertising by academic medical centers. *Archives of Internal Medicine* 165(6):645-651.

Lauer, M. S. 2007. Screening for coronary heart disease: has the time for universal imaging arrived? *Cleveland Clinic Journal of Medicine* 74(9):645-650, 653-654, 656.

Lazar, K. 2008. Legislature votes to crack down on companies' gifts to doctors. *Boston Globe Online*, July 31. http://www.boston.com/news/local/breaking_news/2008/07/legislature_vot.html (accessed August 12, 2008).

LCME (Liaison Committee on Medical Education). 2008. *Accreditation Standards.* http://www.lcme.org/standard.htm (accessed August 12, 2008).

Lee, K., P. Bacchetti, and I. Sim. 2008. Publication of clinical trials supporting successful new drug applications: a literature analysis. *PLoS Medicine* 5(9):e191.

Lemmens, T. 2004. Piercing the veil of corporate secrecy about clinical trials. *Hastings Center Report* 34(5):14-18.

Lemmens, T., and P. B. Miller. 2003. The human subjects trade: ethical and legal issues surrounding recruitment incentives. *Journal of Law, Medicine and Ethics* 31(3):398-418.

Lemmens, T., and P. A. Singer. 1998. Bioethics for clinicians. 17. Conflict of interest in research, education and patient care. *Canadian Medical Association Journal* 159(8):960-965.

Lenzer, J. 2002. Alteplase for stroke: money and optimistic claims buttress the "brain attack" campaign. *British Medical Journal* 324(7339):723-729.

Lenzer, J. 2008. Truly independent research? *British Medical Journal* 337:a1332.

Lesser, L. I., C. B. Ebbeling, M. Goozner, D. Wypij, and D. S. Ludwig. 2007. Relationship between funding source and conclusion among nutrition-related scientific articles. *PLoS Medicine* 4(1):e5.

Lever, A., and S. Z. Lewis. 2008. Conflicts of interest in evidence-based guidelines: issues and solutions. Presentation for the American College of Chest Physicians to the Institute of Medicine Committee on Conflict of Interest in Medical Research, Education, and Practice, Washington, DC, May 22.

Levine, M. 2008. Untitled. Presentation for the American Medical Association to the Institute of Medicine Committee on Conflict of Interest in Medical Research, Education, and Practice, Washington, DC, March 13.

Levinsky, N. G. 2002. Nonfinancial conflicts of interest in research. *New England Journal of Medicine* 347(10):759-761.

Levinson, W., A. Kao, A. M. Kuby, and R. A. Thisted. 2005. The effect of physician disclosure of financial incentives on trust. *Archives of Internal Medicine* 165(6):625-630.

Lexchin, J., L. A. Bero, B. Djulbegovic, and O. Clark. 2003. Pharmaceutical industry sponsorship and research outcome and quality: systematic review. *British Medical Journal* 326(7400):1167-1170.

Lilly (Eli Lilly and Company). 2008. *Lilly Set to Become First Pharmaceutical Research Company to Disclose Physician Payments.* Indianapolis, IN: Lilly. http://newsroom.lilly.com/releasedetail.cfm?ReleaseID=336444 (accessed November 5, 2008).

Lipton, S., E. A. Boyd, and L. A. Bero. 2004. Conflicts of interest in academic research: policies, processes, and attitudes. *Accountability in Research* 11(2):83-102.

Lo, B. 2001. Ethical and policy implications of hospitalist systems. *American Journal of Medicine* 111(9B):48-52.

Lo, B., L. E. Wolf, and A. Berkeley. 2000. Conflict-of-interest policies for investigators in clinical trials. *New England Journal of Medicine* 343(22):1616-1620.

Loftus, P. 2008. Pfizer ends direct funding of courses. *Wall Street Journal*, July 3, B11.

Lohr, K. N. 2004. Rating the strength of scientific evidence: relevance for quality improvement programs. *International Journal for Quality in Health Care* 16(1):9-18.

Lopes, M. J. 2009. Request for Final Promulgation of 105 C.M.R. 970.000. Memorandum to the members of the Public Health Council, Boston, MA. http://www.mass.gov/Eeohhs2/docs/dph/legal/pharmacy_med_device_phc_memo_march12.doc (accessed March 13, 2009).

Lu, C. Y., D. Ross-Degnan, S. B. Soumerai, and S. A. Pearson. 2008. Interventions designed to improve the quality and efficiency of medication use in managed care: a critical review of the literature—2001-2007. *BMC Health Services Research* 8:75.

Lurie, P. 2007. Untitled. Presentation to the Institute of Medicine Committee on Conflict of Interest in Medical Research, Education, and Practice, Washington, DC, November 5.

Lurie, P., C. M. Almeida, N. Stine, A. R. Stine, and S. M. Wolfe. 2006. Financial conflict of interest disclosure and voting patterns at Food and Drug Administration Drug Advisory Committee meetings. *Journal of the American Medical Association* 295(16):1921-1928.

Lurker, N., and B. Caprara. 2005. The sampling subsidy: Pharma can't afford to kill it or continue it. Alternatives are needed now. *Pharmaceutical Executive*, February 2005. http://www.impactrx.com/pdfs/PharmaExec_Feb05_Sampling.pdf (accessed August 27, 2007).

Maatz, C. T. 1992. University physician-researcher conflicts of interest: the inadequacy of current controls and proposed reform. *High Technology Law Journal* 7:137-188.

Mainous, A. G., III, W. J. Hueston, and E. C. Rich. 1995. Patient perceptions of physician acceptance of gifts from the pharmaceutical industry. *Archives of Family Medicine* 4(4):335-339.

Maloney, D. G., A. J. Grillo-Lopez, C. A. White, D. Bodkin, R. J. Schilder, J. A. Neidhart, N. Janakiraman, et al. 1997. IDEC-C2B8 (rituximab) anti-CD20 monoclonal antibody therapy in patients with relapsed low-grade non-Hodgkin's lymphoma. *Blood* 90(6):2188-2195.

Manchanda, P., and P. K. Chintagunta. 2004. Responsiveness of physician prescription behavior to salesforce effort: an individual level analysis. *Marketing Letters* 15(2-3):129-145.

Manchanda, P., and E. Honka. 2005. The effects and role of direct-to-physician marketing in the pharmaceutical industry: an integrative review. *Yale Journal of Health, Policy, Law, and Ethics* 5(2):785-822.

Marco, C. A., and T. A. Schmidt. 2004. Who wrote this paper? Basics of authorship and ethical issues. *Academic Emergency Medicine* 11(1):76-77.

Marco, C. A., J. C. Moskop, R. C. Solomon, J. M. Geiderman, and G. L. Larkin. 2006. Gifts to physicians from the pharmaceutical industry: an ethical analysis. *Annals of Emergency Medicine* 48(5):513-521.

Martinson, B. C., M. S. Anderson, and R. de Vries. 2005. Scientists behaving badly. *Nature* 435(7043):737-738.

Marusič, A., T. Bates, A. Anic, and M. Marusič. 2006. How the structure of contribution disclosure statements affects validity of authorship: a randomized study in a general medical journal. *Current Medical Research and Opinion* 22(6):1035-1044.

Maskell, J. 2007. *Entering the Executive Branch of Government: Potential Conflicts of Interest with Previous Employments and Affiliations.* CRS Report for Congress, Order Code RL31822. Washington, DC: Congressional Research Service. http://www.fas.org/sgp/crs/misc/RL31822.pdf (accessed August 1, 2008).

Masur, H. 2007. From the President: IDSA Practice Guidelines: Valuable, Credible, Flexible. *IDSA News*, January 1. http://www.idsociety.org/newsArticle.aspx?id=5472 (accessed August 19, 2008).

Mathews, A. W. 2005. Ghost story: at medical journals, writers paid by industry play big role. *Wall Street Journal*, December 13, A1, A8.

Matteson, E. L., and T. Bongartz. 2006. Investigation, explanation, and apology for incomplete and erroneous disclosures. *Journal of the American Medical Association* 296(18):2205.

Matz, R. 1996. Inflating physicians' expectations. *Journal of General Internal Medicine* 11(1):62-63.

Mazmanian, P. E. 2007. Theory and evidence to explain guidelines, variation, and risk of unwanted influence. *Journal of Continuing Education in the Health Professions* 27(4):199-200.

Mazzaschi, A. 1990. NIH and ADAMHA's conflict-of-interest guidelines withdrawn. *FASEB Journal* 4(2):137-138.

McCanse, C. 2001. AMA initiative aims to heighten awareness of gift-giving guidelines. *FP Report* 7(9), Leawood, KS: American Academy of Family Physicians. http://www.aafp.org/fpr/20010900/07.html (accessed July 28, 2008).

McClure, S. M., M. K. York, and P. R. Montague. 2004. The neural substrates of reward processing in humans: the modern role of FMRI. *Neuroscientist* 10(3):260-268.

McCormick, B. B., G. Tomlinson, P. Brill-Edwards, and A. S. Detsky. 2001. Effect of restricting contact between pharmaceutical company representatives and internal medicine residents on posttraining attitudes and behavior. *Journal of the American Medical Association* 286(16):1994-1999.

McCrary, S. V., C. B. Anderson, J. Jakovljevic, T. Khan, L. B. McCullough, N. P. Wray, and B. A. Brody. 2000. A national survey of policies on disclosure of conflicts of interest in biomedical research. *New England Journal of Medicine* 343(22):1621-1626.

McCrory, D. C., S. Z. Lewis, J. Heitzer, G. Colice, and W. M. Alberts. 2007. Methodology for lung cancer evidence review and guideline development: ACCP evidence-based clinical practice guidelines (2nd edition). *Chest* 132(3 Suppl.):23S-28S.

McDonagh, A. F. 2001. Phototherapy: from ancient Egypt to the new millennium. *Journal of Perinatology* 21(Suppl. 1):S7-S12.

McFadden, D. W., E. Calvario, and C. Graves. 2007. The devil is in the details: the pharmaceutical industry's use of gifts to physicians as marketing strategy. *Journal of Surgical Research* 140(1):1-5.

McKinney, W. P., D. L. Schiedermayer, N. Lurie, D. E. Simpson, J. L. Goodman, and E. C. Rich. 1990. Attitudes of internal medicine faculty and residents toward professional interaction with pharmaceutical sales representatives. *Journal of the American Medical Association* 264(13):1693-1697.

McLaughlin, J. K., J. D. Boice, Jr., R. E. Tarone, and W. J. Blot. 2007. A rebuttal: secret ties to industry and conflicting interests in cancer research. *American Journal of Industrial Medicine* 50(3):235-236.

McMahon, B. J., R. Neubauer, B. Janis, S. Tucker, and M. Agnew. 2003. Developing and implementing a program of grand rounds for internists that is free of commercial bias. *Annals of Internal Medicine* 139(1):77-78.

McNeil, B., and M. Roberts. 1991. The evolution and current status of conflict of interest regulation in biomedical science. In *Patient Outcomes Research Teams (PORTS): Managing Conflict of Interest*. Washington, DC: National Academy Press.

Medical News Today. 2007. APA Names DSM-V Task Force Members-Leading Experts to Revise Handbook for Diagnosing Mental Disorders, USA. http://www.medicalnewstoday.com/articles/77663.php (accessed September 25, 2008).

MedPAC (Medicare Payment Advisory Commission). 2005a. *Report to the Congress: Medicare Payment Policy*. Washington, DC: MedPAC. http://www.medpac.gov/publications/congressional_reports/Mar05_EntireReport.pdf (accessed September 17, 2008).

MedPAC. 2005b. *Report to the Congress: Physician-Owned Specialty Hospitals*. Washington, DC: MedPAC. http://www.medpac.gov/documents/Mar05_SpecHospitals.pdf (accessed September 17, 2008).

MedPAC. 2005c. Strategies to improve care: pay for performance and information technology. In *Report to the Congress: Medicare Payment Policy*. Washington, DC: MedPAC. http://www.medpac.gov/publications/congressional_reports/Mar05_Ch04.pdf (accessed December 15, 2008).

MedPAC. 2006. *Report to the Congress: Medicare Payment Policy.* Washington, DC: MedPAC. http://www.medpac.gov/documents/jun06_entirereport.pdf (accessed November 18, 2008).

MedPAC. 2007. *Report to the Congress: Promoting Greater Efficiency in Medicare.* Washington, DC: MedPAC. http://www.medpac.gov/documents/jun07_EntireReport.pdf (accessed November 18, 2008).

MedPAC. 2008a. *Public reporting of physicians' financial relationships.* MedPAC public meeting, April 9. Washington, DC: MedPAC. http://www.medpac.gov/transcripts/0408_Public_reporting_phys_relationships_public_pres.pdf (accessed January 13, 2009).

MedPAC. 2008b. *Public Reporting of Physicians' Financial Relationships: Draft Recommendations.* MedPAC public meeting, October 2. Washington, DC: MedPAC. http://www.medpac.gov/transcripts/Public%20reporting_Oct%2008_public.pdf (accessed January 13, 2009).

MedPAC. 2008c. *Public Reporting of Physicians' Financial Relationships: Policy Options.* MedPAC public meeting, September 4. Washington, DC: MedPAC. http://www.medpac.gov/transcripts/Public%20reporting%20physician%20relationships_Sept%2008_public.pdf (accessed January 13, 2009).

MedPAC. 2008d. *Public Reporting of Physicians' Financial Relationships with Drug and Device Manufacturers, Hospitals, and ASCs.* MedPAC public meeting, March 5. Washington, DC: MedPAC. http://www.medpac.gov/transcripts/Public%20reporting_physicians%20relationships_final.pdf (accessed January 13, 2009).

MedPAC. 2009. *Report to the Congress: Medicare Payment Policy.* Washington, DC: MedPAC. http://www.medpac.gov/documents/Mar09_EntireReport.pdf (accessed March 8, 2009).

Melander, H., J. Ahlqvist-Rastad, G. Meijer, and B. Beermann. 2003. Evidence b(i)ased medicine—selective reporting from studies sponsored by pharmaceutical industry: review of studies in new drug applications. *British Medical Journal* 326(7400):1171-1173.

Mello, M. M., B. R. Clarridge, and D. M. Studdert. 2005a. Academic medical centers' standards for clinical-trial agreements with industry. *New England Journal of Medicine* 352(21):2202-2210.

Mello, M. M., B. R. Clarridge, and D. M. Studdert. 2005b. Researchers' views of the acceptability of restrictive provisions in clinical trial agreements with industry sponsors. *Accountability in Research* 12(3):163-191.

Merton, R. K. 1968. *Social Theory and Social Structure.* New York: The Free Press.

MGMA (Medical Group Management Association). 2008. *Specialty Physician Compensation Barely Keeps up with Inflation.* Inglewood, CO: MGMA. http://www.mgma.com/press/article.aspx?id=20662 (accessed September 17, 2008).

Mike, V., A. N. Krauss, and G. S. Ross. 1996. Doctors and the health industry: a case study of transcutaneous oxygen monitoring in neonatal intensive care. *Social Science and Medicine* 42(9):1247-1258.

Millenson, M. 2003. *Getting Doctors to Say Yes to Drugs: The Cost and Quality of Impact of Drug Company Marketing to Physicians.* http://www.bcbs.com/betterknowledge/cost/Drug_Co_Marketing_Report.pdf (accessed June 27, 2007).

Miller, D. P., R. J. Mansfield, J. B. Woods, J. L. Wofford, and W. P. Moran. 2008. The impact of drug samples on prescribing to the uninsured. *Southern Medical Journal* 101(9):888-893.

Miller, G. 2005. Neuroscience. Economic game shows how the brain builds trust. *Science* 308(5718):36.

Mirowski, P., and R. Van Horn. 2005. The contract research organization and the commercialization of scientific research. *Social Studies of Science* 35(4):503-548.

MIT (Massachusetts Institute of Technology). Undated. *What is Coeus?* http://web.mit.edu/coeus/www/coeus_description.htm (accessed November 11, 2008).

Mitchell, J. M. 2008. Do financial incentives linked to ownership of specialty hospitals affect physicians' practice patterns? *Medical Care* 46(7):732-737.

Mitchell, J. M., and E. Scott. 1992. Physician self-referral: empirical evidence and policy implications. *Advances in Health Economics and Health Services Research* 13:27-42.

Moher, D., D. J. Cook, S. Eastwood, I. Olkin, D. Rennie, and D. F. Stroup. 1999. Improving the quality of reports of meta-analyses of randomised controlled trials: the QUOROM statement. Quality of Reporting of Meta-Analyses. *Lancet* 354(9193):1896-1900.

Moher, D., K. F. Schulz, and D. G. Altman. 2001. The CONSORT statement: revised recommendations for improving the quality of reports of parallel-group randomised trials. *Annals of Internal Medicine* 134(8):657-662.

Monmaney, T. 2000. Top medical journal admits 19 lapses of ethics policy. *The Los Angeles Times*, February 24, A1.

Montague, B. T., A. H. Fortin VI, and J. Rosenbaum. 2008. A systematic review of curricula on relationships between residents and the pharmaceutical industry. *Medical Education* 42(3):301-308.

Moore, D. A., D. M. Cain, G. Loewenstein, and M. H. Bazerman. 2005. *Conflicts of Interest: Challenges and Solutions in Business, Law, Medicine, and Public Policy.* New York: Cambridge University Press.

Morgan, M. A., J. Dana, G. Loewenstein, S. Zinberg, and J. Schulkin. 2006. Interactions of doctors with the pharmaceutical industry. *Journal of Medical Ethics* 32(10):559-563.

Moses, H. 2008. Conflict of interest in basic and translational biomedical research. Presentation to the Institute of Medicine Committee on Conflicts of Interest in Medical Research, Education, and Practice, Washington, DC, May 22.

Moses, H., and J. B. Martin. 2001. Academic relationships with industry: a new model for biomedical research. *Journal of the American Medical Association* 285(7):933-935.

Moses, H., E. R. Dorsey, D. H. Matheson, and S. O. Thier. 2005. Financial anatomy of biomedical research. *Journal of the American Medical Association* 294(11):1333-1342.

Mowatt, G., L. Shirran, J. M. Grimshaw, D. Rennie, A. Flanagin, V. Yank, G. MacLennan, P. C. Gotzsche, and L. A. Bero. 2002. Prevalence of honorary and ghost authorship in Cochrane reviews. *Journal of the American Medical Association* 287(21):2769-2771.

Mowery, D. C., R. R. Nelson, B. N. Sampat, and A. A. Ziedonis. 2001. The growth of patenting and licensing by U.S. universities: an assessment of the effects of the Bayh-Dole Act of 1980. *Research Policy* 30:99-119.

Mowery, D. C., R. R. Nelson, B. N. Sampat, and A. A. Ziedonis. 2004. *Ivory Tower and Industrial Innovation: University-Industry Technology Transfer Before and After the Bayh-Dole Act in the United States.* Stanford, CA: Stanford Business Books.

Murphy, M. K., N. A. Black, D. L. Lamping, C. M. McKee, C. F. Sanderson, J. Askham, and T. Marteau. 1998. Consensus development methods, and their use in clinical guideline development. *Health Technology Assessment* 2(3):i-iv, 1-88.

NAAMECC (North American Association of Medical Education and Communication Companies). 2009. *Welcome to NAAMECC.* Birmingham, AL: NAAMECC. http://naamecc.org/ (accessed March 22 2009).

NAAMECC and Coalition for Healthcare Communication. 2008. *Critical Concerns with Accuracy and Validity of "Report 1 of the Council on Ethical and Judicial Affairs: Industry Support of Professional Education in Medicine."* Letter to M. Levine (AMA) and R. Christensen (AMA), May 22. http://www.acme-assn.org/home/NAAMECC_CEJA.pdf (accessed September 25, 2008).

Naghavi, M., E. Falk, H. S. Hecht, M. J. Jamieson, S. Kaul, D. Berman, Z. Fayad, et al. 2006. From vulnerable plaque to vulnerable patient. Part III: Executive summary of the Screening for Heart Attack Prevention and Education (SHAPE) Task Force report. *American Journal of Cardiology* 98(2A):2H-15H.

Nallamothu, B. K., J. Young, H. S. Gurm, G. Pickens, and K. Safavi. 2007. Recent trends in hospital utilization for acute myocardial infarction and coronary revascularization in the United States. *American Journal of Cardiology* 99(6):749-753.

NASS (North American Spine Society). 2007. *Diagnosis and Treatment of Degenerative Lumbar Spinal Stenosis*. Burr Ridge, IL: NASS. p. 133.

NASS. 2008. *Diagnosis and Treatment of Degenerative Lumbar Spondylolisthesis*. Burr Ridge, IL: NASS. p. 131.

NBAC (National Bioethics Advisory Commission). 2001. *Ethical and Policy Issues in Research Involving Human Participants*. Bethesda, MD: NBAC. http://bioethics.georgetown.edu/nbac/human/oversumm.pdf (accessed December 12, 2008).

NEJM (*New England Journal of Medicine*). 2008. *Financial Disclosure & Authorship Form*. http://authors.nejm.org/help/disclosRev.pdf (accessed September 15, 2008).

Ngai, S., J. L. Gold, S. S. Gill, and P. A. Rochon. 2005. Haunted manuscripts: ghost authorship in the medical literature. *Accountability in Research* 12(2):103-114.

NGC (National Guideline Clearinghouse). 2009a. *ACR Practice Guideline for the Performance of Total Body Irradiation*. Rockville, MD: NGC. http://www.guideline.gov/summary/summary.aspx?doc_id=10914&nbr=5694&ss=6&xl=999#s25 (accessed March 9, 2009).

NGC. 2009b. *Assessment: Use of Epidural Steroid Injections to Treat Radicular Lumbosacral Pain*. Report of the Therapeutics and Technology Assessment Subcommittee of the American Academy of Neurology. Rockville, MD: NGC. http://www.guideline.gov/summary/summary.aspx?doc_id=10717&nbr=5580#s25 (accessed January 13, 2009).

NGC. 2009c. *Bronchial Intraepithelial Neoplasia/Early Central Airways Lung Cancer: ACCP Evidence-Based Clinical Practice Guidelines*. Rockville, MD: NGC. http://www.guideline.gov/summary/summary.aspx?doc_id=11414&nbr=5933 (accessed January 13, 2009).

NGC. 2009d. *Clinical Practice Guidelines for the Management of Blastomycosis: 2008 Update by the Infectious Diseases Society of America*. Rockville, MD: NGC. http://www.guideline.gov/summary/summary.aspx?view_id=1&doc_id=12589#s25&nbr=6497&ss=6&xl=999 (accessed April 06, 2009).

NGC. 2009e. *Diagnosis and Treatment of Degenerative Lumbar Spondylolisthesis*. Rockville, MD: NGC. http://www.guideline.gov/summary/summary.aspx?view_id=1&doc_id=12680#s25 (accessed January 13, 2009).

NGC. 2009f. *Management Guidelines for Patients with Thyroid Nodules and Differentiated Thyroid Cancer.* Rockville, MD: NGC. http://www.guideline.gov/summary/summary.aspx?doc_id=9738&nbr=5212#s25 (accessed January 13, 2009).

NGC. 2009g. *Recommended Adult Immunization Schedule: United States, October 2007-September 2008*. Rockville, MD: NGC. http://www.guideline.gov/summary/summary.aspx?doc_id=11679&nbr=006028&string (accessed March 10, 2009).

NGC. 2009h. *Updated Clinical Practice Guidelines for the Prevention and Treatment of Mucositis*. Rockville, MD: NGC. http://www.guidelines.gov/summary/summary.aspx?doc_id=12094&nbr=006223&string=irradiation (accessed January 13, 2009).

NHRPAC (National Human Research Protections Advisory Committee). 2001. *NHRPAC Recommendations on HHS's Draft Interim Guidance on Financial Relationships in Clinical Research*. Washington, DC: NHRPAC. http://www.hhs.gov/ohrp/nhrpac/mtg12-00/finguid.htm (accessed March 10, 2009).

Nicholson, S., M. V. Pauly, A. Y. Wu, J. F. Murray, S. M. Teutsch, and M. L. Berger. 2008. Getting real performance out of pay-for-performance. *Milbank Quarterly* 86(3):435-457.

NIH (National Institutes of Health). 1995. Objectivity in research. In *NIH Guide* 24(25). Bethesda, MD: NIH. http://grants2.nih.gov/grants/guide/notice-files/not95-179.html (accessed February 11, 2009).

NIH. 2002. *Financial Conflict of Interest: Objectivity in Research*. Bethesda, MD: NIH. http://grants1.nih.gov/grants/policy/coi/nih_review.htm (accessed November 12, 2008).

NIH. 2004. *Report of the National Institutes of Health Blue Ribbon Panel on Conflict of Interest Policies*. Bethesda, MD: NIH. http://www.nih.gov/about/ethics_COI_panelreport.pdf (accessed December 29, 2008).

NIH. 2005. *Summary of NIH-Specific Amendments to Conflict of Interest Ethics Regulations*. Bethesda, MD: NIH. http://www.nih.gov/about/ethics/summary_amendments_08252005.htm (accessed November 12, 2008).

NIH. 2007. *Targeted Site Reviews on Financial Conflict of Interest: Observations*. Bethesda, MD: NIH. http://grants.nih.gov/grants/policy/coi/TSR_Observations_2-14-2007.doc (accessed July 17, 2008).

NIH. 2008a. *Frequently Asked Questions: Responsibility of Applicants for Promoting Objectivity in Research for Which PHS Funding Is Sought*. Bethesda, MD: NIH. http://grants.nih.gov/grants/policy/coifaq.htm#a2 (accessed June 23, 2008).

NIH. 2008b. *NIH Announces a New Business Process for Reporting an Identified Financial Conflict of Interest for Grants and/or Cooperative Agreements Beginning October 10, 2008*. NIH announcement Notice NOT-OD-09-001. Bethesda, MD: NIH. http://grants.nih.gov/grants/guide/notice-files/NOT-OD-09-001.html (accessed February 19, 2009).

NIH. 2008c. *Re-Engineering the Clinical Research Enterprise: Clinical Research Policy Analysis and Coordination*. Bethesda, MD: NIH. http://nihroadmap.nih.gov/clinicalresearch/overview-policy.asp (accessed July 3, 2008).

NIH. 2008d. *Re-Engineering the Clinical Research Enterprise: Translational Research*. Bethesda, MD: NIH. http://nihroadmap.nih.gov/clinicalresearch/overview-translational.asp (accessed July 3, 2008).

NIH. Undated. *NIH Consensus Development Program: About Us*. Bethesda, MD: NIH. http://consensus.nih.gov/ABOUTCDP.htm#panel (accessed June 23, 2008).

Nissen, S. E. 2006. President's page: American College of Cardiology fellowship: where ideals and personal responsibility intersect. *Journal of the American College of Cardiology* 47(9):1901-1903.

Nix, M. 2008. Guideline methodology: National Guideline Clearinghouse™ (NGC) data. Presentation to the Institute of Medicine Committee on Conflict of Interest in Medical Research, Education, and Practice, Washington, DC, May 22.

NKF (National Kidney Foundation). 2007. *KDOQI Disclosure and COI Policies*. New York, NY: NKF. http://www.kidney.org/professionals/KDOQI/guidelinesCOI.cfm (accessed February 23, 2009).

NLM (National Library of Medicine). 2007. *Fact Sheet: Conflict of Interest Disclosure and Journal Supplements in MEDLINE®*. Bethesda, MD: NLM. http://www.nlm.nih.gov/pubs/factsheets/supplements.html (accessed February 27, 2009).

Northfield Laboratories. 2006. *Northfield Laboratories Releases Summary Observations from Its Elective Surgery Trial*. http://phx.corporate-ir.net/phoenix.zhtml?c=91374&p=irol-newsArticle&ID=833808&highlight= (accessed October 10, 2008).

NPG (Nature Publishing Group). 2007. Compete, collaborate, compel. *Nature Genetics* 39(8):931. (Editorial.)

NPG. 2008. *Competing Financial Interests*. http://www.nature.com/authors/editorial_policies/competing.html (accessed September 15, 2008).

NRC (National Research Council). 2003. *Sharing Publication-Related Data and Materials: Responsibilities of Authorship in the Life Sciences*. Washington, DC: The National Academies Press.

Nuckols, T. K., Y. W. Lim, B. O. Wynn, S. Mattke, C. H. MacLean, P. Harber, R. H. Brook, et al. 2008. Rigorous development does not ensure that guidelines are acceptable to a panel of knowledgeable providers. *Journal of General Internal Medicine* 23(1):37-44.

O'Brien, M. A., A. D. Oxman, D. A. Davis, R. B. Haynes, N. Freemantle, and E. L. Harvey. 2000. Educational outreach visits: effects on professional practice and health care outcomes. *Cochrane Database of Systematic Reviews* (2):CD000409.

OIG (Office of the Inspector General, U.S. Department of Health and Human Services). 1989. *Financial Arrangements Between Physicians and Health Care Businesses.* Washington, DC: U.S. Department of Health and Human Services. http://www.oig.hhs.gov/oei/reports/oai-12-88-01411.pdf (accessed November 18, 2008).

OIG. 2003. *Compliance Program Guidance for Pharmaceutical Manufacturers.* Washington, DC: U.S. Department of Health and Human Services. http://www.oig.hhs.gov/fraud/docs/complianceguidance/042803pharmacymfgnonfr.pdf (accessed February 13, 2009).

OIG. 2004. *Corporate Integrity Agreement Between the Office of Inspector General of the Department of Health and Human Services and Pfizer, Inc.* Washington, DC: U.S. Department of Health and Human Services. http://www.oig.hhs.gov/fraud/cia/agreements/pfizer_5_11_2004.pdf (accessed December 12, 2008).

OIG. 2005. *Outside Activities of Senior-Level NIH Employees.* Washington, DC: U.S. Department of Health and Human Services. http://oig.hhs.gov/oei/reports/oei-01-04-00150.pdf (accessed November 11, 2008).

OIG. 2007. *Corporate Integrity Agreement Between the Office of Inspector General of Department of Health and Human Services and Jazz Pharmaceuticals, Inc.* Washington, DC: U.S. Department of Health and Human Services. http://oig.hhs.gov/fraud/cia/agreements/Jazz%20CIA.pdf (accessed June 10, 2009).

OIG. 2008. *National Institutes of Health: Conflicts of Interest in Extramural Research.* Washington, DC: U.S. Department of Health and Human Services. http://oig.hhs.gov/oei/reports/oei-03-06-00460.pdf (accessed June 23, 2008).

OIG. 2009. *The Food and Drug Administration's Oversight of Clinical Investigator's Financial Information.* Washington, DC: U.S. Department of Health and Human Services. http://oig.hhs.gov/oei/reports/oei-05-07-00730.pdf (accessed February 27, 2009).

OIG. Undated. *Corporate Integrity Agreements.* Washington, DC: U.S. Department of Health and Human Services. http://www.oig.hhs.gov/fraud/cias.asp (accessed October 29, 2008).

Oncology Congress. 2008. *Educational Grants.* http://www.oncologycongress.com/app/homepage.cfm?appname=100432&moduleID=2147&LinkID=18209 (accessed November 21, 2008).

Oncology Congress. 2009. *Industry-Supported Satellite Symposia Opportunities.* http://www.oncologycongress.com/app/homepage.cfm?appname=100432&moduleID=2147&LinkID=18089 (accessed January 27, 2009).

Oregon DOJ (Department of Justice). 2008a. *AG Hardy Myers Files Judgment Against Merck; Oregon is Lead State in $58 million settlement.* Press release, July 13. Salem: Oregon DOJ. http://www.doj.state.or.us/releases, 2008/rel052008.shtml (accessed September 25, 2008).

Oregon DOJ. 2008b. *AG Myers Files Judgment Against Pfizer for $60 Million Concerning It's Marketing of Drugs Celebrex & Bextra.* Press release, October 22. Salem: Oregon DOJ. http://www.doj.state.or.us/releases/2008/rel102208.shtml (accessed November 13, 2008).

O'Reilly, K. B. 2006. AMA opt-out program will keep prescribing data from drug reps. *American Medical News*, May 22/29. http://www.ama-assn.org/amednews/2006/05/22/prl10522.htm (accessed March 2, 2009).

O'Reilly, K. B. 2008. Drugmakers vow to disclose their payments to physicians. *American Medical News*, November 17. http://www.ama-assn.org/amednews/2008/11/17/prsa1117.htm (accessed December 2, 2008).

ORI (Office of Research Integrity). 2008. *About ORI: History.* Rockville, MD: ORI. http://ori.dhhs.gov/about/history.shtml (accessed February 10, 2009).

Orlowski, J. P., and L. Wateska. 1992. The effects of pharmaceutical firm enticements on physician prescribing patterns. There's no such thing as a free lunch. *Chest* 102(1):270-273.

OTA (Office of Technology Assessment). 1984. *Commercial Biotechnology: An International Analysis.* Report OTA-BA-218. Washington, DC: U.S. Government Printing Office.

OTA. 1986. *Payment for Physician Services: Strategies for Medicare.* Report OTA-H-294. Washington, DC: U.S. Government Printing Office.

OTA. 1994. *Identifying Health Technologies That Work: Searching for Evidence.* Report OTA-H-608. Washington, DC: U.S. Government Printing Office.

Oxman, A. D. 1994. Checklists for review articles. *British Medical Journal* 309(6955): 648-651.

Oxman, A. D., H. J. Schunemann, and A. Fretheim. 2006a. Improving the use of research evidence in guideline development. 2. Priority setting. *Health Research Policy and Systems* 4:14.

Oxman, A. D., H. J. Schunemann, and A. Fretheim. 2006b. Improving the use of research evidence in guideline development. 8. Synthesis and presentation of evidence. *Health Research Policy and Systems* 4:20.

Papanikolaou, G. N., M. S. Baltogianni, D. G. Contopoulos-Ioannidis, A. B. Haidich, I. A. Giannakakis, and J. P. Ioannidis. 2001. Reporting of conflicts of interest in guidelines of preventive and therapeutic interventions. *BMC Medical Research Methodology* 1:3.

Parascandola, M. 2007. A turning point for conflicts of interest: the controversy over the National Academy of Sciences' first conflicts of interest disclosure policy. *Journal of Clinical Oncology* 25(24):3774-3779.

Pear, R. 2008. Long-term fix is elusive in Medicare payments. *The New York Times*, July 13, A18.

Pearson, S. D., K. Kleinman, D. Rusinak, and W. Levinson. 2006. A trial of disclosing physicians' financial incentives to patients. *Archives of Internal Medicine* 166(6):623-628.

Pellegrino, E. D., and A. S. Relman. 1999. Professional medical associations: ethical and practical guidelines. *Journal of the American Medical Association* 282(10):984-986.

Pellegrino, E. D., and D. C. Thomasma. 1993. *Virtues in Medical Practice.* New York: Oxford University Press.

Peppercorn, J., E. Blood, E. Winer, and A. Partridge. 2007. Association between pharmaceutical involvement and outcomes in breast cancer clinical trials. *Cancer* 109(7):1239-1246.

Perkins, H. S. 1995. May the piper take payment and still call the tune? *Journal of General Internal Medicine* 10(11):645-646.

Perlis, R. H., C. S. Perlis, Y. Wu, C. Hwang, M. Joseph, and A. A. Nierenberg. 2005. Industry sponsorship and financial conflict of interest in the reporting of clinical trials in psychiatry. *American Journal of Psychiatry* 162(10):1957-1960.

Perrone, M. 2009. Drugmakers' push boosts 'murky' ailment. *The Associated Press*, February 8. http://abcnews.go.com/Business/WireStory?id=6831203&page=3 (accessed April 8, 2009).

Perry, S. 1982. Special report. The brief life of the National Center for Health Care Technology. *New England Journal of Medicine* 307(17):1095-1100.

Petersen, M. 2003. Science journals tighten rules for disclosure of financial ties. *The New York Times*, September 27, A10.

Pettypiece, S. 2007. Pfizer job cuts may prompt Glaxo, Sanofi to follow. *Bloomberg Online News*, January 23. http://www.bloomberg.com/apps/news?pid=20601087&sid=ag94zZTfJ4h4&refer=home (accessed August 12, 2008).

Pfizer. 2008. *Pfizer Changes Its Funding of Continuing Medical Education in the U.S.* New York, NY: Pfizer. https://www.pfizermededgrants.com/pfizercme/help/CME_Funding_Change_Announcement.html (accessed November 5, 2008).

Pham, H. H., and P. B. Ginsburg. 2007. Unhealthy trends: the future of physician services. *Health Affairs* 26(6):1586-1598.

Pham, H. H., K. J. Devers, J. H. May, and R. Berenson. 2004. Financial pressures spur physician entrepreneurialism. *Health Affairs* 23(2):70-81.

PhRMA (Pharmaceutical Research and Manufacturers of America). 2008. *Code on Interactions with Healthcare Professionals.* Washington, DC: PhRMA. http://www.phrma.org/files/PhRMA%20Marketing%20Code%202008.pdf (accessed August 1, 2008).

Piwowar, H. A., and W. W. Chapman. 2008. A review of journal policies for sharing research data. Proceedings of the ELPUB 2008 Conference on Electronic Publishing, Toronto, Ontario, Canada, June 2008. http://elpub.scix.net/data/works/att/001_elpub2008.content.pdf (accessed October 10, 2008).

Plint, A., D. Moher, K. Schulz, D. Altman, and A. Morrison. 2005. *Does the CONSORT checklist improve the quality of reports of randomized controlled trials? A systematic review*. Paper presented at the Fifth International Congress on Peer Review and Biomedical Publication, Chicago, IL, September 16-18.

Podolsky, S. H., and J. A. Greene. 2008. A historical perspective of pharmaceutical promotion and physician education. *Journal of the American Medical Association* 300(7):831-833.

Poitras, S., J. Avouac, M. Rossignol, B. Avouac, C. Cedraschi, M. Nordin, C. Rousseaux, et al. 2007. A critical appraisal of guidelines for the management of knee osteoarthritis using Appraisal of Guidelines Research and Evaluation criteria. *Arthritis Research & Therapy* 9(6):R126.

PPRC (Physician Payment Review Commission). 1987. *Medicare Physician Payment: An Agenda for Reform: Annual Report to Congress, 1987*. Washington, DC: PPRC.

Pritchard, M. S. 1996. Conflicts of interest: conceptual and normative issues. *Academic Medicine* 71(12):1305-1313.

Psaty, B. M., and R. A. Kronmal. 2008. Reporting mortality findings in trials of rofecoxib for Alzheimer disease or cognitive impairment: a case study based on documents from rofecoxib litigation. *Journal of the American Medical Association* 299(15):1813-1817.

Psaty, B. M., and D. Rennie. 2006. Clinical trial investigators and their prescribing patterns: another dimension to the relationship between physician investigators and the pharmaceutical industry. *Journal of the American Medical Association* 295(23):2787-2790.

Radek, K. A., L. A. Baer, J. Eckhardt, L. A. DiPietro, and C. E. Wade. 2008. Mechanical unloading impairs keratinocyte migration and angiogenesis during cutaneous wound healing. *Journal of Applied Physiology* 104(5):1295-1303.

Randall, D. A. 2007. The high cost of free lunch. *Obstetrics and Gynecology* 110(4):932; author reply 932-933.

Rapp, K. 2003. *New Times, New Ethical Standards: AdvaMed's Revised Code Updates Medtech Business Practices to Meet Modern Demands for Ethical Conduct and Social Responsibility.* http://www.devicelink.com/mx/archive/03/11/rapp.html (accessed March 10, 2009).

Ratanawongsa, N., A. Teherani, and K. E. Hauer. 2005. Third-year medical students' experiences with dying patients during the internal medicine clerkship: a qualitative study of the informal curriculum. *Academic Medicine* 80(7):641-647.

Read, J. L., and P. M. Campbell. 1988. Health care innovation: a progress report. *Health Affairs* 7(3):174-185.

Read, J. L., and K. B. Lee, Jr. 1994. Health care innovation: progress report and focus on biotechnology. *Health Affairs* 13(3):215-225.

Reck, J. 2008. *A Template for Establishing and Administering Prescriber Support and Education Programs: A Collaborative, Service Based Approach for Achieving Maximum Impact.* Hallowell, ME: Prescription Policy Choices. http://www.policychoices.org/documents/AcademicDetailingTemplate.pdf (accessed October 29, 2008).

Relman, A. S. 1984. Dealing with conflicts of interest. *New England Journal of Medicine* 310(18):1182-1183.

Relman, A. S. 2001. Separating continuing medical education from pharmaceutical marketing. *Journal of the American Medical Association* 285(15):2009-2012.

Relman, A. S. 2003. Defending professional independence: ACCME's proposed new guidelines for commercial support of CME. *Journal of the American Medical Association* 289(18):2418-2420.

Relman, A. S. 2008. Industry support of medical education. *Journal of the American Medical Association* 300(9):1071-1073.

Renfrew, M. J., L. Dyson, G. Herbert, A. McFadden, F. McCormick, J. Thomas, and H. Spiby. 2008. Developing evidence-based recommendations in public health—incorporating the views of practitioners, service users and user representatives. *Health Expect* 11(1):3-15.

Rennie, D. 1997. Thyroid storm. *Journal of the American Medical Association* 277(15): 1238-1243.

Rennie, D., V. Yank, and L. Emanuel. 1997. When authorship fails. A proposal to make contributors accountable. *Journal of the American Medical Association* 278(7):579-585.

Rettig, R. 1997. *Health Care in Transition: Technology Assessment in the Private Sector.* Santa Monica, CA: RAND.

Rice, T. 1997. Physician payment policies: impacts and implications. *Annual Review of Public Health* 18:549-565.

Rick, S., and G. Loewenstein. 2008. Intangibility in intertemporal choice. *Philosophical Transactions of the Royal Society of London. Series B: Biological Sciences* 363(1511): 3813-3824.

Ridgeway, J. 1968. *The Closed Corporation: American Universities in Crisis.* New York: Random House.

Riechelmann, R. P., L. Wang, A. O'Carroll, and M. K. Krzyzanowska. 2007. Disclosure of conflicts of interest by authors of clinical trials and editorials in oncology. *Journal of Clinical Oncology* 25(29):4642-4647.

Rising, K., P. Bacchetti, and L. Bero. 2008. Reporting bias in drug trials submitted to the Food and Drug Administration: review of publication and presentation. *PLoS Medicine* 5(11):1561-1570.

Rochon, P. A., J. H. Gurwitz, C. M. Cheung, J. A. Hayes, and T. C. Chalmers. 1994. Evaluating the quality of articles published in journal supplements compared with the quality of those published in the parent journal. *Journal of the American Medical Association* 272(2):108-113.

Rockhold, F. W., and S. Snapinn. 2007. Improving the image of pharmaceutical industry research: transparency is not always clear. *Biopharmaceutical Report* 15(1):2-12. http://www.amstat.org/sections/sbiop/br_winter07.pdf (accessed February 22, 2009).

Rodwin, M. 1996. Physicians' conflicts of interest in HMOs and hospitals. In *Conflicts of Interest in Clinical Practice and Research*, edited by R. G. Spece, D. S. Shimm, and A. E. Buchanan. New York: Oxford University Press.

Rose, J. 2008. Industry influence in the creation of pay-for-performance quality measures. *Quality Management in Health Care* 17(1):27-34.

Rosenthal, E. 2008. Drug makers' push leads to vaccines' fast rise. *The New York Times*, August 20, A1.

Rosenthal, M. B., B. E. Landon, K. Howitt, H. R. Song, and A. M. Epstein. 2007. Climbing up the pay-for-performance learning curve: where are the early adopters now? *Health Affairs* 26(6):1674-1682.

Ross, J. S., P. Lurie, and S. M. Wolfe. 2000. *Medical Education Services Suppliers: A Threat to Physician Education.* Washington, DC: Public Citizen. http://take-back-the-power.org/publications/release.cfm?ID=7142 (accessed October 10, 2008).

Ross, J. S., J. E. Lackner, P. Lurie, C. P. Gross, S. Wolfe, and H. M. Krumholz. 2007. Pharmaceutical company payments to physicians: early experiences with disclosure laws in Vermont and Minnesota. *Journal of the American Medical Association* 297(11):1216-1223.

Ross, J. S., K. P. Hill, D. S. Egilman, and H. M. Krumholz. 2008. Guest authorship and ghostwriting in publications related to rofecoxib: a case study of industry documents from rofecoxib litigation. *Journal of the American Medical Association* 299(15):1800-1812.

Rothman, K. J. 2001. My actual beliefs. *Journal of Clinical Epidemiology* 54(12):1275; author reply 1276-1277.

Roughead, E. E., K. J. Harvey, and A. L. Gilbert. 1998. Commercial detailing techniques used by pharmaceutical representatives to influence prescribing. *Australian and New Zealand Journal of Medicine* 28(3):306-310.

Sackett, D., S. Straus, S. Richardson, W. Rosenberg, and R. B. Haynes. 2000. *Evidence-Based Medicine: How to Practice and Teach EBM* (2nd edition). London: Churchill Livingstone.

SACME (Society for Academic Continuing Medical Education). 2007. *Survey for 2006: Descriptive Results.* SACME Biennial Survey, January. Birmingham, AL: SACME. http://www.sacme.org/site/sacme/assets/pdf/BS_results_2006.pdf (accessed October 10, 2008).

SACME. 2008a. *About Us.* Birmingham, AL: SACME. http://www.sacme.org/index.cfm?usecookieval=false&pagepath=About_Us&id=1017 (accessed November 21, 2008).

SACME. 2008b. *SACME Response to ACCME Call for Comment on Limiting Interactions Between Accredited Providers and Commercial Interests over Commercial Support with Industry.* Birmingham, AL: SACME. http://www.sacme.org/site/sacme/assets/pdf/SACME_Response_to_ACCME_Calls_for_Comment_9-2008.pdf (accessed December 2, 2008).

Sade, R. M. 2007. A national survey of physician-industry relationships. *New England Journal of Medicine* 357(5):507; author reply 508.

Sadek, H., and Z. Henderson. 2004. It's all in the details: delivering the right information to the right rep at the right time can greatly increase sales force effectiveness. *Pharmaceutical Executive*, October. http://www.imshealth.com/vgn/images/portal/cit_40000873/2/10/71263609PE_All_in_the_Details.pdf (accessed June 27, 2007).

Sage, W. M. 2007. Some principles require principals: why banning "conflicts of interest" won't solve incentive problems in biomedical research. *Texas Law Review* 85:1413-1463.

Sagsveen, M. G. 2008. Untitled. Presentation for the American Academy of Neurology to the Institute of Medicine Committee on Conflict of Interest in Medical Research, Education, and Practice, Washington, DC, May 22.

Salsberg, E. 2008. Addressing healthcare workforce issues for the future. Statement before the Committee on Health, Education, Labor, and Pensions (HELP), U.S. Senate, February 12. http://www.aamc.org/advocacy/library/workforce/testimony/2008/021208.pdf (accessed April 10, 2009).

Sampat, B. N. 2006. Patenting and US academic research in the 20th century: the world before and after Bayh-Dole. *Research Policy* 35(6):772-789.

San Miguel, J. F., R. Schlag, N. K. Khuageva, M. A. Dimopoulos, O. Shpilberg, M. Kropff, I. Spicka, et al. 2008. Bortezomib plus melphalan and prednisone for initial treatment of multiple myeloma. *New England Journal of Medicine* 359(9):906-917.

Sawka, A. M., and L. Thabane. 2003. Effect of industry sponsorship on the results of biomedical research. *Journal of the American Medical Association* 289(19):2502-2503; author reply 2503.

Schacht, W. H. 2008. *The Bayh-Dole Act: Selected Issues in Patent Policy and the Commercialization of Technology.* CRS Report for Congress, Order Code RL32076. Washington, DC: Congressional Research Service. http://assets.opencrs.com/rpts/RL32076_20080403.pdf (accessed December 15, 2008).

Schneider, C., and A. Young. 2008. Emory puts heat on researcher. *The Atlanta Journal-Constitution*, October 5, A1.

Schneider, J. A., V. Arora, K. Kasza, R. Van Harrison, and H. Humphrey. 2006. Residents' perceptions over time of pharmaceutical industry interactions and gifts and the effect of an educational intervention. *Academic Medicine* 81(7):595-602.

Schroter, S., J. Morris, S. Chaudhry, R. Smith, and H. Barratt. 2004. Does the type of competing interest statement affect readers' perceptions of the credibility of research? Randomised trial. *British Medical Journal* 328(7442):742-743.

Schünemann, H. 2008. Systematic reviews and other strategies to protect against bias in guidelines development. Presentation to the Institute of Medicine Committee on Conflict of Interest in Medical Research, Education, and Practice, Washington, DC, May 22.

Schünemann, H., A. Fretheim, and A. D. Oxman. 2006. Improving the use of research evidence in guideline development. 1. Guidelines for guidelines. *Health Research Policy and Systems* 4:13.

Schwartz, L., S. Woloshin, and R. Moynihan. 2008. Who's watching the watch dogs? *British Medical Journal (Clinical Research Edition)* 337:a2535.

Schwitzer, G., G. Mudur, D. Henry, A. Wilson, M. Goozner, M. Simbra, M. Sweet, and K. A. Baverstock. 2005. What are the roles and responsibilities of the media in disseminating health information? *PLoS Medicine* 2(7):e215.

Seidenberg, R. 1971. Advertising and abuse of drugs. *New England Journal of Medicine* 284(14):789-790.

Severinghaus, J. W. 2007. Takuo Aoyagi: discovery of pulse oximetry. *Anesthesia and Analgesia* 105(6 Suppl.):S1-S4, table of contents.

SGIM (Society of General and Internal Medicine). 2006. *Policy on Acceptance and Disclosure of External Funds.* Washington, DC: SGIM. http://www.sgim.org/userfiles/file/SocietyInfo/ExternalFundsPolicyJan2006.pdf (accessed December 15, 2008).

Shaneyfelt, T. M., M. F. Mayo-Smith, and J. Rothwangl. 1999. Are guidelines following guidelines? The methodological quality of clinical practice guidelines in the peer-reviewed medical literature. *Journal of the American Medical Association* 281(20):1900-1905.

Shapiro, D. 2004. Drug companies get too close for med school's comfort. *The New York Times*, January 20, F5.

Shea, B. J., J. M. Grimshaw, G. A. Wells, M. Boers, N. Andersson, C. Hamel, A. C. Porter, et al. 2007. Development of AMSTAR: a measurement tool to assess the methodological quality of systematic reviews. *BMC Medical Research Methodology* 7:10.

Shekelle, P. G., S. H. Woolf, M. Eccles, and J. Grimshaw. 1999. Clinical guidelines: developing guidelines. *British Medical Journal* 318(7183):593-596.

Shelton, S. 2008. Emory will punish psychiatrist Nemeroff: chairmanship taken away, outside income to be vetted. *The Atlanta Journal-Constitution*, December 23, Metro News, 4B. http://www.ajc.com/services/content/printedition/2008/12/23/nemeroff.html (accessed February 19, 2009).

Sherman, T. 2008. Cardiologist will settle fraud case: UMDNJ gave him job for referring patients. *The Star-Ledger*, July 1, p. 16.

Shiffman, R. N., P. Shekelle, J. M. Overhage, J. Slutsky, J. Grimshaw, and A. M. Deshpande. 2003. Standardized reporting of clinical practice guidelines: a proposal from the Conference on Guideline Standardization. *Annals of Internal Medicine* 139(6):493-498.

Shuchman, M. 2007. Commercializing clinical trials—risks and benefits of the CRO boom. *New England Journal of Medicine* 357(14):1365-1368.

Sierles, F. S., A. C. Brodkey, L. M. Cleary, F. A. McCurdy, M. Mintz, J. Frank, D. J. Lynn, et al. 2005. Medical students' exposure to and attitudes about drug company interactions: a national survey. *Journal of the American Medical Association* 294(9):1034-1042.

Sigworth, S. K., M. D. Nettleman, and G. M. Cohen. 2001. Pharmaceutical branding of resident physicians. *Journal of the American Medical Association* 286(9):1024-1025.

Silverstein, F. E., G. Faich, J. L. Goldstein, L. S. Simon, T. Pincus, A. Whelton, R. Makuch, et al. 2000. Gastrointestinal toxicity with celecoxib vs nonsteroidal anti-inflammatory drugs for osteoarthritis and rheumatoid arthritis: the CLASS study: a randomized controlled trial. Celecoxib Long-Term Arthritis Safety Study. *Journal of the American Medical Association* 284(10):1247-1255.

Simon, S. R., S. R. Majumdar, L. A. Prosser, S. Salem-Schatz, C. Warner, K. Kleinman, I. Miroshnik, et al. 2005. Group versus individual academic detailing to improve the use of antihypertensive medications in primary care: a cluster-randomized controlled trial. *American Journal of Medicine* 118(5):521-528.

Sismondo, S. 2008. Pharmaceutical company funding and its consequences: a qualitative systematic review. *Contemporary Clinical Trials* 29(2):109-113.

Sloan, F. A., J. R. Rattliff, and M. A. Hall. 2007. Effects of state managed care patient protection laws on physician satisfaction. *Medical Care Research and Review* 64(5):585-599.

Smith, D. 1992. *Paying for Medicare: The Politics of Reform*. New York: Aldine de Gruyter.

Smith, S. 2006. Article urging heart exams shows conflicting interests. *Boston Globe*, July 25, A1.

Smulders, Y. M., and A. Thijs. 2007. The influence of the pharmaceutical industry on treatment guidelines. *Nederlands Tijdschrift voor Geneeskunde* 151(44):2429-2431. (In Dutch.)

Snyder, L., and C. Leffler. 2005. Ethics manual: fifth edition. *Annals of Internal Medicine* 142(7):560-582.

Sollitto, S., S. Hoffman, M. Mehlman, R. J. Lederman, S. J. Youngner, and M. M. Lederman. 2003. Intrinsic conflicts of interest in clinical research: a need for disclosure. *Kennedy Institute of Ethics Journal* 13(2):83-91.

Solomon, D. H., L. Van Houten, R. J. Glynn, L. Baden, K. Curtis, H. Schrager, and J. Avorn. 2001. Academic detailing to improve use of broad-spectrum antibiotics at an academic medical center. *Archives of Internal Medicine* 161(15):1897-1902.

Sorrell, W. H. 2008. *Pharmaceutical Marketing Disclosures: Report of Vermont Attorney General William H. Sorrell on Payments to Physicians*. Montpelier, VT: Vermont Office of the Attorney General. http://www.atg.state.vt.us/upload/1215544954_2008_Pharmaceutical_Marketing_Disclosures_Report.pdf (accessed September 17, 2008).

Soumerai, S. B., and J. Avorn. 1990. Principles of educational outreach ("academic detailing") to improve clinical decision making. *Journal of the American Medical Association* 263(4):549-556.

Sox, H. C., and D. Rennie. 2008. Seeding trials: just say "no." *Annals of Internal Medicine* 149(4):279-280.

Stanczyk, J., C. Ospelt, and S. Gay. 2008. Is there a future for small molecule drugs in the treatment of rheumatic diseases? *Current Opinion in Rheumatology* 20(3):257-262.

Stanford University. Undated. *Stanford Research Administration: Conflict of Interest*. http://dor.stanford.edu/Resources/coi.html (accessed March 21, 2009).

Stanford University School of Medicine. 2006. *Stanford Industry Interactions Policy.* http://med.stanford.edu/coi/siip/documents/siip_policy_aug06.pdf (accessed September 15, 2008).

Stanford University School of Medicine. 2008. *Continuing Medical Education (CME) Commercial Support Policy.* http://cme.stanford.edu/documents/cme_commercial_support_policy.pdf (accessed September 15, 2008).

Stark, A. 2000. *Conflict of Interest in American Public Life.* Cambridge, MA: Harvard University Press.

Steinberg, E. P., and B. R. Luce. 2005. Evidence based? Caveat emptor! *Health Affairs* 24(1):80-92.

Steinbrook, R. 2005. Commercial support and continuing medical education. *New England Journal of Medicine* 352(6):534-535.

Steinbrook, R. 2006. For sale: physicians' prescribing data. *New England Journal of Medicine* 354(26):2745-2747.

Steinbrook, R. 2007. Guidance for guidelines. *New England Journal of Medicine* 356(4): 331-333.

Steinbrook, R. 2008a. Disclosure of industry payments to physicians. *New England Journal of Medicine* 359(6):559-561.

Steinbrook, R. 2008b. Financial support of continuing medical education. *Journal of the American Medical Association* 299(9):1060-1062.

Steinbrook, R. 2008c. The Gelsinger case. In *The Oxford Textbook of Clinical Research Ethics*, edited by E. J. Emanuel, C. Grady, R. A. Crouch, R. Lie, F. Miller and D. Wendler. New York: Oxford University Press.

Steinman, M. A. 2008. Conflict of interest in graduate and undergraduate medical education. Presentation to the Institute of Medicine Committee on Conflict of Interest in Medical Research, Education, and Practice, Washington, DC, January 21.

Steinman, M. A., M. G. Shlipak, and S. J. McPhee. 2001. Of principles and pens: attitudes and practices of medicine housestaff toward pharmaceutical industry promotions. *American Journal of Medicine* 110(7):551-557.

Steinman, M. A., L. A. Bero, M. M. Chren, and C. S. Landefeld. 2006. Narrative review: the promotion of gabapentin: an analysis of internal industry documents. *Annals of Internal Medicine* 145(4):284-293.

Steinman, M. A., G. M. Harper, M. M. Chren, C. S. Landefeld, and L. A. Bero. 2007. Characteristics and impact of drug detailing for gabapentin. *PLoS Medicine* 4(4):e134.

Steneck, N. H. 1984. Commentary: the university and research ethics. *Science, Technology, & Human Values* 9(4):6-15.

Stievater, D. N., A. Petersen, and R. Bhatia. 2006. Sewing up new sales. *Pharmaceutical Executive*, September. http://www.impactrx.com/pdfs/Sewing_Up_Sales_PharmaExec10_26_06.pdf (accessed August 27, 2007).

Stolberg, S. G. 1999. The biotech death of Jesse Gelsinger. *NYT Magazine*, November 28, pp. 136-140, 149-150.

Stolberg, S. G. 2000. Biomedicine is receiving new scrutiny as scientists become entrepreneurs. *The New York Times*, February 20, Sec. 1, p. 26.

Stossel, T. P. 2005. Regulating academic-industrial research relationships—solving problems or stifling progress? *New England Journal of Medicine* 353(10):1060-1065.

Stossel, T. P. 2007. Regulation of financial conflicts of interest in medical practice and medical research: a damaging solution in search of a problem. *Perspectives in Biology and Medicine* 50(1):54-71.

Stossel, T. P. 2008. Has the hunt for conflicts of interest gone too far? Yes. *British Medical Journal* 336(7642):476.

Stotland, N. 2008. APA responds to Sen. Grassley. *Psychiatric News* 43(17):3.

Streiffer, R. 2006. Academic freedom and academic-industry relationships in biotechnology. *Kennedy Institute of Ethics Journal* 16(2):129-149.

Stroup, D. F., J. A. Berlin, S. C. Morton, I. Olkin, G. D. Williamson, D. Rennie, D. Moher, et al. 2000. Meta-analysis of observational studies in epidemiology: a proposal for reporting. Meta-Analysis of Observational Studies in Epidemiology (MOOSE) group. *Journal of the American Medical Association* 283(15):2008-2012.

Studdert, D. M., M. M. Mello, and T. A. Brennan. 2004. Financial conflicts of interest in physicians' relationships with the pharmaceutical industry—self-regulation in the shadow of federal prosecution. *New England Journal of Medicine* 351(18):1891-1900.

Sulmasy, D. P., M. G. Bloche, J. M. Mitchell, and J. Hadley. 2000. Physicians' ethical beliefs about cost-control arrangements. *Archives of Internal Medicine* 160(5):649-657.

Suwa, K. 2003. Pulse oximeters: personal recollections of the past and hopes for the future. *Journal of Anesthesia* 17(4):267-269.

Swann, J. P. 1988. *Academic Scientists and the Pharmaceutical Industry*. Baltimore, MD: The Johns Hopkins University Press.

Symm, B., M. Averitt, S. N. Forjuoh, and C. Preece. 2006. Effects of using free sample medications on the prescribing practices of family physicians. *Journal of the American Board of Family Medicine* 19(5):443-449.

Takhar, J., D. Dixon, J. Donahue, B. Marlow, C. Campbell, I. Silver, J. Eadie, et al. 2007. Developing an instrument to measure bias in CME. *Journal of Continuing Education in the Health Professions* 27(2):118-123.

Tanaka, M., and S. Watanabe. 1994. Overwintering in the Antarctica as an analog for long term manned spaceflight. *Advances in Space Research* 14(8):423-430.

Tcheng, J. E., D. E. Kandzari, C. L. Grines, D. A. Cox, M. B. Effron, E. Garcia, J. J. Griffin, et al. 2003. Benefits and risks of abciximab use in primary angioplasty for acute myocardial infarction: the Controlled Abciximab and Device Investigation to Lower Late Angioplasty Complications (CADILLAC) trial. *Circulation* 108(11):1316-1323.

Tenaglia, M., and P. Angelastro. 2005. No margin for error. *Pharmaceutical Executive*, September. http://www.amundsengroup.com/images/nomarginforerror.pdf (accessed August 27, 2007).

Tereskerz, P. M., and J. Moreno. 2005. Ten steps to developing a national agenda to address financial conflicts of interest in industry sponsored clinical research. *Accountability in Research* 12(2):139-155.

Thayer, A. 2005. Insulin: in Top Pharmaceuticals: a look at drugs that changed the world. *Chemical & Engineering News* 83(25):3.

Thompson, D. F. 1993. Understanding financial conflicts of interest. *New England Journal of Medicine* 329(8):573-576.

Thrasher, K., and M. Franklin. 1999. Minnesota sets the pace: medical technology started with a pacemaker. *Minnesota Technolog*, November/December. http://technolog.it.umn.edu/technolog/novdec99/pacemaker.html (accessed July 15, 2008).

Tovino, S. A. 2007. Functional neuroimaging and the law: trends and directions for future scholarship. *American Journal of Bioethics* 7(9):44-56.

Trachtman, H. 2003. The death of common sense. *American Journal of Bioethics* 3(3): W31-W32.

Tregear, M. 2007. *Guideline Heterogeneity*. Workshop—Part 2, ECRI Institute, August 27 Presentation at the Fourth Annual Guidelines International Network Meeting, Toronto on August 22-25.

Tu, H. T., and P. B. Ginsburg. 2006. *Losing Ground: Physician Income, 1995-2003*. Tracking Report 15. Washington, DC: Center for Studying Health System Change, pp. 1-8.

Tunis, S. R., D. B. Stryer, and C. M. Clancy. 2003. Practical clinical trials: increasing the value of clinical research for decision making in clinical and health policy. *Journal of the American Medical Association* 290(12):1624-1632.

Turner, E. H., A. M. Matthews, E. Linardatos, R. A. Tell, and R. Rosenthal. 2008. Selective publication of antidepressant trials and its influence on apparent efficacy. *New England Journal of Medicine* 358(3):252-260.

Turton, F. E., and L. Snyder. 2007. Physician-industry relations. *Annals of Internal Medicine* 146(6):469.

Ubel, P. A., R. M. Arnold, G. P. Gramelspacher, R. B. Hoppe, C. S. Landefeld, W. Levinson, W. Tierney, and S. W. Tolle. 1995. Acceptance of external funds by physician organizations: issues and policy options. *Journal of General Internal Medicine* 10(11):624-630.

Ubel, P. A., C. Jepson, and D. A. Asch. 2003. Misperceptions about beta-blockers and diuretics: a national survey of primary care physicians. *Journal of General Internal Medicine* 18(12):977-983.

University of California. 2008. *Health Care Vendor Relations Policy*. Oakland, CA: University of California. http://www.ucop.edu/ucophome/coordrev/policy/PP031208Policy.pdf (accessed December 12, 2008).

University of Louisville. 2008. *University of Louisville Health Care Policy on Vendors*. Louisville, KY: University of Louisville. http://louisville.edu/medschool/dean/docs/VendorPolicy%20Approved.pdf (accessed December 31, 2008).

University of Massachusetts. 2008. *Vendor Relations Policy Frequently Asked Questions (FAQs)*. http://www.amsascorecard.org/documents/0000/0027/FAQs_UMM_Policy_2-2008.doc (accessed December 31, 2008).

University of Michigan. 2005. *Conflicts of Interest and Conflicts of Commitment*. Standard Practice Guide (Number 201.65-1). Ann Arbor: University of Michigan. http://spg.umich.edu/pdf/201.65-1.pdf (accessed July 11, 2008).

University of Michigan Health System. 2007. *UMHHC Policy 07-01-045: Drug Samples in UMHHC*. Ann Arbor: University of Michigan Health System. http://www.imapny.org/usr_doc/Drug_Sample_PolicyM4.pdf (accessed October 7, 2008).

University of Minnesota. 2008. *Potential Conflicts of Interest: A Course for University of Minnesota Researchers*. St. Paul, MN: University of Minnesota. http://cflegacy.research.umn.edu/coi/index.shtml (accessed March 21, 2009).

University of Pittsburgh. 2007. *Industry Interactions Policy*. Pittsburgh, PA: University of Pittsburgh. http://www.ogc.pitt.edu/publications/IndustryRelationshipsPolicy.pdf (accessed October 7, 2008).

University of Rochester. 2006. *University of Rochester Policy on Institutional Conflict of Interest in Research Activities*. Rochester, NY: University of Rochester. http://www.rochester.edu/ORPA/policies/COIresearch.pdf (accessed January 13, 2009).

University of Washington. 2008. *State Ethics Act of 2005—Impact on UW Policy*. Seattle: University of Washington. http://www.washington.edu/research/main.php?page=stateEthicsAct (accessed October 21, 2008).

University of Wisconsin. 2008. *Showcase: Campus-Wide Change Efforts*. Madison: University of Wisconsin. http://www.oqi.wisc.edu/Showcase/Portals/0/CampusWideChange.pdf (accessed January 13, 2009).

USPHS (U.S. Public Health Service Commissioned Corps). 1995. Objectivity in research; final rule. *Federal Register* 60(132):35810-35819.

USPSTF (U.S. Preventive Services Task Force). 2007a. Screening for lipid disorders in children: U.S. Preventive Services Task Force recommendation statement. *Pediatrics* 120(1):e215-e219.

USPSTF. 2007b. *Screening for Lipid Disorders in Children: U.S. Preventive Services Task Force Recommendation Statement*. Rockville, MD: Agency for Healthcare Research and Quality. http://www.ahrq.gov/clinic/uspstf07/chlipid/chlipidrs.htm (accessed March 21, 2009).

USPSTF. 2007c. *Screening for Sickle Cell Disease in Newborns: U.S. Preventive Services Task Force Recommendation Statement*. Rockville, MD: Agency for Healthcare Research and Quality. http://www.ahrq.gov/clinic/uspstf07/sicklecell/sicklers.htm (accessed April 25, 2008).

USPSTF. 2008. *Methods and Background: U.S. Preventive Services Task Force*. Rockville, MD: Agency for Healthcare Research and Quality. http://www.ahrq.gov/clinic/uspstf08/methods/procmanual.htm (accessed April 10, 2009).

van Eijk, M. E., J. Avorn, A. J. Porsius, and A. de Boer. 2001. Reducing prescribing of highly anticholinergic antidepressants for elderly people: randomised trial of group versus individual academic detailing. *British Medical Journal* 322(7287):654-657.

Varley, C. K., M. D. Jibson, M. McCarthy, and S. Benjamin. 2005. A survey of the interactions between psychiatry residency programs and the pharmaceutical industry. *Academic Psychiatry* 29(1):40-46.

Verkerk, K., H. Van Veenendaal, J. L. Severens, E. J. Hendriks, and J. S. Burgers. 2006. Considered judgement in evidence-based guideline development. *International Journal for Quality in Health Care* 18(5):365-369.

Vesely, R. 2005. Kaiser doctors conflict-of-interest policy tightened. *Oakland Tribune*, April 27.

Vogeli, C., R. Yucel, E. Bendavid, L. M. Jones, M. S. Anderson, K. S. Louis, and E. G. Campbell. 2006. Data withholding and the next generation of scientists: results of a national survey. *Academic Medicine* 81(2):128-136.

von Elm, E., D. G. Altman, M. Egger, S. J. Pocock, P. C. Gotzsche, and J. P. Vandenbroucke. 2007. The Strengthening the Reporting of Observational Studies in Epidemiology (STROBE) statement: guidelines for reporting observational studies. *PLoS Medicine* 4(10):e296.

Vreman, H. J., R. J. Wong, J. R. Murdock, and D. K. Stevenson. 2008. Standardized bench method for evaluating the efficacy of phototherapy devices. *Acta Paediatrica* 97(3): 308-316.

Wager, E. 2007. Authors, ghosts, damned lies, and statisticians. *PLoS Medicine* 4(1): e34-e35.

Walker, L. 2001. *ROI for Meetings Beats Detailing and DTC*. http://meetingsnet.com/medicalmeetings/meetings_roi_meetings_beats/ (accessed September 25, 2008).

Wall, L. L., and D. Brown. 2007. The high cost of free lunch. *Obstetrics and Gynecology* 110(1):169-173.

Wallack, T. 2008. Tied up over disclosure: life sciences firms anxious about rules on gifts to doctors. *The Boston Globe*, August 13, C1.

WAME (World Association of Medical Editors). 2008. *WAME Recommendations on Publication Ethics Policies for Medical Journals*. http://www.wame.org/resources/publication-ethics-policies-for-medical-journals#conflicts (accessed December 2, 2008).

Warlow, C. 2007. No ghosts here please. *Practical Neurology* 7(2):72-73.

Warner, T. D., and J. P. Gluck. 2003. What do we really know about conflicts of interest in biomedical research? *Psychopharmacology* 171(1):36-46.

Warner, T. D., and L. W. Roberts. 2004. Scientific integrity, fidelity and conflicts of interest in research. *Current Opinion in Psychiatry* 17:381-385.

Wartman, S. A. 2007. *The Academic Health Center: Evolving Organizational Models*. Washington, DC: Association of Academic Health Centers. http://www.aahcdc.org/policy/reddot/AAHC_Evolving_Organizational_Models.pdf (accessed August 12, 2008).

Waters, R. 2006. J&J sued by Texas in whistleblower case on marketing (update1). *Bloomberg Online News*, December 28. http://www.bloomberg.com/apps/news?pid=20601202&sid=a2mpCNBojB2I&refer=healthcare (accessed April 25, 2008).

Watson, P. Y., A. K. Khandelwal, J. L. Musial, and J. D. Buckley. 2005. Resident and faculty perceptions of conflict of interest in medical education. *Journal of General Internal Medicine* 20(4):357-359.

Weber, M. 2006. *Medicine and Conflicts of Interest: Creating a New Morality.* http://www.medicalprogresstoday.com/spotlight/spotlight_indarchive.php?id=1399 (accessed October 10, 2008).

Wegman, A., D. van der Windt, M. van Tulder, W. Stalman, and T. de Vries. 2004. Nonsteroidal antiinflammatory drugs or acetaminophen for osteoarthritis of the hip or knee? A systematic review of evidence and guidelines. *Journal of Rheumatology* 31(2):344-354.

Weinfurt, K. P., J. Y. Friedman, J. S. Allsbrook, M. A. Dinan, M. A. Hall, and J. Sugarman. 2006a. Views of potential research participants on financial conflicts of interest: barriers and opportunities for effective disclosure. *Journal of General Internal Medicine* 21(9):901-906.

Weinfurt, K. P., M. A. Dinan, J. S. Allsbrook, J. Y. Friedman, M. A. Hall, K. A. Schulman, and J. Sugarman. 2006b. Policies of academic medical centers for disclosing financial conflicts of interest to potential research participants. *Academic Medicine* 81(2):113-118.

Weinfurt, K. P., J. Y. Friedman, M. A. Dinan, J. S. Allsbrook, M. A. Hall, J. K. Dhillon, and J. Sugarman. 2006c. Disclosing conflicts of interest in clinical research: views of institutional review boards, conflict of interest committees, and investigators. *Journal of Law, Medicine and Ethics* 34(3):581-591, 481.

Weinfurt, K. P., M. A. Hall, M. A. Dinan, V. DePuy, J. Y. Friedman, J. S. Allsbrook, and J. Sugarman. 2008a. Effects of disclosing financial interests on attitudes toward clinical research. *Journal of General Internal Medicine* 23(6):860-866.

Weinfurt, K. P., M. A. Hall, J. Y. Friedman, C. Hardy, A. K. Fortune-Greeley, J. S. Lawlor, J. S. Allsbrook, L. Lin, K. A. Schulman, and J. Sugarman. 2008b. Effects of disclosing financial interests on participation in medical research: a randomized vignette trial. *American Heart Journal* 156(4):689-697.

Weinfurt, K. P., D. M. Seils, J. P. Tzeng, L. Lin, K. A. Schulman, and R. M. Califf. 2008c. Consistency of financial interest disclosures in the biomedical literature: the case of coronary stents. *PLoS ONE* 3(5):e2128.

Weinmann, S., M. Koesters, and T. Becker. 2007. Effects of implementation of psychiatric guidelines on provider performance and patient outcome: systematic review. *Acta Psychiatrica Scandinavica* 115(6):420-433.

Weiss, R. 2005. NIH clears most researchers in conflict-of-interest probe. *The Washington Post*, February 23, A1.

Wellman, H. R. 1967. Memorandum to the faculty and staff of the University of California on the university-wide statement on conflicts of interest. http://www.ucop.edu/ucophome/coordrev/policy/10-05-67.html (accessed July 29, 2008).

Wennberg, J. E. 2003. The more things change . . .: the federal government's role in the evaluative sciences. *Health Affairs* Suppl. Web Exclusives:W3-308–W3-310.

Werhane, P., and J. Doering. 1995. Conflicts of interest and conflicts of commitment. *Professional Ethics* 4(3-4):47-81.

Whelan, E. 2008. 'Conflict' chills research. *The Washington Times*, April 8, A19.

Whittington, C. J., T. Kendall, P. Fonagy, D. Cottrell, A. Cotgrove, and E. Boddington. 2004. Selective serotonin reuptake inhibitors in childhood depression: systematic review of published versus unpublished data. *Lancet* 363(9418):1341-1345.

Willman, D. 2004. The National Institutes of Health: public servant or private marketer? *Los Angeles Times*, December 22, A1.

Willman, D. 2006. NIH audit criticizes scientist's dealings. *Los Angeles Times*, September 10, A1.

Wilson, J. W., C. M. Ott, K. Honer zu Bentrup, R. Ramamurthy, L. Quick, S. Porwollik, P. Cheng, et al. 2007. Space flight alters bacterial gene expression and virulence and reveals a role for global regulator Hfq. *Proceedings of the National Academy of Sciences of the United States of America* 104(41):16299-16304.

Wimsatt, L., A. Trice, and R. Decker. 2005. *Federal Demonstration Partnership: Fall 2005 Faculty Burden.* http://thefdp.org/Faculty_Burden_Survey.pdf (accessed July 2, 2008).

Witkin, K. B. 1997. Using pilot studies to chart a course in clinical research. *Medical Device & Diagnostic Indaustry Magazine*, June. http://www.devicelink.com/mddi/archive/97/06/018.html (accessed March 2, 2009).

WMS (Wisconsin Medical Society). 2008. *Wisconsin Medical Society Board Passes New Physician Gift Policy.* Press release, October 16. Madison, WI: WMS. http://www.wisconsinmedicalsociety.org/publications_and_media/press_releases (accessed October 29, 2008).

Woolf, S. H., R. Grol, A. Hutchinson, M. Eccles, and J. Grimshaw. 1999. Clinical guidelines: potential benefits, limitations, and harms of clinical guidelines. *British Medical Journal* 318(7182):527-530.

Woolley, K. L., J. A. Ely, M. J. Woolley, L. Findlay, F. A. Lynch, Y. Choi, and J. M. McDonald. 2006. Declaration of medical writing assistance in international peer-reviewed publications. *Journal of the American Medical Association* 296(8):932-934.

Wright, J. M., T. L. Perry, K. L. Bassett, and G. K. Chambers. 2001. Reporting of 6-month vs 12-month data in a clinical trial of celecoxib. *Journal of the American Medical Association* 286(19):2398-2400.

Yank, V., D. Rennie, and L. A. Bero. 2007. Financial ties and concordance between results and conclusions in meta-analyses: retrospective cohort study. *British Medical Journal* 335(7631):1202-1205.

Zarin, D. A., T. Tse, and N. C. Ide. 2005. Trial registration at ClinicalTrials.gov between May and October 2005. *New England Journal of Medicine* 353(26):2779-2787.

Zerhouni, E. 2007. Untitled. Presentation to the Institute of Medicine Committee on Conflicts of Interest in Medical Research, Education, and Practice, Washington, DC, November 6.

Zerhouni, E. 2008. NIH response to OIG findings and recommendations. Appendix to the Office of Inspector General Report. In *National Institutes of Health: Conflicts of Interest in Intramural Research*. Bethesda, MD: National Institutes of Health. http://oig.hhs.gov/oei/reports/oei-03-06-00460.pdf (accessed June 23, 2008).

Zipkin, D. A., and M. A. Steinman. 2005. Interactions between pharmaceutical representatives and doctors in training. A thematic review. *Journal of General Internal Medicine* 20(8):777-786.

A

Study Activities

During 2006, the Institute of Medicine's (IOM's) Board on Health Sciences Policy began to discuss threats to public trust in biomedical research and medicine created by certain types of financial relationships between pharmaceutical, medical device, and biotechnology companies and researchers based in universities and federal agencies. As the discussion expanded, others expressed concerns about conflicts of interest in medical education, especially continuing medical education. The IOM was also approached about whether it would examine financial relationships and conflicts of interest as they affect the publication of research and the development of clinical practice guidelines.

In response, the IOM developed a proposal for a broad-ranging study that would examine conflicts of interest across medical research, medical education, clinical practice, and practice guideline development. It secured funding for the study from both public and private sources and appointed a 17-member committee to oversee the study. The charge to the committee was to develop a consensus report that would

- examine and describe conflicts of interest involving health care professionals and industry in different contexts, including, for example, the conduct of research, the education of health care professionals, the development of practice guidelines, the provision of patient care, and the management of academic and other institutions;
- propose principles to inform the design of policies, guidelines, and other tools to identify and manage conflicts of interest in these contexts without damaging constructive collaboration with industry; and
- consider methods to disseminate, promote, implement, and evaluate these principles and policies.

The committee met six times between November 2007 and October 2008. It held public sessions at its first four meetings to hear views from a wide range of experts and interested parties. The May 2008 meeting included a workshop on conflict of interest issues in basic research and another on conflict of interest issues in the development of clinical practice guidelines. The agendas for the public meetings are listed below. The committee also invited written statements of views from approximately 50 additional organizations; those that submitted statements are listed.

INSTITUTE OF MEDICINE
COMMITTEE ON CONFLICT OF INTEREST IN MEDICAL RESEARCH, EDUCATION, AND PRACTICE

Keck Center of the National Academies
November 5–6, 2007—Open Sessions

November 5

3:00 **Welcome and Introductions**
Bernard Lo, M.D., Committee Chair

3:10 **Overview of Conflicts of Interest in Medical Research, Education,** and Practice
Robert Steinbrook, M.D., National Correspondent, *New England Journal of Medicine*
Eric Campbell, Ph.D., Associate Professor, Institute for Health Policy, Massachusetts General Hospital, and Harvard University
Greg Koski, M.D., Ph.D., Senior Scientist, Institute for Health Policy, Massachusetts General Hospital, and Harvard University
Peter Lurie, M.D., M.P.H., Deputy Director, Public Citizen's Health Research Group

Discussion

5:00 **Adjourn**

November 6

8:30 **Welcome and Introductions**

8:35 **Perspectives from Industry**
Garry A. Neil, M.D., Group President, Johnson & Johnson

8:50 Discussion with Study Sponsor
Christine Cassel, M.D., President, American Board on Internal Medicine Foundation

9:05 Conflict of Interest in Medical Research
Cary P. Gross, M.D., Associate Professor of Medicine, Yale University
David Korn, M.D., Senior Vice President for Biomedical and Health Sciences Research, Association of American Medical Colleges

Discussion

10:10 Break

10:30 Conceptual Issues in Conflict of Interest
Ezekiel J. Emanuel, M.D., Ph.D., Chair, Department of Bioethics, Magnuson Clinical Center, National Institutes of Health

Discussion

11:10 Discussion with Study Sponsor
Elias A. Zerhouni, M.D., Director, National Institutes of Health

Noon Adjourn

INSTITUTE OF MEDICINE COMMITTEE ON CONFLICT OF INTEREST IN MEDICAL RESEARCH, EDUCATION, AND PRACTICE

Keck Center of the National Academies
January 21, 2008—Open Session

1:00 Welcome, Introductions, and Statement About the Meeting
Bernard Lo, M.D., Committee Chair

1:10 Conflict of Interest in Medical Education
Suzanne Fletcher, M.D., M.Sc., Professor Emerita of Ambulatory Care and Prevention, Harvard Medical School
Michael Steinman, M.D. (*by conference call*), Assistant Professor of Medicine, San Francisco Veterans Affairs Medical Center and University of California, San Francisco

Discussion

2:10 **Conflict of Interest in Medical Education**
Murray Kopelow, M.D., Chief Executive, Accreditation Council for Continuing Medical Education
Ingrid Philibert, M.H.A., M.B.A., Senior Vice President, Department of Field Activities, Accreditation Council for Graduate Medical Education
F. Daniel Duffy, M.D., Senior Adviser to the President, American Board of Medical Specialties

Discussion

3:10 **Break**

3:30 **Perspectives from Industry**
Paul Citron, Ph.D., Retired, Vice President for Technology Policy and Academic Affairs, Medtronic
Cathryn Clary, M.D., Vice President, U.S. External Medical Affairs, Pfizer, Inc.

Discussion

4:15 **General Discussion**

5:00 **Adjourn**

INSTITUTE OF MEDICINE COMMITTEE ON CONFLICT OF INTEREST IN MEDICAL RESEARCH, EDUCATION, AND PRACTICE

Board Room, National Academy of Sciences
March 13, 2008—Open Session

8:15 **Welcome and Chair's Statement**
Bernard Lo, M.D., Committee Chair

8:30 **Statements from Organizations**
Consumers Union
Gail Shearer, Director, Health Policy Analysis
John Santa, M.D., Consultant and Associate Professor, Oregon Health Sciences University and Portland State University

Center for Science in the Public Interest
Merrill Goozner, Director, Integrity in Science

Alpha-One
John Walsh, President

Questions and Discussion

9:25 **Statements from Organizations**
Pharmaceutical Research and Manufacturers Association
Alan Goldhammer, Ph.D., Deputy Vice President, Regulatory Affairs

AdvaMed (Advanced Medical Devices Association)
Kris Rapp, Vice President, Global Ethics & Compliance for Hospira, Inc.

BIO (Biotechnology Industry Organization)
Jonca Bull, M.D., Director, Clinical and Regulatory Affairs, Genentech

North American Association of Medical Education and Communication Companies
Karen M. Overstreet, Ed.D., R.Ph., Past President and President, Indicia Medical Education, LLC

Questions and Discussion

10:25 **Break**

10:45 **Lessons Learned I: Developing and Implementing Medical School Conflict-of-Interest Policies**
Philip A. Pizzo, M.D., Carl and Elizabeth Naumann Dean and Professor of Pediatrics and of Microbiology and Immunology, Stanford University School of Medicine

Joseph B. Martin, M.D., Ph.D., Edward R. and Anne G. Lefler Professor of Neurobiology, and Dean, Harvard Medical School, 1997–2007

Questions and Discussion

Follow-up Questions and Discussion for Earlier Panels

12:00 **Lunch break**

1:00 **Statements from Organizations**
American Medical Association
Mark A. Levine, M.D., Chair, Council of Ethical and Judicial Affairs

American College of Physicians
Joel S. Levine, M.D., Chair, Board of Regents and Senior Associate Dean for Clinical Affairs, University of Colorado School of Medicine

American Psychiatric Association
Carolyn B. Robinowitz, M.D., President and Clinical Professor of Psychiatry at Georgetown and George Washington Universities

American College of Cardiology
John C. Lewin, M.D., C.E.O.
Sidney C. Smith Jr., M.D., Professor of Medicine and Director, Center for Cardiovascular Science and Medicine, University of North Carolina, Chapel Hill

American Medical Student Association
Brian Palmer, M.D., M.P.H., Past President and Psychiatry Resident, Massachusetts General Hospital/McLean Hospital

Questions and Discussion

2:30 **Break**

3:00 **Lessons Learned II: Developing and Implementing Conflict-of-Interest Policies**
David Korn, M.D., Senior Vice President for Biomedical and Health Sciences Research Association of American Medical Colleges
Leo Furcht, M.D., Past President, Federation of American Societies for Experimental Biology and Allen Pardee, Professor and Head of Laboratory Medicine and Pathology, University of Minnesota School of Medicine
Harold C. Sox, M.D., International Committee of Medical Journal Editors, and Editor, *Annals of Internal Medicine*

Questions and Discussion

4:15 Continued Questions and Discussion and Public Comment

5:00 Adjourn

Organizations Submitting Written Statements
In addition to the organizations presenting statements during the March meeting, the following organizations provided written statements to the committee:

Accreditation Council for Continuing Medical Education
Alliance for Continuing Medical Education
Alzheimer's Association
American Academy of Family Physicians
American Academy of Ophthalmology
American Academy of Orthopedic Surgeons
American Academy of Pediatrics
American Board of Medical Specialties
American Society of Hematology
American Thoracic Society
Coalition for Healthcare Communication
Infectious Diseases Society of America
National Kidney Foundation
North American Spine Society
Society for Academic Continuing Medical Education

INSTITUTE OF MEDICINE
COMMITTEE ON CONFLICT OF INTEREST IN MEDICAL RESEARCH, EDUCATION, AND PRACTICE

Lecture Room, National Academy of Sciences
May 22, 2008—Open Session

Conflict of Interest in Basic and Translational Research

8:15 Welcome, Introductions, and Chair's Statement
Bernard Lo, M.D., Committee Chair

8:35 Additional Perspectives on Professional Society Policies
Kenneth Kaushansky, M.D., President, American Society of Hematology and Chair and Helen M. Ranney Professor, Department of Medicine, University of California, San Diego

9:00 **Perspectives on Financial Relationships and Conflicts of Interest in Basic and Early-Stage Translational Research: Part 1**
Leslie Z. Benet, Ph.D., Professor, Department of Biopharmaceutical Sciences, University of California, San Francisco
Gail Cassell, Ph.D., Vice President, Scientific Affairs, and Distinguished Lilly Research Scholar for Infectious Diseases, Eli Lilly and Company
Edward Benz, M.D., (*by telephone*), President, Dana-Farber Cancer Institute

Discussion

10:10 **Break**

10:30 **Perspectives on Financial Relationships and Conflicts of Interest in Basic and Early-Stage Translational Research: Part 2**
Hamilton Moses III, M.D., Chair, The Alerion Institute
Leo Furcht, M.D., Past President, Federation of American Societies for Experimental Biology and Allen Pardee, Professor and Head of Lab Medicine and Pathology, University of Minnesota School of Medicine

Discussion

11:25 **Financial Disclosures and Trust in Health Care Professionals**
Mark Hall, J.D., Professor of Law and Public Health, Wake Forest University School of Law
Kevin Weinfurt, Ph.D., Associate Professor of Psychiatry and Behavioral Sciences, and of Psychology and Neuroscience, Duke Clinical Research Institute

Discussion

Noon **Lunch break**

Conflict of Interest in Clinical Practice Guidelines

1:00 **Welcome, Introductions, and Chair's Statement**
Bernard Lo, M.D., Committee Chair

1:15 **Individual and Organizational Financial Relationships with Industry**
Elizabeth Boyd, Ph.D., Assistant Vice President for Research, Compliance and Policy, University of Arizona

Discussant: Mary Nix, M.S., Health Scientist Administrator, National Guideline Clearinghouse, Agency for Healthcare Research and Quality

Discussion

2:00 **Organizational Policies, Practices, and Challenges in Developing and Implementing Conflict-of-Interest and Related Policies**
Dina Michels, Esq., Vice President and General Counsel, American Society of Clinical Oncology
Murray Sagsveen, J.D., General Counsel, American Academy of Neurology
Sidney C. Smith, Jr., M.D., American College of Cardiology, and Professor of Medicine and Director, Academic Center for Cardiovascular Disease
Mary Barton, M.D., M.P.P., Scientific Director, U.S. Preventive Services Task Force, and University of North Carolina

Discussants:
Fran Visco, President, National Breast Cancer Coalition
Alvin Lever, M.A., C.E.O., American College of Chest Physicians
Sandra Zelman Lewis, Ph.D., Assistant Vice President, American College of Chest Physicians
Henry Masur, M.D., Chief, Department of Critical Care Medicine, National Institutes of Health Clinical Center
John C. Ring, M.D., Director, Policy Research and Development, American Heart Association

3:00 **Break**

3:20 **Continued Discussion of Organizational Policies and Practices**

4:00 **Systematic Reviews and Other Strategies to Protect Against Bias in Guidelines Development**
Holger Schunemann, M.D., Ph.D., Associate Professor of Medicine, University of Buffalo, and Italian National Cancer Institute, Rome, Italy

Discussion (all participants)

5:00 Public Comments

5:30 Adjourn

B

U.S. Public Health Service Regulations: Objectivity in Research (42 CFR 50)

TITLE 42—PUBLIC HEALTH
CHAPTER I—PUBLIC HEALTH SERVICE,
DEPARTMENT OF HEALTH AND HUMAN SERVICES

SUBCHAPTER D—GRANTS
PART 50—POLICIES OF GENERAL APPLICABILITY

Subpart F–Responsibility of Applicants for Promoting Objectivity in Research for Which PHS Funding Is Sought

Sec. 50.601 — Purpose.

This subpart promotes objectivity in research by establishing standards to ensure there is no reasonable expectation that the design, conduct, or reporting of research funded under PHS [Public Health Service] grants or cooperative agreements will be biased by any conflicting financial interest of an Investigator.

Sec. 50.602 — Applicability.

This subpart is applicable to each Institution that applies for PHS grants or cooperative agreements for research and, through the implementation of this subpart by each Institution, to each Investigator participating in such research (see Sec. 50.604(a)); provided that this subpart does not apply to SBIR [Small Business Innovation Research] Program Phase I applications. In those few cases where an individual, rather than an institution, is an applicant for PHS grants or cooperative agreements for research, PHS Awarding Components will make case-by-case determinations on the steps to be taken to ensure that the design, conduct, and reporting of the research will not be biased by any conflicting financial interest of the individual. [p35816]

Sec. 50.603 — Definitions.

As used in this subpart:

HHS means the United States Department of Health and Human Services, and any components of the Department to which the authority involved may be delegated.

Institution means any domestic or foreign, public or private, entity or organization (excluding a Federal agency).

Investigator means the principal investigator and any other person who is responsible for the design, conduct, or reporting of research funded by PHS, or proposed for such funding. For purposes of the requirements of this subpart relating to financial interests, "Investigator" includes the Investigator's spouse and dependent children.

PHS means the Public Health Service, an operating division of the U.S. Department of Health and Human Services, and any components of the PHS to which the authority involved may be delegated.

PHS Awarding Component means the organizational unit of the PHS that funds the research that is subject to this subpart.

Public Health Service Act or PHS Act means the statute codified at 42 U.S.C. 201 et seq.

Research means a systematic investigation designed to develop or contribute to generalizable knowledge relating broadly to public health, including behavioral and social-sciences research. The term encompasses basic and applied research and product development. As used in this subpart, the term includes any such activity for which research funding is available from a PHS Awarding Component through a grant or cooperative agreement, whether authorized under the PHS Act or other statutory authority.

Significant Financial Interest means anything of monetary value, including but not limited to, salary or other payments for services (e.g., consulting fees or honoraria); equity interests (e.g., stocks, stock options or other ownership interests); and intellectual property rights (e.g., patents, copyrights and royalties from such rights). The term does not include:

(1) Salary, royalties, or other remuneration from the applicant institution;

(2) Any ownership interests in the institution, if the institution is an applicant under the SBIR Program;

(3) Income from seminars, lectures, or teaching engagements sponsored by public or nonprofit entities;

(4) Income from service on advisory committees or review panels for public or nonprofit entities;

(5) An equity interest that when aggregated for the Investigator and the Investigator's spouse and dependent children, meets both of the following tests: Does not exceed $10,000 in value as determined through reference to public prices or other reasonable measures of fair market value, and does not represent more than a five percent ownership interest in any single entity; or

(6) Salary, royalties or other payments that when aggregated for the Investigator and the Investigator's spouse and dependent children over the next twelve months, are not expected to exceed $10,000.

Small Business Innovation Research (SBIR) Program means the extramural research program for small business that is established by the Awarding Components of the Public Health Service and certain other Federal agencies under Pub. L. 97-219, the Small Business Innovation Development Act, as amended. For purposes of this subpart, the term SBIR Program includes the Small Business Technology Transfer (STTR) Program, which was established by Pub. L. 102-564.

Sec. 50.604 — Institutional responsibility regarding conflicting interests of investigators.

Each Institution must:

(a) Maintain an appropriate written, enforced policy on conflict of interest that complies with this subpart and inform each Investigator of that policy, the Investigator's reporting responsibilities, and of these regulations. If the Institution carries out the PHS-funded research through subgrantees, contractors, or collaborators, the Institution must take reasonable steps to ensure that Investigators working for such entities comply with this subpart, either by requiring those Investigators to comply with the Institution's policy or by requiring the entities to provide assurances to the Institution that will enable the Institution to comply with this subpart.

(b) Designate an institutional official(s) to solicit and review financial disclosure statements from each Investigator who is planning to participate in PHS-funded research.

(c)(1) Require that by the time an application is submitted to PHS each Investigator who is planning to participate in the PHS-funded research has submitted to the designated official(s) a listing of his/her known Significant Financial Interests (and those of his/her spouse and dependent children):

(i) That would reasonably appear to be affected by the research for which PHS funding is sought; and

(ii) In entities whose financial interests would reasonably appear to be affected by the research.

(2) All financial disclosures must be updated during the period of the award, either on an annual basis or as new reportable Significant Financial Interests are obtained.

(d) Provide guidelines consistent with this subpart for the designated official(s) to identify conflicting interests and take such actions as necessary to ensure that such conflicting interests will be managed, reduced, or eliminated.

(e) Maintain records of all financial disclosures and all actions taken by the Institution with respect to each conflicting interest for at least three years from the date of submission of the final expenditures report or, where applicable, from other dates specified in 45 CFR 74.53(b) for different situations.

(f) Establish adequate enforcement mechanisms and provide for sanctions where appropriate.

(g) Certify, in each application for the funding to which this subpart applies, that:

(1) There is an effect at that Institution a written and enforced administrative process to identify and manage, reduce or eliminate conflicting interests

with respect to all research projects for which funding is sought from the PHS,

(2) Prior to the Institution's expenditure of any funds under the award, the Institution will report to the PHS Awarding Component the existence of a conflicting interest (but not the nature of the interest or other details) found by the institution and assure that the interest has been managed, reduced or eliminated in accordance with this subpart; and, for any interest that the Institution identifies as conflicting subsequent to the Institution's initial report under the award, the report will be made and the conflicting interest managed, reduced, or eliminated, at least on an interim basis, within sixty days of that identification;

(3) The Institution agrees to make information available, upon request, to the HHS regarding all conflicting interests identified by the Institution and how those interests have been managed, reduced, or eliminated to protect the research from bias; and

(4) The Institution will otherwise comply with this subpart. [p35817]

Sec. 50.605 — Management of conflicting interests.

(a) The designated official(s) must: Review all financial disclosures; and determine whether a conflict of interest exists and, if so, determine what actions should be taken by the institution to manage, reduce or eliminate such conflict of interest. A conflict of interest exists when the designated official(s) reasonably determines that a Significant Financial Interest could directly and significantly affect the design, conduct, or reporting of the PHS-funded research. Examples of conditions or restrictions that might be imposed to manage conflicts of interest include, but are not limited to:

(1) Public disclosure of significant financial interests;

(2) Monitoring of research by independent reviewers;

(3) Modification of the research plan;

(4) Disqualification from participation in all or a portion of the research funded by the PHS;

(5) Divestiture of significant financial interests; or

(6) Severance of relationships that create actual or potential conflicts.

(b) In addition to the types of conflicting financial interests described in this paragraph that must be managed, reduced, or eliminated, an Institution may require the management of other conflicting financial interests, as the Institution deems appropriate.

Sec. 50.606 — Remedies.

(a) If the failure of an Investigator to comply with the conflict of interest policy of the Institution has biased the design, conduct, or reporting of the PHS-funded research, the Institution must promptly notify the PHS Awarding Component of the corrective action taken or to be taken. The PHS Awarding Component will consider the situation and, as necessary, take appropriate action, or refer the matter to the Institution for further action, which may include directions to the Institution on how to maintain appropriate objectivity in the funded project.

(b) The HHS may at any time inquire into the Institutional procedures and actions regarding conflicting financial interests in PHS-funded research, including a requirement for submission of, or review on site, all records pertinent to compliance with this subpart. To the extent permitted by law, HHS will maintain the confidentiality of all records of financial interests. On the basis of its review of records and/or other information that may be available, the PHS Awarding Component may decide that a particular conflict of interest will bias the objectivity of the PHS-funded research to such an extent that further corrective action is needed or that the Institution has not managed, reduced, or eliminated the conflict of interest in accordance with this subpart. The PHS Awarding Component may determine that suspension of funding under 45 CFR 74.62 is necessary until the matter is resolved.

(c) In any case in which the HHS determines that a PHS-funded project of clinical research whose purpose is to evaluate the safety or effectiveness of a drug, medical device, or treatment has been designed, conducted, or reported by an Investigator with a conflicting interest that was not disclosed or managed as required by this subpart, the Institution must require the Investigator(s) involved to disclose the conflicting interest in each public presentation of the results of the research.

Sec. 50.607 — Other HHS regulations that apply.

Several other regulations and policies apply to this subpart.

They include, but are not necessarily limited to:

42 CFR Part 50, Subpart D–Public Health Service grant appeals procedure

45 CFR Part 16–Procedures of the Departmental Grant Appeals Board

45 CFR Part 74–Uniform Administrative Requirements for Awards and Subawards to Institutions of Higher Education, Hospitals, Other Non-Profit Organizations, and Commercial Organizations; and Certain Grants and Agreements with States, Local Governments and Indian Tribal Governments

45 CFR Part 76–Government-wide debarment and suspension (non-procurement)

45 CFR Part 79–Program Fraud Civil Remedies

45 CFR Part 92–Uniform Administrative Requirements for Grants and Cooperative Agreements to State and Local Governments

C

Conflict of Interest in Four Professions: A Comparative Analysis

Michael Davis and Josephine Johnston***

This paper presents a selective survey of the ways in which important professions other than medicine understand and regulate conflicts of interest. The professions evaluated here—law (lawyers), accountancy (certified public accountants [CPAs]), architecture, and engineering—each differ from medicine in having clients or employers rather than patients as the focus of concern. The difference is not simply one of terminology. A client or an employer is not necessarily human. Many are corporations or governments. Even the human clients differ from patients. With some exceptions (e.g., clients accused of crimes), they are typically healthy, calm, and relatively well-informed about the service to be provided; they are seldom as vulnerable as a physician's patient typically is. A client or employer simply asks that something be done (a building put up, a machine designed, a contract drawn, or a company audited). Emergencies are much rarer in these professions than they are in medicine, and time to think through a problem is more plentiful. Because of their relative sophistication and bargaining strength (compared both with patients and with the professional in question), clients or employers need not readily consent to accept the conflicts disclosed to them; they are more likely to insist that a conflict be avoided or resolved or to use the conflict to better the bargain. In other words, law, ac-

* Michael Davis, Ph.D., is a senior fellow within the Center for Study of Ethics in the Professions and a professor of philosophy in the Humanities Department, Illinois Institute of Technology.

** Josephine Johnston, L.L.B., is a research scholar at the Hastings Center, Garrison, New York.

counting, architecture, and engineering are professions in which one might expect much less concern with conflicts of interest than in medicine.

Although these are the chief differences between medicine and the professions discussed here, they are not the only ones. These other professions differ substantially in size from medicine—and from each other. Physicians outnumber architects in the United States by about 10 to 1, engineers outnumber physicians by about 3 to 1, and the numbers of individuals in the other professions fall somewhere in between. Importantly, only one profession, engineering, does much that physicians would recognize as scientific research.

The professions evaluated here were chosen because none is a close analogue of medicine. Medicine tends to be the model for adjacent professions (osteopathy, dentistry, pharmacy, nursing, and so on). The comparison of medicine with an adjacent profession would provide less contrast and therefore less understanding of conflict of interest as a general problem for professions. All of the professions discussed here have substantial experience with employment in large organizations. Two of the professions—engineering and accounting—have a long history of employment in such organizations. Only a small minority of engineers has ever been self-employed in the way that most physicians, except those in research and teaching, were until recently. Even self-employed architects, lawyers, and accountants often work for and in large organizations in a way that physicians have only recently begun to do in large numbers. Looking at how these nonmedical professions respond to the conflicts of interest that are more likely to arise in large organizations should help physicians both look critically at present arrangements and anticipate the future. Finally, these professions all recognize conflicts of interest as posing a threat to the integrity of the profession and have developed ethics rules to address the threat.

TERMINOLOGY

"Conflict of interest" is not an old term. The first court case to use it in something like the sense that is now standard occurred in 1949.[1] Federal legislation first addressed conflict of interest in the late 1950s.[2] The *Index of Legal Periodicals* had no heading for "conflict of interest" until 1967; *Black's Law Dictionary* had none until 1979. No ordinary dictionary of English seems to have had an entry for "conflict of interest" before 1971. The term also began to appear in codes of ethics in the 1970s, although related terms, such as "adverse interest," "conflicting interest," "bias,"

[1] *In re Equitable Office Bldg. Corp.*, D.C.N.Y., 83 F. Supp. 531.

[2] Staff report of the Antitrust Subcommittee (Subcommittee No. 5) of House Judiciary Committee, 85th Cong., 2d sess., Federal Conflict of Interest Legislation (Comm. Print 1958).

"prejudice," and the like appeared in codes much earlier.[3] This short history may explain, at least in part, the variation in how the term is used among professions. We are all trying to keep pace with the usage.

The term "conflict of interest" is not self-explanatory but is an idiom or term of art (a term designed to pick out a phenomenon until then lacking a suitable name). For the professions discussed here, the term groups together a range of scenarios in which the professional judgment of the individual in question risks being compromised.[4] These professions do not use explicit definitions of "conflict of interest" but instead describe in their codes a variety of situations that fall under the heading "conflict of interest" and that must either be avoided or managed in specified ways. For example, the definitions section of the American Bar Association's (ABA's) *Model Rules of Professional Conduct* includes definitions of "informed consent" and "fraud" but not "conflict of interest."[5] Instead, situations labeled conflicts of interest are described in the *Model Rules*.[6] Similarly, the American Institute of Certified Public Accountants' (AICPA's) *Code of Professional Conduct* includes a definition of some of the terms used in its conflict of interest rules, such as "immediate family" but not "conflict of interest." In fact, AICPA's Code does not use the term "conflict of interest" at all, speaking instead of various threats to "independence" and "objectivity," including the threat posed by certain financial interests.[7]

The major concern uniting the professions' use of the term is to protect the judgment of individual professionals from undue influence, whether the risk arises from gifts or kickbacks; an individual's personal (generally financial) interests; or the interests of family members, colleagues, or current and former clients. In some of the professions, a situation—for example, the representation of both plaintiff and defendant in the same legal case—is labeled a conflict of interest when it would be described as a conflict of obligations or responsibilities in the report to which this paper is an appendix (see Chapter 2) because neither obligation would be considered secondary to the other.

For all of the professions discussed in this paper, a certain sort of expert

---

[3] Neil R. Luebke, "Conflict of Interest as a Moral Category," *Business and Professional Ethics Journal* 1987; 6 (Spring): 66–81.

[4] Michael Davis, "Conflict of Interest Revisited," *Business and Professional Ethics Journal* 1993; 12 (Winter): 21–41.

[5] American Bar Association, Model Rules for Professional Conduct: Rules 1.0. www.abanet.org/cpr/mrpc/rule_1_0.html.

[6] American Bar Association, Model Rules for Professional Conduct: Rules 1.7–1.10. www.abanet.org/cpr/mrpc/mrpc_toc.html.

[7] The American Institute of Certified Public Accountants, AICPA Code of Professional Responsibility: Section 100—Independence, Integrity, and Objectivity. www.aicpa.org/About/code/sec100.htm.

and trustworthy judgment in individual situations (the judgment characteristic of the profession) is what makes members of the profession useful. A conflict of interest makes that judgment unreliable just when reliability is needed. A conflict of interest is therefore always considered a threat to the good that the profession seeks to achieve and is often also a threat to the profession's reputation. That is what makes having a conflict of interest a serious concern in professional ethics.

The next four sections of this paper consider in detail how the four professions on our list understand conflict of interest, respond to it, and why. The final section summarizes and compares the professions and identifies approaches from which medical research, education, and practice might learn.

LAWYERS

The main legal professions—lawyers and judges—have traditionally taken conflict of interest very seriously. Because justice is to be fairly meted out, interests that might cause a judge to be or appear to be partial are also generally prohibited. Although lawyers owe obligations to the legal system and the public, their primary obligation is to their clients; interests that might interfere with this obligation are generally to be avoided. The legal professions have some of the strictest rules about conflict of interest and have a long history of examining and enforcing those rules. In the interests of space, the focus here is on lawyers because their work, in most respects, is more like that of physicians than is the work of judges. (Judges are more like physicians serving on drug and device approval panels or as authors of review articles, whose charge is to weigh all the evidence and reach a reasoned and impartial decision.[8])

In legal practice, conflicts of interest are conceptualized in the context of the attorney-client relationship, which is protected by very strong obligations of loyalty and confidentiality. Broadly speaking, two kinds of conflict are understood to arise in that relationship: first, conflicts between the interests of two or more clients (whether they be current clients or a current client and a former client) and, second, conflicts between the interests of one or more clients and the personal interests of the attorney.

The first kind of conflict is created by the act of entering into a certain attorney-client relationship. For that reason, lawyers routinely conduct "conflicts checks" before taking on a new client or a new file from an existing client. The second kind of conflict can be created by either enter-

[8] For an example of rules of professional conduct for judges, see New York State Commission on Judicial Conduct, Rules of Conduct, at http://www.scjc.state.ny.us/Legal%20Authorities/rgjc.htm. Judicial ethics emphasizes independence.

ing into a new attorney-client relationship; taking on a new file from an existing client; or taking on a personal interest, including but not limited to a financial interest. In part, because the conflict of interest of one lawyer is, as a general principle, imputed to all lawyers working in the same firm or group practice, procedures, internal databases, and software have been developed to assist large firms in identifying possible conflicts of interest. So, for example, a lawyer who marries will immediately report that change of status to his firm along with the spouse's investments, family connections, employer, and the like. In some cases, law firms have staff dedicated to monitoring conflicts of interest, including, according to one New York City law firm partner whom we spoke with, general counsel whose risk management responsibilities include conflict of interest issues. Lawyers also use letters of engagement to carefully specify which of the firm's lawyers will be working for the client on the particular matter to avoid or make more manageable any future conflict of interest.

For the first kind of conflict, the analogy with medicine is not particularly strong: physicians are not generally constrained from taking on new patients because of their loyalty to other (current or former) patients, although analogous problems concerning confidentiality may arise when one physician serves several members of the same family. The analogy becomes somewhat stronger if one thinks of a pharmaceutical company or a device manufacturer with whom a physician has a financial relationship as one "client" and one or more patients as the other "client."

The legal profession's management of the second kind of conflict—a conflict between a lawyer's personal interests and the interests of a client—could provide more direct instruction to medicine, insofar as there is a concern that physicians' financial and other relationships with industry might lead physicians to make clinical decisions that they would not have made but for those financial or other relationships.

Furthermore, the legal profession's general attitude toward conflict of interest might be instructive for medicine. Conflicts of interest are understood to be a common feature of legal practice for which the profession has developed norms, rules, and procedures. Censure attaches not to finding oneself in a position in which agreeing to represent a client would create a conflict of interest (all lawyers are in this position from time to time, even though they try to avoid it) but to agreeing to represent that client without properly addressing the conflict of interest.

Lawyers share some similarities with physicians. Until recently, many lawyers worked alone or in small group practices. Lawyers are under a strong obligation of fidelity to their individual clients; and although some clients are large companies or sophisticated and powerful individuals, many are vulnerable individuals, including people who are in trouble with the law, are victims of physical harm or abuse, or are making major decisions that can have a lasting impact on their lives and the lives of their families (e.g., buying or selling property, making a will, or adopting a child). However, although some lawyers represent clients with a compromised decision-making ability, lawyers do not routinely deal with clients whose decision-making ability may be medically impaired.

In the United States, as in most other common-law jurisdictions, a lawyer (often called an attorney) may conduct all aspects of litigation (including court appearances); may represent clients in negotiations; may give legal advice; and may prepare contracts, wills, and other legal documents. The specific criteria for admission to the bar are set by each state: candidates must generally hold a law degree (J.D.) from an accredited law school; pass that state's bar examination; and in all but three jurisdictions, pass the Multistate Professional Responsibility Examination, which is a 2-hour-long multiple-choice test that includes questions about conflict of interest.[9]

To be accredited, American law schools are required to provide substantial instruction to all J.D. students in the values, rules, and responsibilities of the legal profession, including instruction in the identification and management of conflicts of interest.[10] Law professors themselves are subject to any conflict of interest policies of their own institutions. In keeping with the Association of American Law Schools' 2003 *Statement of Good Practices by Law Professors in the Discharge of Their Ethical and Professional Responsibilities*, law professors are obligated in publications and presentations to "disclose the material facts relating to receipt of direct or indirect payment for, or any personal economic interest in, any covered activity that the professor undertakes in a professorial capacity."[11]

To maintain the license to practice law, 41 U.S. states require completion of a prescribed number of hours of continuing legal education (CLE), and 36 of these states mandate the inclusion of professional responsibility (also called "legal ethics"), including in some states "elimination of bias."[12] Providers of mandatory CLE, which can be law schools, law firms (which offer CLE only to lawyers in-house or to outside lawyers as well), or private companies, must individually be accredited by each state's CLE accrediting authority. Mandatory CLE can be funded in a number of ways: it may be provided for a fee or it may be offered for free by the ABA, by state bar

[9] American Bar Association, Bar Admissions Basic Overview. www.abanet.org/legaled/baradmissions/basicoverview.html.

[10] American Bar Association, 2007–2008 Standards for Approval of Law Schools, Interpretation 302-9. www.abanet.org/legaled/standards/standards.html.

[11] Association of American Law Schools, Statement of Good Practices by Law Professors in the Discharge of Their Ethical and Professional Responsibilities, 2003. www.aals.org/about_handbook_sgp_eth.php.

[12] American Bar Association, Summary of MCLE Jurisdiction Requirements. www.abanet.org/cle/mcleview.html.

associations, or by law firms. (One lawyer with whom we spoke noted that large malpractice firms sometimes sponsor CLE.) The lawyer or the lawyer's employer pays the fee. Providers are required to offer tuition assistance to unemployed attorneys, attorneys working in the public sector, and those in a financial hardship situation. Lawyers seem unconcerned about the prospect of commercial interests being involved with CLE—they even allow corporate sponsorship at CLE events. Of course, in general, commercial providers of CLE are not potential clients or adverse parties but simply the makers of the tools or the providers of the services that lawyers use in the course of their work.

As a result of these requirements, virtually all, if not all, U.S. lawyers have received instruction on the identification and management of conflicts of interest, and many continue to address this issue in their CLE. Because the legal profession has developed considerable case law, detailed rules (described below), and legal scholarship (two or three dozen articles per year) addressing lawyers' conflicts of interest, there is much for American law students and lawyers to learn.

Canons, Model Codes, and Model Rules

Although local bar associations began to appear in the United States in the late 19th century, most U.S. lawyers at the time were only informally controlled by reputation and peer pressure. The ABA was founded in 1878; and one of its first major initiatives became, in 1908, the Canons of Professional Ethics, developed in response to a perceived need to promote and vouch for the integrity (or reliability) of lawyers generally.[13] Initially there were 32 canons, and the number of canons eventually expanded to 47. The individual canons were fairly brief (the briefest is one sentence of two dozen words, whereas the longest is a few paragraphs). They were not accompanied by further guidance or detailed explanation, as is found in modern codes of legal ethics. Nevertheless, they were influential. By 1924, virtually every state and local bar association had adopted the canons.[14]

A number of the canons are relevant to conflict of interest, although it was the sixth canon (titled Adverse Influences and Conflicting Interests) that addressed the issue directly. Canon 6 consisted of three short paragraphs, and although it was fairly unsophisticated and incomplete, it captured the major conflict of interest issues that attorneys face even today. It attempted

[13] Ted Schneyer, How Things Have Changed: Contrasting the Regulatory Environment of the Canons and the Model Rules. www.abanet.org/cpr/schneyer.pdf.

[14] James M. Altman, "Considering the ABA's 1908 Canons of Ethics," *Fordham Law Review* 2003; 71: 2395–2524, at 2396, quoting Report of the Standing Committee on Professional Ethics and Grievances, *American Bar Association Report* 1924; 49: at 466, 467.

a definition of client-client conflict of interest as a conflict of obligation ("when, in behalf of one client, it is his duty to contend for that which duty to another client requires him to oppose"), identified client loyalty and confidentiality as two values threatened by conflict of interest, identified the particular problems of concurrent and subsequent representation of conflicting clients, and proposed one remedy for concurrent representation (disclosure followed by informed consent).[15] Other canons dealt with related conflict of interest issues, including a prohibition on a lawyer purchasing an interest in the subject that is a matter of litigation and a requirement that contingency fee arrangements be supervised by the court to prevent unjust charges.

Fifteen amendments to the canons (none related to Canon 6) were adopted before the ABA developed a new code, the *Model Code of Professional Responsibility*, in 1969.[16] The *Model Code* was a far more detailed document than the canons. It contained nine "canons" (described as "axiomatic norms"). These doubled as section titles. Each canon was followed by a series of Ethical Considerations and Disciplinary Rules. The Ethical Considerations were described as "aspirational in character," representing the objectives toward which all lawyers should strive. The Disciplinary Rules were, unlike the Ethical Considerations, mandatory and set "the minimum level of conduct below which no lawyer can fall without being subject to disciplinary action."

Conflict of interest was mainly addressed in Canon 5 of the *Model Code*, which states: "A Lawyer Should Exercise Independent Professional Judgment on Behalf of a Client." The first of the 24 Ethical Considerations for Canon 5 explains that

> [The] professional judgment of a lawyer should be exercised, within the bounds of the law, solely for the benefit of his client and free of compromising influences and loyalties. Neither his personal interests, the interests of other clients, nor the desires of third persons should be permitted to dilute his loyalty to his client.

The seven Disciplinary Rules describe a mix of situations in which a conflict of interest is prohibited outright and situations in which the interest is permissible only after the conflict of interest is fully disclosed to and informed consent is received from the client or clients in question.

Although the states more or less uniformly adopted the *Model Code*, it was soon abandoned.[17] In 1983, the ABA adopted a replacement. One theory about why the *Model Code* was so quickly replaced is that it mixed

---

[15] American Bar Association Canons of Ethics, Canon 6.

[16] American Bar Association, Model Code of Professional Responsibility, 1983. www.law.cornell.edu/ethics/aba/mcpr/MCPR.HTM.

[17] Charles W. Wolfram, *Modern Legal Ethics*, West Publishing, 1986.

minimum standards of conduct permitted under the law with ethical rules intended to set higher standards and therefore was perceived as confusing ethics with law (and, in the process, reducing ethical standards).[18] In its report to the ABA recommending the adoption of a new code of professional responsibility, the Kutak Commission on Evaluation and Professional Standards cited a steady increase in concern about professional ethics, including Supreme Court cases, statutes and regulations, opinions of the ABA's Committee on Ethics and Professional Responsibility, and reports and articles, as leading it to reconsider the *Model Code*.[19] The commission ultimately concluded that amendments would not suffice to address this increased concern, and so, just 15 years after adopting the *Model Code*, the ABA replaced it with the *Model Rules of Professional Conduct*. The states were slow to adopt the *Model Rules*, although today all states but California, Maine, and New York have professional conduct rules that follow the format of the *Model Rules*. (New York still follows the *Model Code*, and California and Maine have developed their own rules.)[20]

The *Model Rules* are fairly detailed, clustered under eight headings, and accompanied by lengthy comments. The *Model Rules* most closely related to conflict of interest fall under the heading "Client-Lawyer Relationship" and are described in the following sections.

Rule 1.7. Conflict of Interest: Current Clients

Rule 1.7[21] begins with a strong statement of general principle, followed by a description of the circumstances in which the general principle does not apply. The general principle is that a lawyer "shall not represent a client if the representation involves a concurrent conflict of interest." A concurrent conflict of interest is defined as the situation in which the representation of one client will be directly adverse to that of another client (conflict of obligation) or there is a "significant risk" that representing one client will be "materially limited" by the lawyer's responsibilities to another client, a former client, or a third party or by the personal interest of the lawyer (true conflict of interest). However, the lawyer may proceed

---

[18] Robert P. Lawry, "The Law and Ethics of Lawyers' Conflicts of Interest," in Thomas Murray and Josephine Johnston (eds.), *Ethical Issues in Financial Conflicts of Interest in Biomedical Research*, forthcoming.

[19] American Bar Association Commission on Evaluation of Professional Standards (Robert J. Kutak Chairman), "Model Rules of Professional Conduct: Discussion Draft," January 20, 1980. www.abanet.org/cpr/mrpc/kutak_1-80.pdf.

[20] American Bar Association website, ABA Model Rules of Professional Conduct: State Adoption of Model Rules. www.abanet.org/cpr/mrpc/model_rules.html.

[21] American Bar Association, Model Rules for Professional Conduct: Rule 1.7. www.abanet.org/cpr/mrpc/rule_1_7.html.

despite this conflict with the written informed consent of each client and provided that so proceeding (1) is not prohibited by law and (2) will not involve representing two opposing parties in litigation and (3) provided that the lawyer "reasonably believes" that he or she can provide competent and diligent representation to both clients. (The *Model Rules* define "reasonably believes" in both subjective and objective terms: the lawyer must actually believe, and the belief must be reasonable.)

Rule 1.7 is accompanied by a comment, which is 35 paragraphs long.[22] Its second paragraph describes the process that lawyers must go through under the rule: they must

> 1) clearly identify the client or clients; 2) determine whether a conflict of interest exists; 3) decide whether the representation may be undertaken despite the existence of a conflict, i.e., whether the client's consent could be an appropriate cure; and 4) if so, consult with the clients affected under paragraph (a) [any clients affected by a concurrent conflict of interest] and obtain their informed consent, confirmed in writing.

Determining whether a conflict of interest exists often involves some judgment (although the comment casts the net fairly widely to include cases both of "direct adverseness" and of "significant risk that a lawyer's ability [to act for the client] will be materially limited"). The key judgment here, however, is whether the conflict is "consentable"—bearing in mind that the presumption is that a lawyer must not represent opposing parties in litigation or where prohibited by law. The rationale for the division between consentable and nonconsentable seems to be that some conflicts of interest are too risky for the client or profession—for example, the lawyer might appear to a reasonable outsider to be taking egregious advantage of the client for the lawyer's personal benefit (even though the lawyer is not).

Paragraph 14 of the comment for Rule 1.7 begins by noting that although clients may ordinarily consent to representation notwithstanding a conflict, "some conflicts are nonconsentable, meaning that the lawyer cannot properly ask for . . . agreement or provide representation on the basis of the client's consent." Although it is long, the comment provides little additional guidance on how to determine whether a conflict is consentable other than to note at Paragraph 15 that representation is prohibited if the lawyer "cannot reasonably conclude that [he or she] will be able to provide competent and diligent representation." The next two rules provide more specific guidance.

[22] American Bar Association, Model Rules for Professional Conduct: Rule 1.7 Comment. www.abanet.org/cpr/mrpc/rule_1_7_comm.html.

Rule 1.8. Conflict of Interest: Current Clients: Specific Rules

Rule 1.8[23] adds to the general principles contained in Rule 1.7 10 classes of conflict of interest situations, some of which may be resolved with the consent of the client (and sometimes subject to other protective measures) and some of which cannot be resolved even with consent. Rule 1.8 therefore helps lawyers to determine when a conflict may be consentable.

Conflict of interest situations that are not consentable include

- soliciting or preparing an instrument to receive a substantial gift from a client unless the client is a relative,
- negotiating literary or media rights that would substantially rely on information relating to the representation,
- providing financial assistance to a client for litigation except where the client is indigent or where litigation costs will be repaid under a contingency agreement or lien, and
- having sexual relations with a client unless the sexual relationship preceded the attorney-client relationship.

Conflict of interest situations that are in principle consentable (provided that other conditions are met, such as advising the client of the desirability of seeking independent legal counsel) include

- entering into a business transaction with a client,
- knowingly acquiring an ownership or other interest that is adverse to a client,
- using information about one client to another client's disadvantage,
- accepting compensation for representing a client from a third party, and
- representing two or more clients in an aggregated settlement or agreement (for example, both parties in a friendly divorce).

In such situations, provided that full disclosure is followed by valid informed consent, a lawyer might reasonably be able to argue that an "arm's-length transaction" took place (something not possible in the nonconsentable situations), that is, that the client was fully able to look after its own interests without relying on the lawyer.

[23] American Bar Association, Model Rules for Professional Conduct: Rule 1.8. www.abanet.org/cpr/mrpc/rule_1_8.html.

Rule 1.9. Duties to Former Clients

Rule 1.9[24] provides that a lawyer should not agree to represent a person if the lawyer has previously represented a client in the same or a related matter and the interests of the new person are materially adverse to the interests of the former client, unless the lawyer has the written informed consent of the former client. (The requirement of "written" consent assures both a record, in case of a later dispute, and more formality at the time that consent is given.) The same rule applies when a lawyer knowingly takes on a new client whose interests are materially adverse to the interests of a former or a current client of that lawyer's former firm and about whom the lawyer has acquired protected information. This rule is designed to respond to lawyer mobility and to ensure that lawyers do not bring with them conflicts of interest from their previous firms without the consent of the former client.

In contrast to the first two parts of Rule 1.9, which allow the lawyer to represent the new client with the informed consent of the former client, the third part of Rule 1.9 (which concerns loyalty rather than conflict of interest) provides that information about former clients cannot be used to the disadvantage of the former client unless use of that information is otherwise allowed in the rules (that is, loyalty to the client continues after the representation ends). Like Rule 1.8, therefore, Rule 1.9 distinguishes between conflict of interest situations that are low risk enough to be resolved by informed consent and those that are nonconsentable because the risk is too high to be resolved by disclosure and consent or the problem is more serious than conflict of interest (conscious disloyalty).

Rule 1.10. Imputation of Conflicts of Interest: General Rule

Rule 1.10[25] is extremely important today when so many lawyers practice in large firms rather than as sole practitioners. Under the rule, the conflicts of interest of one lawyer in a firm are imputed to all lawyers in the firm: "a firm of lawyers is essentially one lawyer for purposes of the rules governing loyalty to the client."[26] The rule prohibits a member of a law firm from knowingly representing a client that any one of them practicing alone would be prohibited from representing under Rules 1.7 and 1.9, unless the prohibition is based on a personal interest of the lawyer and "does

[24] American Bar Association, Model Rules for Professional Conduct: Rule 1.9. www.abanet.org/cpr/mrpc/rule_1_9.html.

[25] American Bar Association, Model Rules for Professional Conduct: Rule 1.10. www.abanet.org/cpr/mrpc/rule_1_10.html.

[26] American Bar Association, Model Rules for Professional Conduct: Rule 1.10. comment, www.abanet.org/cpr/mrpc/rule_1_10_comm.html.

not present a significant risk of materially limiting the representation of the client by the remaining lawyers in the firm." Disqualification under the rule may be waived with the consent of the affected client (and subject to the prohibitions contained in Rule 1.7).

Rule 1.10 is strict and can be very burdensome for large law firms. Law firms have devised methods for "screening" lawyers within firms as a way of managing conflicts of interest (discussed in more detail below), but it is important to note that screens (which in other professions or arenas might be described as "firewalls") are not discussed in the *Model Rules*, except in limited situations involving former government lawyers.

In addition to these codes of ethics, case law has developed over several centuries to deal with lawyers' conflicts of interest (under various names). In the United States, this case law is helpfully summarized in the American Law Institute's *Restatement of the Law Governing Lawyers*.[27] Chapter 8 of that document analyzes conflicts of interest in general, including conflicts between a lawyer and a client, among current clients, between a lawyer and a former client, and because of the lawyer's obligation to a third person. This case law complicates matters for lawyers, since they must follow both the rules (explicitly or implicitly) laid down in those cases and the ABA's ethical rules. At the same time, the case law effectively addresses the malpractice liability of lawyers who fail to resolve a conflict of interest adequately and provides civil remedies for this malpractice, including damages paid to harmed clients or third parties and disqualification from continuing to represent a client in a particular matter.

The combined effect of the case law described in the restatement of the law governing lawyers and the ethical rules of each jurisdiction is that lawyers who fail to avoid conflicts of interest or to manage them adequately can be sued for malpractice, forced to pay monetary damages, disqualified by a judge from representing a client, or some combination of these. They can also lose their fee or receive only a reduced fee and face disciplinary action by the state bar (including disbarment). Although conflicts of interest are, in the first instance, to be identified by individual practitioners, local bars and the courts can become involved at later stages if those conflicts have not been properly managed. In this way, lawyers rely on self-regulation backed by the threat of professional and legal sanctions.

In fact, few lawyers are disciplined and even fewer are disbarred. A 2006 ABA survey found that of over 120,000 complaints filed against lawyers on any issue, only 3.5 percent led to formal discipline and less than 0.5

[27] Charles W Wolfram (ed.), *Restatement of the Law Third, The Law Governing Lawyers*, American Law Institute, 2000.

percent led to disbarment.[28] Although data on the numbers of allegations or findings of improper management of conflict of interest are not available at the federal level, some data are available at the state level. For example, between 2002 and 2006, sanctions for conflict of interest were imposed in only 11 percent of 530 cases, only 1 of which resulted in revocation of the license to practice (other sanctions were suspensions and reprimands).[29]

Conflict of Interest Management: Key Issues for Lawyers

Although the bar's system of conflict of interest management is well developed, it is not without its critics or its thorny issues. For example, despite the large number of cases, articles, and the detailed codes or rules, the legal profession's management of conflict of interest is still described as "abstruse," "arcane," and "intractable."[30] According to law professor Kevin McMunigal, however, the primary problem in the law's conflict of interest doctrine is a failure to recognize the regulation of conflict of interest as a kind of risk management and not prevention of direct harm. This failure leads the legal profession to use harm rules, which punish lawyers who harm clients, and risk rules, which aim to prevent harm to clients indirectly by keeping lawyers out of risky situations or by otherwise managing conflicts of interest but without engaging the all important question: How much risk is too much?

McMunigal gives the example of a lawyer in a high-profile criminal case who early on accepts a lucrative book deal to write about the case. When the prosecution offers to settle the case (an option, McMunigal adds, that would clearly be in the client's best interests), the lawyer advises her client to reject the settlement. McMunigal argues that the risky situation of the book deal (with the temptation being to take the case to trial to ensure publicity and probably help future book sales) probably led the lawyer to give bad legal advice (which would be harmful if it was followed). However, as McMunigal sees it, the legal profession uses the language of conflict of interest to describe and address both the risky situation and the harmful action. If the legal profession could more clearly separate harm rules—for example, rules against lawyers providing bad legal advice or against lawyers entering into unfair business deals with their clients—from risk rules—for example, rules prohibiting a lawyer from preparing an instrument by which

[28] American Bar Association, Survey on Lawyer Discipline Systems: 2006. www.abanet.org/cpr/discipline/sold/home.html.

[29] Michigan Attorney Discipline Board, Annual Reports 2000–2006, Appendix B (in each annual report). www.adbmich.org/ANNUALRPT.HTM.

[30] Kevin C. McMunigal, "Conflict of Interests as Risk Analysis," in Michael Davis and Andrew Stark (eds.), *Conflict of Interest in the Professions*, New York: Oxford University Press, 2001.

the lawyer will receive a gift from the client or rules against accepting book deals based on cases—then, McMunigal argues, the legal profession would also avoid confusion about the goals of and justification for each kind of rule.[31]

McMunigal suggests that conflict of interest rules should be understood as being restricted to governing risky situations, leaving rules against breaching confidentiality or against providing incompetent advice to deal with situations in which actual harm has resulted (and in which the causal chain can be proved). In the medical context, conflict of interest rules could therefore focus on identifying and governing situations in which the risk of tainted judgment is considered unacceptably high. The rules invoked to deal with actual harm to patients (other than harm to trust in their physicians and the profession in general) would allege not conflict of interest but inappropriate practice, bias, breach of confidentiality, or the like. Another consequence of sharply distinguishing between risk and actual harm would be to make unnecessary the distinction between "actual" and "potential" conflicts of interest, which McMunigal considers to be a distinction of little practical use.

In his analysis of the legal profession's management of conflicts of interest, law professor Robert Lawry focuses on a different kind of problem.[32] He sees a gradual lessening of professional standards to allow for the greater mobility of lawyers, which is at least partially justified by an appeal to the increased sophistication of some clients. One reason for this reduction in standards is, as mentioned above, the mixing over time of ethics (a guide to good professional behavior) and law (minimum standards by which to police the profession). Another reason is the reality of modern legal practice, where lawyers move from town to town and firm to firm. Yet another reason that exceptions to conflict of interest rules and methods for managing conflicts of interest have developed is to allow medium to large firms to serve many clients, some of whom will, from time to time, have both opposing interests and an interest in relying on lawyers who know them.

---

[31] Consider the debate over financial conflicts of interest in biomedical research: there is some confusion about whether the goal of conflict of interest rules is to identify cases of actual harm (usually bias) or to reduce the risk of harm (Shira Lipton, Elizabeth Boyd, and Lisa Bero, "Conflicts of Interest in Academic Research: Policies, Processes, and Attitudes," *Accountability in Research* 2004; 11(2): 83–102). The parties can end talking past each another, with one side asking for proof that harm was caused in this or that case by a conflict of interest before agreeing to the rules and the other side appealing to intuitive ideas about risk or to data showing correlations between conflicts of interest and bad outcomes in aggregates to justify prohibitions or other measures.

[32] Robert P. Lawry, "The Law and Ethics of Lawyers' Conflicts of Interest," in Thomas H. Murray and Josephine Johnston (eds.), *Ethical Issues in Financial Conflicts of Interest in Biomedical Research*, Baltimore (MD): Johns Hopkins University Press, forthcoming.

Screens, Chinese Walls, and Cones of Silence

One major mechanism for managing conflicts of interest with concurrent clients is through the use of screens (also known as "firewalls," "Chinese walls," or "cones of silence"). Screens are mechanisms by which lawyers working on one matter are prohibited from certain kinds of communication with lawyers in the same firm working on a conflicting matter. The prohibition is sometimes augmented by placing the lawyers in separate locations (on different floors or in different buildings), controls on e-mail and file access, and the like. Some screens are simply matters of honor; some involve real walls. Screens cannot change a nonconsentable conflict into a consentable one. Instead, screens are used "to encourage clients to consent to a loyalty conflict."[33]

Lawry sees screens as further evidence of erosion in lawyers' conflict of interest standards. Lawyers were introduced to the idea of screens in 1975 by Formal Opinion 342 of the ABA's Standing Committee on Ethics, which argued that former government lawyers should be permitted to work for a firm doing business with the government if they are screened within the firm from files that they worked on while they were in government. Without such screens, it was argued, "good lawyers would avoid government work, to the detriment of the common good." This principle, which was developed for government lawyers and which is discussed only in the *Model Rules* (and comments) in reference to government lawyers, is now routinely extended to private lawyers. Lawry reports that 22 of 51 jurisdictions allow screening without the consent of the former client.[34] Screens have also received some recognition in the courts and are endorsed in the restatement of the law governing lawyers as a way of dealing with conflicts created by lawyers switching firms. Reasonable people will likely continue to disagree about whether screens are a sign of eroding legal ethics or evidence that legal practitioners are both committed to legal ethics and capable of creating effective management systems. Nevertheless, the debate shows that lawyers are engaging with the fundamental question of how to balance the risks of conflict of interest in such situations against the benefits of tolerating the conflict if it is properly managed.

ACCOUNTANTS

As in other professions, much work in accounting can be conducted by uncertified (or unlicensed) individuals, but some accounting functions

[33] Susan R. Martyn, "Visions of the Eternal Law Firm: The Future of Law Firm Screens," *South Carolina Law Review* 1994; 45(1): 937–959.

[34] Thomas D. Morgan and Ronald D. Rotunda, *Selected Standards on Professional Responsibility*, New York: Foundation Press, 2006.

can be carried out only by a certified accountant. Certified accountants in the United States are: (1) CPAs, who are licensed by their state to provide auditing and attestation services; (2) certified internal auditors, who mostly provide their services directly to their employers; or (3) certified management accountants and certified business accountants, who, although they deal with the public, cannot audit public companies. Each of these certifications is issued by a professional body that maintains a code of ethics and that examines applicants on the basis of that code of ethics as well as on the basis of their technical skills. Individuals may carry more than one certification, but only licensed CPAs can perform the mandatory audits of publicly traded U.S. companies. CPAs are the focus of this discussion because of their prominent public role and their recent struggles to manage conflicts of interest.

Like lawyers, CPAs have clients—the companies that hire them to prepare their financial statements—but like architects and engineers and unlike lawyers, CPAs are wary of going too far in acting in their clients' interests. Lawyers, particularly during litigation, must primarily attend to their client's interests, leaving it to opposing counsel or the judge to find the flaws in their argument or weaknesses in the client's case. CPAs, in contrast, are obliged to put the public interest first when they perform an audit or attestation; they are not allowed to withhold or ignore negative information; indeed, part of their job is to seek out such information.[35] The rationale for privileging the public interest is that shareholders and other investors rely on the work of CPAs when they make decisions about whether and how to invest their money. Thus, although a company will engage and pay a CPA (often through an accounting firm) to perform its audits, both the company and the public are the beneficiaries of the CPA's work. The public benefits from having financial information that it can rely on. The company benefits from the public's ability to trust the company's financial reports.

Unlike a physician's patients, the accountant's clients are frequently sophisticated individuals or businesses; few are physically or mentally compromised. Although the matters entrusted to the accountant are seldom trivial, they are not literally life and death.

---

[35] That said, they are not generally required to blow the whistle on their clients by reporting fraud to outside agencies (Leonard J. Brooks, "Conflict of Interest in the Accounting Profession," in Michael Davis and Andrew Stark (eds.), *Conflict of Interest in the Professions*, New York: Oxford University Press, 2001). They are only required by law to report fraud to the client's senior management and its audit committee, a subcommittee of the client's board of directors that itself is under strict reporting requirements (Section 10A(1)(b) of the Securities Exchange Act of 1934 and American Institute of Certified Public Accountants, Statement on Auditing Standards: No. 99, Considerations of Fraud in a Financial Audit Statement).

Licenses and Professional Membership

As in other professions, professional accounting societies were developed to ensure clients that people holding themselves out as accountants met minimal levels of education, competence, and ethical conduct.[36] Today, professional accounting societies do not license accountants—that function has been taken over by the state-designated accountancy boards—but the professional societies provide guidance on many issues, from technical accounting standards to ethics. Clients, who rely on accountants to provide specialized services and advice, may find some reassurance in the imprimatur of good standing in a professional society.

AICPA is a voluntary association. Although all CPAs must be licensed by their state boards of accountancy (or the equivalent), they are not obliged to be members of their state or national CPA organizations. Membership in good standing of the state or national CPA organization can, however, enhance the reputation of the CPA. (AICPA provides marketing tool kits to its members.)

The specific requirements for the CPA license vary somewhat from state to state, but all states require that individuals pass the Uniform Certified Public Accountant examination, which was developed and which is maintained by AICPA and which is administered by the National Association of State Boards of Accountancy. Questions about professional ethics are included in the Uniform Certified Public Accountant examination and are based on AICPA's *Code of Professional Conduct.*

Many state licensing boards require continuing professional education (CPE) that includes ethics or professional conduct. These state boards prescribe CPE course requirements, but the courses are offered to CPAs by approved companies (sometimes called "sponsors") for a fee. Some attention is paid to the independence of the CPE programs and their sponsors. In New York, for example, CPE can be offered only by sponsors that have been approved by the New York Department of Education, which requires sponsors to have a "direct interest in offering courses on a regular basis" and will not approve "programs devoted to the promotion of particular products or services" or "[i]nsurance, pension, investment, software and other offerings primarily promotional or informational in nature."[37]

---

[36] Leonard J. Brooks, "Conflict of Interest in the Accounting Profession," in Michael Davis and Andrew Stark (eds.), *Conflict of Interest in the Professions*, New York: Oxford University Press, 2001.

[37] The University of New York, The State Education Department, State Board of Public Accountancy, Instructions for Completing Application for Continuing Education Sponsor Agreement. www.op.nysed.gov/cpa-mcesponsorapplication.pdf.

CPE is offered by a range of sponsors, including universities and private companies.[38]

Accountancy After Enron

In addition to understanding and following AICPA's *Code of Professional Conduct* (described in more detail below), CPAs need to be aware of and follow the rules of their state board of accountancy; the ethics standards of their state CPA organization (if they are members); any applicable state laws; and any applicable federal laws, notably, the Public Company Accounting Reform and Investor Protection Act of 2002.[39] This act, commonly known as the Sarbanes-Oxley Act, was passed in response to a number of corporate and accounting scandals in the late 1990s and early 2000s. Before passage of the act, the largest accounting firms had diversified their practices to the extent that audits were a small part of the services that they provided to their clients. Considered key to gaining insight into the client's business, audit prices steadily declined while other services increased in profitability. As a business school professor at the University of Saskatchewan puts it, "Clients became sophisticated purchasers, shopping around for the best deal and putting intense pressure on audit prices, and thus on profits . . . some companies [clients] began to resort to a practice known as 'opinion shopping.'"[40] Accounting firms were soon offering consulting services to audit clients that brought in far more than the audit fee, and therefore, "the auditors did not want to do anything to rock the boat with clients, potentially jeopardizing their chief source of income."[41]

This tension between auditing and consulting was identified and critiqued before the Enron scandal, but it was only after the collapse of Enron and WorldCom that practices and codes of conduct changed to address it. Boyd calls Enron "the 'smoking gun' evidence, indicating that the profession had reached a stage where commercial interests simply overwhelmed allegiance to professional integrity." Policy makers were not content to leave it to accounting firms or AICPA to address the issue. They chose to pass legislation—the Sarbanes-Oxley Act—to restore the reliability of the public company audit process.

Subject to certain preapprovals, Section 201 of the Sarbanes-Oxley Act prohibits auditors from providing a number of other services contemporaneous to the audit, including bookkeeping, management functions,

---

[38] See the registry of the National Registry of CPE Sponsors. http://registry.nasbatools.com/display_page.

[39] Sarbanes-Oxley Act of 2002. http://thomas.loc.gov/cgi-bin/query/z?c107:H.R.3763.ENR.

[40] Colin Boyd, "The Structural Origins of Conflicts of Interest in the Accounting Profession," *Business Ethics Quarterly* 2004; 14(3): 377–398.

[41] Arthur Levitt, *Take on the Street*, New York: Pantheon Books, 2002.

investment advice, investment banking services, and legal services. The act also creates the Public Company Accounting Oversight Board (PCAOB) to oversee CPA practice in relation to public companies. Under Section 103 of the act, PCAOB has established standards and rules on a variety of issues, including ethics, that apply to registered public accounting firms preparing and issuing audit reports as required by the act or the rules of the Securities and Exchange Commission.

PCAOB's conflict of interest rules are designed to preserve the independence of the accounting firm.[42] Rule 3520 states: "a registered public accounting firm and its associated persons must be independent of the firm's audit client throughout the audit and professional engagement period." Rules 3521, 3522, and 3523 describe situations in which an accounting firm cannot be considered independent, for example, if the firm provides a service or product to the audit client for a contingent fee or a commission, if the firm provides assistance in planning or tax advice on certain types of potentially abusive tax transactions to an audit client, or if the firm provides any tax services to certain persons in a financial reporting oversight role at an audit client or to immediate family members of such persons.

Violation of the PCAOB rules can lead to an investigation by PCAOB. Following a hearing, sanctions can be imposed, including (1) revoking a firm's registration; (2) barring an individual from participating in audits of public companies; (3) monetary penalties; and (4) remedial measures, such as training, the implementation of new quality control procedures, or the appointment of an independent monitor.[43] PCAOB's website reports that 3 of the 17 disciplinary proceedings before PCAOB over the past 3 years have found "independence" violations.

There has been some criticism that the post-Enron measures are too burdensome,[44] with others countering that the measures fail to do enough to end auditor-client "coziness."[45] Either way, this legislation and accompanying rules and sanctions serve as a cautionary tale. They installed the external regulation of a profession that apparently had not sufficiently regulated its own conflicts of interest. Since the Sarbanes-Oxley Act was passed, AICPA and state CPA societies have strengthened their codes of conduct, an example of a change in law forcing a tightening of ethical standards.

---

[42] Public Company Accounting Oversight Board, Bylaws and Rules—Rules—Professional Standards, Section 3. www.pcaobus.org/Rules/Rules_of_the_Board/Section_3.pdf.

[43] Section 105(b)(4) of the Sarbanes-Oxley Act of 2002.

[44] Jonathan D. Glater, "Here It Comes: The Sarbanes-Oxley Backlash," *New York Times*, April 17, 2005.

[45] Richard L. Kaplan, "The Mother of All Conflicts: Auditors and Their Clients," *Iowa Journal of Corporate Law* 2004; 29: 363–383.

AICPA Code of Professional Conduct

The current version of the AICPA *Code of Professional Conduct*[46] emphasizes independence and objectivity. The AICPA *Code of Professional Conduct* is divided into principles and rules. The six principles are expressed in a sentence or two. Each principle is clarified by up to five subparagraphs. The dozen rules that follow the principles are also expressed in one or two sentences but are followed by more detailed guidance in the form of Interpretations of Rules of Conduct and Ethics Rulings (rather like the American Medical Association's [AMA's] Opinions).

AICPA's professional ethics committee adopted Interpretations of Rules of Conduct "after exposure to state societies, state boards, practice units and other interested parties." The Interpretations of Rules of Conduct are intended "to provide guidelines as to the scope and application of the Rules but are not intended to limit such scope or application." Ethics rulings are formal rulings made by AICPA's professional ethics committee applying the rules and their interpretations to a particular set of facts. AICPA members who depart from ethics rulings in similar circumstances will be "requested to justify such departures."[47]

Two of the Code's principles bear on conflict of interest. The first, titled Integrity, states that "to maintain and broaden public confidence, members should perform all professional responsibilities with the highest sense of integrity" and includes a reference to observing the principles of objectivity and independence in its final subparagraph. The other relevant principle, titled the Public Interest, requires members "to act in a way that will serve the public interest, honor the public trust, and demonstrate commitment to professionalism." Acknowledging that members may encounter conflicting pressures, this principle advises that, when resolving such conflicts, members recall that when they "fulfill their responsibility to the public, clients' and employers' interests are best served."[48]

Although these two principles clearly bear on conflict of interest, it is the fourth principle (titled Objectivity and Independence) that addresses conflict of interest most directly. It states: "A member should maintain objectivity and be free of conflicts of interest in discharging professional re-

---

[46] The American Institute of Certified Public Accountants, AICPA Code of Professional Responsibility. www.aicpa.org/About/code/index.html.

[47] The American Institute of Certified Public Accountants, AICPA Code of Professional Responsibility: Introduction, Other Guidance. www.aicpa.org/About/code/othguid.htm.

[48] The American Institute of Certified Public Accountants, AICPA Code of Professional Responsibility: Section 53, Article II, The Public Interest, and Section 54, Article III, Integrity. www.aicpa.org/About/code/sec50.htm.

sponsibilities. A member in public practice should be independent in fact and appearance when providing auditing and other attestation services."[49]

The general rule, therefore, is that all CPAs should always be free of conflicts of interest. An even higher standard is set for CPAs in public practice. That is, when a CPA is performing certain services in public practice, the CPA should maintain objectivity in appearance as well as in fact. Public practice is defined as the performance for a client of accounting, tax, personal financial planning, litigation support, and other professional services for which practice standards are promulgated by AICPA. (The closest medical equivalent to a CPA's public practice is a physician's publication of research or the testimonials or other public statements that an individuals makes as a physician.)

Four subparagraphs follow this principle. The first discusses, in a fairly philosophical way, objectivity (describing it as "a state of mind" and imposing the obligation to be "impartial, intellectually honest, and free of conflicts of interest") and then independence ("precludes relationships that may appear to impair a member's objectivity in rendering attestation services"). After noting the variety of roles that an accountant might play in society, including teaching, the second subclause states: "Regardless of service or capacity, members should protect the integrity of their work, maintain objectivity, and avoid any subordination of their judgment." The principle is thus fairly strict: CPAs should at no time enter into relationships that might even appear to impair their objectivity. The third subclause focuses on accountants working in public practice, stating that to protect their independence (the appearance of objectivity), they should be continually assessing "client relationships and public responsibility" and "should be independent in fact and appearance." The effect of this subparagraph is to require constant vigilance of the possible impact of interactions with clients on the CPA's (actual and apparent) commitment to the public interest. The fourth subclause applies to members not in public practice (e.g., members employed by a company rather than acting as an external accountant or auditor). That subclass concedes that CPAs not in public practice "cannot maintain the appearance of independence" but nevertheless imposes on them "the responsibility to maintain objectivity in rendering professional services."

More detail in the form of rules, interpretations, and ethics rulings follow at Sections 101 (Independence) and 102 (Integrity and Objectivity).[50]

---

[49] The American Institute of Certified Public Accountants, AICPA Code of Professional Responsibility: Section 55, Article IV, Objectivity and Independence. www.aicpa.org/About/code/et_55.html.

[50] The American Institute of Certified Public Accountants, AICPA Code of Professional Responsibility: Section 100, Independence, Integrity, and Objectivity. www.aicpa.org/About/code/sec100.htm.

Section 101 begins with the rule that a member in public practice shall be independent according to the standards set by state boards, state CPA institutes, the U.S. Securities and Exchange Commission, and PCAOB, among others. The interpretation for this rule then describes the circumstances under which independence will be considered impaired. Situations of impairment include the following: when the accountant, during the period of professional engagement, holds or commits to acquiring a financial interest in the client; when the accountant has a loan to or from the client or in some circumstances when the accounting firm, one of its partners, or a partner's immediate family members hold an ownership stake in the client; and when the accountant's firm or a partner or employee of the firm was simultaneously a director, officer, or employee of the client. (The last prohibition applies not simply during the period of the professional engagement but during the whole period covered by the financial statements being prepared by the accountant.) When in doubt about whether a particular circumstance might cause independence to be questioned, the section asks that members "evaluate whether that circumstance would lead a reasonable person aware of all the relevant facts to conclude that there is an unacceptable *threat* to the member's and the firm's independence" (emphasis added).

Fourteen additional interpretations follow, and that number is far too many to cover in any detail here. It will be enough to note here that the net cast is fairly wide. Section 101 captures a number of situations involving the accountant; the firm; colleagues; family members; close relatives; or current or previous financial, employment, ownership, or management relationships with the client. The interpretations also differentiate between direct financial interests (such as ownership and investment interests) and indirect financial interests, including some holdings through mutual funds. In one of the Ethics Rules accompanying Section 101, the question of the CPA's acceptance of gifts or entertainment from a client is posed. The answer is that the acceptance of gifts or entertainment from a client that the CPA is auditing will be considered to impair objectivity, unless the value is "clearly insignificant to the recipient." The ethics ruling is less restrictive when the client is not an "attest client" (i.e., one for whom the CPA performs auditing or other attestation services), although even in such cases the CPA is required to assess whether accepting the gift is reasonable, given the nature, value, timing, and frequency of the gift.

The overall aim of the independence rule and its interpretations and ethics rulings at Section 101 is to ensure that audits of companies will be carried out by accountants and accountancy firms who provide no other financial services to the company, are not investors in or directors of the company, do not and have not recently worked for the company, have no other financial or other ties to the company, and are otherwise free of any appearance suggesting to a reasonable person a loss of objectivity. Despite its detail, this section has been criticized for failing to address one particular threat to independence (and objectivity): the significance of the client company's audit fees to the bottom line of the accountant or the firm.[51] One observer points out that Arthur Andersen's Houston, Texas, office received $1 million per week from Enron while it was auditing the company: "[The] livelihoods of several audit partners and several hundred audit firm employees depend[ed] on keeping a client happy."

Section 102 (Integrity and Objectivity) is far briefer than Section 101 and applies to all CPAs in all of their work (i.e., not simply to CPAs performing audits). It begins with the rule that "in the performance of any professional service a member shall maintain objectivity and integrity, shall be free of conflicts of interest, and shall not knowingly misrepresent facts or subordinate his or her judgment to others." Although the rule is concerned with the misrepresentation of fact as well as conflict of interest, the interpretations for the rule offer a definition of conflict of interest: "a conflict of interest may occur if a member performs a professional service for a client or employer and the member or his or her firm has a relationship with another person, entity, product, or service that could, in the member's professional judgment, be viewed by the client, employer, or other appropriate parties as impairing the member's objectivity." Note that the relationship need not be financial or familial, and it need not actually impair the CPA's objectivity—it is enough that it could, in the member's judgment, appear to impair his or her objectivity.

In contrast to Section 101, which provides no way to manage the impairments to independence that it covers, Section 102 suggests that disclosure and consent may be acceptable ways to manage conflicts of interest "if the *member* believes that the professional service can be performed with objectivity, and the relationship is disclosed to and consent is obtained from such client, employer, or other appropriate parties" (emphasis added). The interpretation explicitly states that concern about independence in certain professional engagements, such as audits and reviews, as expressed in the previous rule (Section 101), cannot be addressed by disclosure and consent. The discussion ends with an explicitly nonexhaustive list of situations that ought to raise independence concerns, including when the CPA has a significant financial interest in or is on the management of a company that is a major competitor of the client for which he or she performs management consulting services, when the CPA is asked to perform litigation services for a case filed against one of his or her clients, or when a CPA provides services for several members of the same family with opposing interests.

[51] David Cotton, "Fixing CPA Ethics Can Be an Inside Job," *Washington Post*, October 20, 2002. P. B2.

These are all situations in which the usual public reliance on the auditor's work is absent.

Enforcement of Ethics Rules

The AICPA *Code of Professional Conduct* focuses on the impact of existing and preexisting relationships (whether of the accountant, firm, colleagues, and sometimes, members of the family) on the accountant's objectivity and independence. Objectivity and independence are particularly protected when the accountant is auditing a client for the public's benefit. When offering any service except external auditing, a CPA might be able to disclose a conflict of interest to the client and proceed with the client's consent, but this option is simply not available in a public audit (or other attestation) situation. The reason for the focus on independence from clients (a matter of appearance), from the CPA's personal interests, and from the interests of the CPA's firm, colleagues, and family during audits (and other attestation services) in particular is that a CPA performing an external audit has a primary obligation to the public. Indeed, the second principle in the *Code of Professional Conduct*, titled The Public Interest, states that the public relies "on the objectivity and integrity of certified public accountants to maintain the orderly functioning of commerce."

The rules and practices of CPAs, therefore, are fairly strict when it comes to preserving independence and avoiding even the appearance of conflict of interest. It is important to note, however, that like architects and engineers but unlike lawyers, accountants are able to work for competing clients, often but not always with the knowledge and consent of both parties.[52] The rationale for this difference is that accountants are able to perform an audit of one client without disclosing (or even relying on) information about the other. It would be much harder for a lawyer to adequately represent two competing clients without using the confidential information of one against or in favor of the other.

The preamble to the AICPA *Code of Professional Conduct* neatly describes how it is enforced: "Compliance with the *Code of Professional Conduct* . . . depends primarily on members' understanding and voluntary actions, secondarily on reinforcement by peers and public opinion, and ultimately on disciplinary proceedings, when necessary, against members who fail to comply with the Rules."

Members of AICPA are on notice that they must be prepared to justify any departure that they make from the *Code of Professional Conduct.*

---

[52] Leonard J. Brooks, "Conflict of Interest in the Accounting Profession," in Michael Davis and Andrew Stark (eds.), *Conflict of Interest in the Professions*, New York: Oxford University Press, 2001.

AIPCA's Professional Ethics Executive Committee interprets and enforces the AICPA *Code of Professional Conduct.* The committee investigates allegations of unethical conduct by both its members and the members of almost all state CPA organizations through its Joint Ethics Enforcement Program (JEEP).[53] JEEP has existed since the 1970s and was created in recognition of the fact that the codes of many state CPA societies are identical or similar to the provisions of the AICPA *Code of Professional Conduct* and that it is common for a CPA to be a member of both AICPA and one or more state societies. JEEP therefore provides an efficient mechanism for enforcing ethics rules consistently across the United States.

Violations of the *Code of Professional Conduct* can result in a CPA being expelled, suspended for a period of 1 or 2 years from AICPA or from the local CPA society, directed to complete specified CPE courses, or directed to take other action (e.g., submit subsequent work papers for continued monitoring). All decisions to expel or suspend a CPA are made public through publication on AICPA's website. Very few of these decisions (just 4 of over 150) during the past 3 years included a finding of a breach of the rules regarding independence. AICPA can also publicly admonish a member who has violated the *Code of Professional Conduct.* AICPA's ethics committee can also conclude, upon investigation, that there is no evidence of a violation of the *Code of Professional Conduct* and therefore dismiss the case or simply close a case for lack of evidence or some other reason.[54]

The enforcement mechanisms of suspension, expulsion, and public admonishment seem designed to place the public and colleagues on notice that the CPA does not comply with the *Code of Professional Conduct* and to publicly embarrass the CPA, whereas requiring completion of CPE courses or submitting reports and work papers seems to aim to reeducate the CPA. Because a CPA does not need to be a member of AICPA or a state CPA organization, a finding of violation of AICPA's *Code of Professional Conduct* is not itself sufficient to withdraw the CPA's license to practice. Only the state licensing boards can suspend or revoke a CPA's license.

One important lesson from the recent history of public accountancy is that a failure to address conflicts of interest led to federal regulation of conflict of interest in one important aspect of CPA practice: the auditing of publicly listed companies. Investor confidence in the objectivity and independence of auditors and therefore in the truthfulness of public companies'

---

[53] The American Institute of Certified Public Accountants, Professional Ethics Executive Committee, Fact Sheet 2004–2005. www.aicpa.org/download/ethics/ethics-committee-fact-sheet.pdf.

[54] The American Institute of Certified Public Accountants website, Ethics Enforcement. www.aicpa.org/About/code/sec100.htm.www.aicpa.org/Professional+Resources/Professiona+Ethics+Code+of+Professional+Conduct/Professional+Ethics/Ethics+Enforcement/defin_sanction.htm.

financial statements was considered an important enough goal—given the huge financial stakes involved—to warrant federal legislation and the establishment of a federal oversight body, the PCAOB. A second important lesson is that maintaining objective and independent judgment is not easy. Accountants primarily maintain their objectivity by avoiding most situations that present a conflict of interest. They also maintain their independence by avoiding most situations that could reasonably appear to present a conflict of interest.

ARCHITECTURE

During the decade and a half before World War I, AMA organized medicine as a modern profession. Among the milestones in that process were not only the rethinking of medical education (set forth in the 1910 Flexner Report) but also the abandonment in 1903 of AMA's mandatory *Code of Ethics* of 1847 for the "suggestive and advisory" *Principles of Medical Ethics*. That was followed in 1912 by the abandonment of the 1903 principles for another code (with the same name) binding on all physicians (and surgeons). At about that time (1909), the American Institute of Architects (AIA) adopted its first code of ethics. That code applied only to members of the organization and not to all architects, but the code (like AMA's 1847 code) was binding on all architects. The AIA kept this feature when it adopted a new code in 1977, one organized—like the ABA's 1969 code (which was to be abandoned soon after)—into canons (broad statements of principle), ethical standards (more specific goals that AIA members should aspire to), rules (mandatory standards, the violation of which would justify formal discipline, including expulsion from the AIA), and commentary (when necessary to avoid a common misinterpretation of a rule).[55]

The 1909 AIA code reached all architects, not just AIA members, through its adoption by state licensing boards as local standards of practice. That simple arrangement ended in the 1970s, when the courts declared the AIA's code to be an unreasonable restraint on trade. While the AIA was rewriting its code to avoid another lawsuit (a process that did not end until 1990), the National Council of Architecture Registration Boards (NCARB) wrote its own code.[56]

Because the states' licensure of architecture is generally similar to the states' licensure of accountants (and, in some states, lawyers), continuing education requirements are also similar. Courses must be accredited to satisfy the continuing education requirements. The AIA itself offers some online courses that satisfy continuing education credit. Some of these courses

[55] See www.aia.org/SiteObjects/files/codeofethics.pdf.

[56] See www.architects.org/emplibrary/NCARB.pdf.

are now prepared by suppliers.[57] So far, supplier-prepared courses do not seem to be a problem. One reason that they are not may be that architects' specifications (the equivalent of a physician's prescription) typically either state a generic requirement or take the form "brand *x* or its equivalent." Another reason that supplier courses are not a problem may be that they do not include a trip to some ideal location, lavish entertainment, or other gifts. The course itself must be valuable enough to repay architects for their time and for lost opportunities to take other courses.

NCARB on Conflict of Interest

Architects resemble physicians, lawyers, and accountants in not being able to practice (that is, advertise, sign drawings, or otherwise publicly present themselves as architects) without registering as one (that is, being given a state license to practice). Beginning in 1919, registration boards have maintained a nonprofit group to provide a number of services to the profession: a standardized test for admission into the profession, standards for work experiences that a new graduate of an accredited architectural program should have before licensure (Intern Development Program), self-administered continuing education courses, and so on. NCARB's code of ethics (*Rules of Conduct*) is just one of these services. Adopted in 1977 (and amended since), the *Rules of Conduct* are designed to provide hard-edged rules for discipline (once a state board adopts them). Besides the nominal "Rules"—five titles numbered with Arabic numerals—the code includes (1) actual rules under each rule (numbered with a decimal), (2) a brief commentary after most of these rules, and (3) a long introduction (40 percent of the entire 10-page code). Although the NCARB code does set a somewhat lower standard than the (shorter) AIA code, it generally does so by silence rather than by providing a formal rule significantly different from the corresponding AIA rule. The AIA issues ethics opinions much as AMA does; NCARB does not. A state registration board may, however, issue an opinion as part of disciplinary action against a particular architect.

Conflict of interest is plainly important in the practice of architecture. The second of the five major divisions in NCARB's *Rules of Conduct* is titled Conflict of Interest; the third major division, although it is titled Full Disclosure, is in part (Rule 3.1) about responding to conflict of interest. The other divisions of the code—Competence (Division 1), Compliance with Law (Division 4), and Professional Conduct (Division 5)—have no connection with conflict of interest.

The overall strategy in these provisions is clear. Conflict of interest

[57] See, for example, www.gp.com/build/paperless/education.html (a course offered by Georgia-Pacific).

should generally be avoided, but when avoidance is not possible or at least not reasonable, the conflict must be fully disclosed to all appropriate parties and their consent must be won before the architect can proceed. Interestingly, the term "conflict of interest" is not used in any of the specific rules; its definition is, in effect, the rules under that title. All of the relevant rules (including Rule 3.1) are (primarily) concerned with financial interests. There are four rules under Rule 2, Conflict of Interest.

Rule 2.1 applies to ordinary compensation for services. An architect "shall not accept compensation for services from more than one party on a project unless the circumstances are fully disclosed to and agreed to . . . by all interested parties." Both disclosure and agreement are to be "in writing." The commentary explains that architects may sometimes find it hard to avoid receiving payment from two parties—for example, when ordering a large number of windows from a supplier later produces a rebate check. The architect cannot simply accept the rebate (even if it comes as a surprise) but must first inform the client (and other interested parties) of the payment and the reason for it. The architect cannot accept the payment unless at least the client (and any other interested party) approves. The commentary explains that the "bifurcated loyalty" that such a rebate threatens is "unacceptable unless all parties have understood it and accepted it." The commentary does not limit the "parties" to the client. This is because in many architectural projects several parties may be affected by the payment, such as the engineering firm typically present at any large project, the developer (who may be the immediate client but who is, in fact, a stand-in for the ultimate owner), the ultimate owner (who may be one or more individuals or a legal entity), and even the contractor or subcontractor who must work with the rebated supplies. The commentary can even be interpreted as including the window supplier's competitors among those who must be informed of the payment and the reason for it. They are certainly "interested parties." They are at a competitive disadvantage if they are not also making such rebates.

Behind Rule 2.1 is a conception of architects as having a relatively settled loyalty to the client that everyone dealing with the client relies on. An unusual payment (such as the rebate described above) unsettles the situation. There is no question here of the supplier buying the architect's loyalty with the rebate (as there would be if the payment were a bribe or kickback). The problem is that "money talks," and even architects cannot gauge how much they will listen the next time that they place an order of that sort. Their judgment that their professional judgment will not be affected is not relevant. That, too, is now under suspicion.

Disclosure of the payment makes it possible for all interested parties to redefine their relationship to the architect to take account of this unusual feature. The client may, for example, require the architect to hand over the entire rebate (as well as ask other suppliers whether they will meet the competition). However, because the architect's fee is often a percentage of the total cost of the project, this solution may not be the best. It would create a "perverse incentive." The architect would, in effect, be punished for saving the client money. The architect would have an incentive to avoid suppliers who give rebates. The client might then prefer to split the rebate with the architect, or they might work out some more complicated arrangement—of which all interested parties should be made aware to ensure that their trust in the architect's judgment is not misplaced.

Rule 2.2 concerns financial interests apart from payments, for example, stock in a potential supplier or a loan to a contractor. The architect must assess whether the interest (direct or indirect) is "substantial enough to influence his or her judgment in the performance of professional services" (whether or not it does or would in fact influence it). Architects thus have some discretion under this rule (as they do not under Rule 2.1). The rationale for allowing some discretion (concerning whether an interest is substantial enough) is that avoiding all financial interests seems too much to ask. For example, an architect with money in a large investment fund that holds a few shares of stock in one of the companies she or he is dealing with has an interest in that company. Is revealing such an interest worth the trouble? Should architects be required to avoid investing in any fund that might (on a given day) invest in a potential supplier? That seems too much to require, so long as the architect reveals any interest substantial enough to affect her or his judgment. Of course, when in doubt, the architect should reveal the interest. Rule 2.2 seems to work because it governs only interests other than payments, because architects seldom invest in suppliers and because most architects work in a small world (mostly developers or builders rather than individual clients) in which a substantial investment in a supplier would soon be known.

If the interest is enough to influence the judgment, the architect must fully disclose it in writing to the client or employer (thus creating a paper trail). If the client or employer objects to the business association or the financial interest, the architect must either terminate it or offer to give up the commission or employment. The client or employer may have good reason to accept the bifurcated loyalty that the business association or financial interest in question creates, but the decision is the client's or the employer's (or both, when an architect has both a client, the person who has hired the firm, and an employer, the architectural firm). That decision should be made only with all the relevant facts laid before the decision maker in a form that the decision maker can understand. If the architect is unwilling to make full disclosure, she or he must resign from the job. There is no middle way (no way to manage the conflict) without full disclosure and consent.

Rules 2.3 applies to any payment made in return for specifying or endorsing a supplier. Strictly speaking, this rule does not concern conflict of interest but concerns bribes, kickbacks, and other side payments that buy the architect's judgment. Architects are simply forbidden to solicit or accept such payments. The brief commentary notes that this rule is "absolute"; that is, it admits of no exception, even when all the relevant parties would agree to the payment after full disclosure. So, for example, an architect cannot have an agreement with a supplier that she or he will recommend a certain window frame even if she or he fully informs the clients of that agreement and the clients say, "Fine." Why? Although many of the payments in question are in fact illegal, the rule is indifferent to their legality. Even legal payments for specifying or endorsing a supplier (say, lending one's name to an advertising campaign) are forbidden. What explains this striking departure from architecture's standard strategy of allowing conflict of interest when the relevant parties consent after full disclosure?

The answer seems to be this: conflict of interest threatens professional judgment. It makes it less reliable than it would otherwise be. Sometimes such threats cannot be avoided or cannot be avoided at reasonable cost. Those relying on the architect's judgment then have the right to weigh the costs and benefits and decide whether to take the risk. In contrast, an agreement to specify or endorse a product does not threaten professional judgment. It does something much more dramatic. The architect has, in this respect, signed away judgment. By the agreement, the architect gives up future judgment of the appropriateness of the product in question. The agreement with the supplier prejudges the matter. The architect cannot both claim the power of an architect in that respect (the right to use her or his judgment to decide what is appropriate in that case) and follow an agreement prejudging the case.

Side payments for endorsement are also, in one respect, unnecessary. The client or employer derives no benefit whatsoever from them, and (generally) the architect does not need them to survive or prosper. They are simply not an essential part of practicing architecture.

This explanation of Rule 2.3 treats it as something other than a rule concerned with conflict of interest. Selling one's judgment does not, in general, create a conflict of interest (that is, it does not threaten professional judgment). However, sometimes it does. For example, if Person A is paid to endorse a product as part of an advertising campaign, Person A will have a greater tendency to specify that product than he or she otherwise would. That tendency is what makes Rule 2.3 in part a rule concerned with conflict of interest. Forbidding endorsements for pay eliminates one sort of conflict of interest.

Rule 2.4 concerns the architect acting as adjudicator, that is, as the interpreter of building contract documents or the judge of contract performance. When acting in this role, an architect is to "render decisions impartially, favoring neither party in the dispute." The commentary makes clear that it is customary in the construction industry for the architect, even though he or she is paid by the owner and owes loyalty to the owner, to settle disputes between the owner and a contractor, subcontractor, or supplier concerning whether work has been performed as the contract requires or whether the contract requires this or that. When acting in this capacity, the architect must (according to NCARB) act impartially. If the architect does not believe himself or herself to be capable of acting in that way, he or she "may appropriately decline to act in those two roles" (as the agent of the owner and as a judge between the owner and an adversary). The architect's role in such circumstances has a threat to independent judgment built into it (an interest but not a "special" interest). Both architects and those they work with are aware of that threat to independent judgment. They have traditionally tolerated it since the alternative is whatever delay is necessarily consequent on seeking a truly impartial judge far from the work site. Nonetheless, the architect must at least believe himself or herself to be able to render impartial judgment. If the threat to impartiality is significant enough that the architect doubts his or her own judgment, the architect may (and, indeed, should) decline. Interestingly, the rule is not satisfied if the architect merely believes himself or herself to be impartial; the architect must actually render an impartial decision. If the decision is obviously biased, the architect would be subject to discipline under the rule, even though the architect believed himself or herself to be impartial.

Like Rule 2.3, Rule 2.4 is an absolute rule (although the commentary does not say that explicitly). The rationale for its absoluteness is also much the same as that for Rule 2.3. The point of asking the architect to judge between the owner and those working on a site is to receive quickly (something approaching) impartial judgment (a judgment informed by the architect's knowledge of construction, the documents, and local custom). If the architect were known to be partial, his or her value as a judge would be much reduced. The rule preserves the usefulness of architects in settling such disputes (an efficiency serving everyone's interests in the long run). Like Rule 2.3, Rule 2.4 is (primarily) concerned not with conflict of interest, strictly speaking, but with something closely related, that is, the typical outcome of judgment free of conflict of interest (as well as of bias and prejudice): an impartial decision.

The last of NCARB's conflict of interest rules is Rule 3.1. It requires an architect making a "public statement on architectural questions" (that is, speaking publicly in a professional capacity) to "disclose when he or she is being compensated for making such statement or when he or she has an economic interest in the issue." So, for example, an architect paid by a developer to testify on behalf of a project would have to state that she or he is being so paid. An architect writing a journal article on behalf of a certain manufacturer's product would have to disclose ownership of even a single share of stock in that company. For public statements, the standard of disclosure is more demanding than for statements to client, employer, or other private person. (The term "substantial enough" in Rule 2.2 has no counterpart in Rule 3.1.) The commentary explains why the standard is so demanding: to preserve "the probity which the public expects of the architectural profession," architects are "not allowed under the circumstances described in the rule to disguise the fact that they are not speaking on the particular issue as an independent professional but as a professional engaged to act on behalf of a client" or with a judgment perhaps arising from the wrong sort of interest (a private interest rather than the public interest). The public is entitled to know that the architect might have a certain bias (or even that, from the public's perspective, might seem to have a certain bias), a legitimate bias if it is disclosed but otherwise an illegitimate bias. If architects routinely made public statements in the service of clients without acknowledging that service or in the service of a private interest (however small) without acknowledging that service, their public statements would eventually lose the power that comes from their being thought to be independent. The public statements would be regarded as unreliable (as, indeed, they would be).

This rationale is as interesting for what it leaves out as for what it includes. Like most professions, architecture recognizes itself as having an obligation to serve the public interest (an obligation that may not belong in hard-edged rules but appears, for example, in Canon II of the AIA code). The NCARB commentary might therefore have appealed to this obligation in support of a rule governing public statements (protecting the public). Instead, the commentary appeals to the interest that the profession itself has in maintaining its reliability ("the probity the public expects") both to explain and support the rule.

AIA on Conflict of Interest

The NCARB rules just discussed are the hard-edged rules concerning conflict of interest that state registration boards use to decide whether to discipline a licensed architect. We turn now to the AIA's code. Like AMA, the AIA is a voluntary organization. Also like AMA, it no longer is an organization to which a majority of the profession belongs. Yet, just as no AMA member wants AMA to discipline her or him, so no AIA member wants the AIA to discipline her or him. An AIA member charged with wrongdoing will generally hire a lawyer to present her or his side at the National Ethics Council (NEC) and, if the AIA member loses there, may seek redress in the courts. At least as much as physicians, architects live by their reputations. For that reason, an NEC-appointed hearing officer collects evidence and the full NEC (minus the hearing officer) decides the case in secret. However, for any serious discipline (censure, suspension, or expulsion), the ultimate decision is made public (the architect's name disappears from the membership role, and the architect can no longer be listed as an AIA member). The NEC publishes its decision in the form of a judicial opinion, stating the facts found, the penalty, and the rationale for it, without identifying the parties. The NEC also issues interpretations of the code (Advisory Opinions).[58]

The AIA code (2007) is about half the length of NCARB's and devotes proportionally much less space to conflict of interest. Canon III (Obligations to the Client) provides the overall framework for conflict of interest. AIA members should "exercise unprejudiced and unbiased judgment when performing all professional services." Ethical Standard 3.2 (titled Conflict of Interest) simply states the general strategy for avoiding tendencies to bias and prejudice. Members should "avoid conflicts of interest in their professional practices and fully disclose all unavoidable conflicts as they arise." There are only two disciplinary rules under this ethical standard. The second rule, Rule 3.202 (render decisions impartially), merely restates NCARB's Rule 2.2 (with a briefer commentary), but the first rule, Rule 3.201, adds something new.

Rule 3.201 prohibits AIA members from rendering professional services if their "professional judgment could be affected by responsibilities to another project or person, or by [their own] interests." The only exception to this prohibition is (the usual) "unless all those who rely on the Member's judgment consent after full disclosure." Rule 3.201 understands "interest" as including more than financial interest. Any "responsibility" to another project or person that could affect a member's judgment is an interest for the purposes of this rule (as is any self-interest, even if it is not financial or familial). The commentary underscores the point. The rule is, it says, "intended to embrace the full range of situations that may present a Member with a conflict between his interests or responsibilities and the interests of others." The commentary goes on to give an equally wide reading of "all those who rely." Those entitled to disclosure "may include a client, owner, employee, contractor, or others who rely on or are affected by the Member's professional judgment." An AIA member who cannot appropriately disclose a "conflict directly to the affected person must take steps to ensure that disclosure is made by another means." (Direct disclosure may not be possible because the client is, for example, an individual who is out of town or an organization whose officers are hard to reach; sending notice is not equivalent to "appropriate disclosure.") If a member cannot make adequate disclosure of a conflict of interest (directly or indirectly), he or she cannot render the professional services in question. The member must decline or withdraw.

In addition to the rules under Rule 3.2, there are at least two rules in

---

[58] For either, see www.aia.org/about_ethics#nec.

Canon II (Obligations to the Public) that are (at least in part) concerned with conflict of interest. Rule 2.103 forbids an AIA member from serving in a public capacity to "accept payments or gifts which are intended to influence their judgment." This rule covers bribes (payments made in exchange for some future illegal service) but not kickbacks (a payment for a referral or some other favor already done). The rules cover more than bribes, for example, a dinner or a gift of theater tickets of whatever value given with the intention of influencing judgment. This additional coverage is what justifies discussion of this rule as concerned with conflict of interest.

This is another absolute rule. It is nonetheless unusual in one respect. It is the intention of the payer or giver, not its likely consequence or the recipient's intention, that determines whether the payment or gift is prohibited. The rationale for this approach to payments and gifts is obvious. An architect serving in a public capacity will, in the ordinary course of life, receive many payments and gifts. Prohibiting them all would be unreasonable, but some should be prohibited. For example, no one wants to forbid a gift from the architect's mother or brother-in-law that is part of the normal exchange of gifts among family members. (Such gifts would seldom be given with the intent of influencing the architect's professional judgment.) In contrast, the AIA would, presumably, want to prohibit a gift from a potential developer hoping to reduce the hostility of an architect toward a project that he or she has in mind when that architect is a member of the local planning commission.

Rule 2.301 is concerned with public statements on architectural issues. It is (almost) identical to NCARB's Rule 3.1. Although there is no commentary, its placement under the canon concerned with obligations to the public suggests that its rationale is a bit different. Architects perform a useful service whenever they inform the public of their judgments on architectural issues. They perform a useful service whether they speak disinterestedly or on behalf of a client or interest. However, the service performed is different. Rule 2.301 requires architects to make clear which service they are performing so that their audience, the public, can evaluate it using the appropriate criteria. The underlying rationale is not so much to protect independent judgment as it is not to mislead the public concerning what it may reasonably expect of the judgments offered. The public's trust in what architects say depends in part on knowing who they are working for when they say it.

ENGINEERING

Engineering and medicine have historically been very different professions. Engineers have, for example, generally worked in large organizations, beginning with the army; physicians (like architects) have, until recently, generally worked alone or in small practices (with or without an affiliation with a nearby hospital). Those who employ engineers tend to be the rich and the powerful, not the sick or the wounded. When a work of engineering fails, the result may be hundreds or even thousands of deaths—typically of people of whom the engineers knows little—not, as in conventional medicine, just one person, a patient, known to the physician. (Of course, when physicians advise the Food and Drug Administration [FDA] or a drug manufacturer, the analogy with engineering is much closer.) For these reasons (and others), many of the conflicts of interest that engineers have thought about over the last century lack an exact analogue in medicine. They are nonetheless worth considering in detail because they illustrate how a profession can work from a basic understanding of conflict of interest to a system of detailed rules likely to be of use to practitioners in what would otherwise be situations hard to navigate. To understand the system of rules, it is important to understand something of the institutions in which they are embedded.

Background Institutions

Engineering is divided into four major disciplines (as well as many smaller ones): civil, mechanical, electrical, and chemical. These are more closely related to each other than medicine is to such other health care disciplines, such as dentistry or osteopathy. That is, they are generally taught in departments of the same school; the curricula are similar, especially in the first 2 undergraduate years; the schools have the same accreditation body (ABET, Inc.);[59] and students receive the same first degree upon graduation, a B.S. (with different majors). Nonetheless, engineering has never created the equivalent of AMA. Instead, there are five major societies. One each for the major disciplines: the American Society of Civil Engineers (ASCE), the American Society of Mechanical Engineers (ASME), the Institute of Electrical and Electronic Engineers (IEEE), and the American Institute of Chemical Engineers (AIChE). The fifth major society, the National Society of Professional Engineers (NSPE), cuts across these four. Its members are (primarily) Professional Engineers (PEs). A PE is an engineer (of any discipline) licensed by a state (in much the way that lawyers, CPAs, architects, and physicians are), but only about a fifth of all U.S. engineers are so licensed. The rest, who work in large organizations, do not need a license to practice because of what is known as "the industrial exemption." Although they are not PEs, they

[59] ABET was formerly the American Board for Engineering and Technology; the name change to ABET, Inc., reflects its expansion into new areas.

are full members of the engineering profession.[60] The five major societies (along with many of the smaller ones) frequently cooperate ad hoc as well as maintain many permanent bodies, of which ABET is among the oldest and the most important.

This complexity reappears in the codes of ethics governing engineers. Except for a brief period a half century ago, each of the five major societies has had its own code (as have many of the smaller societies); and, as if this were not enough ethical complexity for one profession, ABET (or its predecessor) has had a separate code (which has not been amended since 1977),[61] one that most engineering societies have endorsed.

Although the relationship among these codes is complex, it is not muddled. The NSPE code[62] is designed (like architecture's NCARB code) primarily for adoption by state licensing boards. Its rules are supposed to be appropriate for use in a disciplinary hearing. In contrast, the ABET code is designed to guide individual engineers. ABET has no enforcement procedure whatsoever (and does not even have a committee to issue advisory opinions) and, apparently, no interest in having its code enforced through any formal procedure. The ABET code thus functions much as the AIA's Ethical Standards do and should therefore be more demanding that the NSPE code. In fact, today it is as often less demanding than more demanding.

Until the 1980s, ABET's code was clearly the most important in engineering. Most engineering societies, including two of the major ones (ASME and ASCE), had adopted it as their own (either the 1977 version or one of its predecessors). In the last decade, however, its importance has declined dramatically. Some societies have amended their codes now and then, to the point that there are now important differences between those codes and ABET's code. Some of the differences arise from the adoption of provisions that the NSPE adopted; some arise from local innovations (which other societies may or may not have followed). In addition, some societies (most notably, the IEEE) have abandoned the ABET code altogether.

The NSPE code now seems destined to become the de facto standard of the profession (in part because the ABET code has gone so long without

[60] Because most engineers are unlicensed, most continuing education depends on employers or on individual engineers. Large employers generally have their own internal technical courses (which the employer funds). Some continuing education goes on in universities as degree programs, certificate programs, or specific technical courses. Most large employers pay for an engineer's continued technical education. Engineers may also be trained by a supplier, once the employer has contracted for some new product (such as software). Most states require PEs to take accredited continuing education courses. Accreditation of such courses is handled much as it is in accounting, architecture, and law.

[61] See http://ethics.iit.edu/codes/coe/accreditation.board.engineering.tech.a.html (Code); http://ethics.iit.edu/codes/coe/accreditation.board.engineering.tech.b.html (Guidelines).

[62] See www.nspe.org/ethics/.

amendment and the IEEE code lacks sufficient detail to provide much guidance). The NSPE code is now much more often reprinted at the back of a text in engineering ethics than any other code. Although it is distinct from ABET's code, NSPE's code resembles it in layout and language because both derive from the "unity code" of a half century ago. Only the IEEE has an independent code (2000)[63]—which some other engineering societies, including the AIChE (2002), have followed. The IEEE code is quite short (260 words) and applies to IEEE members (not to engineers), an important distinction because many IEEE members are not engineers but are computer scientists, physicists, mathematicians, or the like.

This survey confines its review of engineering's methods of dealing with conflict of interest to three codes, those of the IEEE, the NSPE, and ABET, the most important (and distinctive) in U.S. engineering. For all the small differences among these three codes, there is a fundamental agreement about how to deal with conflict of interest.

IEEE Code

The one sentence on conflict of interest in the IEEE code expresses that fundamental agreement succinctly. IEEE members are to "avoid real or perceived conflicts of interest whenever possible, and to disclose them to affected parties when they do exist." The IEEE strategy for dealing with conflict of interest (avoidance whenever possible and disclosure whenever avoidance is not possible or has failed) is similar to that identified for architects but nonetheless differs in two important respects. First, the requirement of avoidance applies not only to "real" conflicts of interest but also to "perceived" ones. Perception—that is, the appearance—of a conflict of interest is treated as being just as bad as the reality. The underlying idea seems to be that an engineer's professional judgment (or, rather, an IEEE member's professional judgment) should be above suspicion. Even perceived conflicts should therefore be avoided (whatever the underlying reality about the interests in question). The underlying reality does not matter to those who would like to rely on an engineer—until it is disclosed and the false appearance is dispelled.

The second important respect in which the IEEE strategy differs from that identified for architects is that there is no indication of what is to be done after disclosure (for example, there is no requirement of consent before continuing). The other engineering codes do provide guidance concerning this question, although the particulars vary a good deal, depending on the circumstances in question. The IEEE has a committee to prepare guidelines to supplement its code.

[63] See www.ieee.org/portal/pages/iportals/aboutus/ethics/code.html.

NSPE Code

The NSPE code is divided into three main parts: a brief, four-sentence preamble; the body of the code, which consists of Part I. Fundamental Canons, Part II. Rules of Practice, and Part III. Professional Obligations; and an addendum (which may be ignored here) that quotes a 1978 federal court decision on competitive bidding and the response of the NSPE Executive Committee. The fundamental canons (about 3 percent of the code) contains three sentences relevant to conflict of interest (in language dating from one of the first engineering codes): "Engineers, in the fulfillment of their professional duties, shall: . . . 3) Issue public statements only in an objective and truthful manner. 4) Act for each employer or client as faithful agents or trustees. 5) Avoid deceptive acts."

The Rules of Practice (which accounts for a quarter of the code's 2,400 words) has six main rules, each of which corresponds to one of the Fundamental Canons. The specific rules under a rule (designated with lowercase letters) are applications or elaborations of the prefacing rule. There are 3 rules under Rule II.3, 5 under Rule II.4, and 2 under Rule II.5, for 10 rules in all. All but two of these (Rules II.3a and II.3b) concern conflict of interest (more or less). In addition, Professional Obligations (about 40 percent of the code) contains six more rules related to conflict of interest. In all, about a fifth of the entire code is concerned with conflict of interest. Apparently, the NSPE takes conflict of interest very seriously. A detailed review of the provisions shows that they cover a surprisingly large number of specific issues.

Rules of Practice

Rule II.3c forbids engineers from issuing "statements, criticisms, or arguments on technical matters that are inspired or paid for by interested parties, unless they [the engineers] have prefaced their comments by explicitly identifying the interested parties on whose behalf they are speaking, and by revealing the existence of any interest the engineers may have in the matters." Although Rule II.3c is similar to NCARB's Rule 3.1 (and AIA Rule 2.301), Rule II.3c differs in one striking respect. The engineer must not only reveal payment for a statement, criticism, or argument but even inspiration, presumably something more than NCARB's "financial interest." Although a financial interest might "inspire" a statement, so might friendship, the urging of a relative, or some other connection unrelated to compensation or financial interest. Although the language is vague, it is obviously meant to sweep wide (something that we might not expect in a code designed for discipline rather than for personal guidance). Why is there such a demanding rule?

For an engineer, the rationale for Rule II.3c is pretty straightforward. Because the rule is under Section 3, it concerns public statements. Engineers view the public much as physicians view patients. Engineers are—as Fundamental Canon 1 puts it—to "[h]old paramount the safety, health, and welfare of the public." There is no official definition of "public"; there is even some debate about the exact boundaries of the public, for example, whether the public includes employees of one's client or employer. The most popular view, though, seems to be that the public includes all those who, owing to a lack of knowledge, power, or opportunity, are unable to protect themselves fully from what engineers do. What engineers call "the public" is (more or less) as dependent on engineering judgment as the physician's patient is dependent on the physician's judgment.

Insofar as what engineers say in public may be influenced by an interested party other than the public, the public needs to know about that influence if it is to decide the appropriate weight to give the statement. The engineer, of course, tries to speak "in an objective and truthful manner" (as Canon 3 requires). If the engineer is not trying to do that, he or she should not speak at all (or, at least, not claim to speak as an engineer). However, if an engineer is aware of an influence that might (but also might not) undermine his or her ability to speak in an objective and truthful manner, he or she must warn the public of that danger to objectivity. There is nothing wrong with issuing public statements in the service of a client or an employer (as long as the statements are objective and truthful). There is, however, something wrong with an engineer giving the impression that he or she is doing something else, that is, expressing independent professional judgment (one independent of an employer, client, or other interested party) when it is not. An engineer must not give a false impression if he or she can reasonably avoid it. Experience and common sense suggest that an engineer may easily avoid giving that false impression by explicitly stating what he or she is doing as he or she begins the public statement in question.

All the rules under the next heading (Rule II.4) are concerned with protecting the client or the employer, not the public. The strategy for dealing with conflict of interest is much the same as that expressed in Rule II.3c. Rule II.4a explicitly uses the term "conflict of interest." Engineers are supposed to "disclose all known or potential conflicts of interest that could influence or appear to influence their judgment or the quality of their services." There is no requirement to avoid those that can be avoided. The rule seems to be concerned with those conflicts that cannot be (or that perhaps just have not been) avoided. Rule II.4a makes something like the distinction between the IEEE's "real" and "perceived" conflicts of interest, that is, between conflicts of interest that "could" influence and those that merely "could appear" to influence a judgment (or the quality of service). There is, however, a new distinction, that between "known" conflicts of interest and those that are merely "potential." Although the distinction seems confused (should not the contrast be between "actual" and "potential" or between "known" and "unknown"?), the intent of the language seems to be clear enough: again (as in Rule II.3c), to sweep as widely as possible. Rule II.4a bars such excuses as, "I didn't know it was a conflict of interest" and "It was only a potential conflict of interest." Lastly, there is no attempt to distinguish financial interests from other kinds of interests. The rule applies to any conflict of interest whatsoever.

Rules II.4b and II.4c are similar to NCARB's Rules 2.1 and 2.2. They make avoidance the standard response to a conflict of interest. Rule II.4b forbids engineers from accepting "compensation, financial or otherwise, from more than one party for services on the same project, or for services pertaining to the same project, unless the circumstances are fully disclosed and agreed to by all interested parties." Rule II.4c forbids engineers from soliciting or accepting "financial or other valuable consideration, directly or indirectly, from outside agents in connection with the work for which they are responsible." The only significant difference between these two rules and the corresponding NCARB rules is (again) a wider sweep. Rule II.4b concerns compensation "financial or otherwise"; Rule II.4c concerns "other valuable consideration" as well as just "financial" ("directly or indirectly" solicited or accepted). So, a dinner, help finding another job, an all-expenses-paid trip to Jamaica, and a free course in some engineering subject, although they are not strictly financial compensation for work on a project (or "pertaining to the same project"), would clearly be close enough to require disclosure under Rule II.4b if they were, for example, offered in the way of offering thanks for favors done on a project. Similarly, although such things might not count as financial considerations, they still seem to count as consideration enough to be forbidden under Rule II.4c (coming from "outside agents").

The last two rules under Rule II.4 concern possible clashes between the engineer's obligations to the public and obligations to a client or an employer. Rule II.4d forbids engineers in public service as members, advisors, or employees of a governmental or a quasigovernmental body or department to "participate in decisions with respect to services solicited or provided by them or their organizations in private or public engineering practice." Engineers in public service are to recuse themselves whenever they, their employer, or their client has an interest in a decision. The client or employer may be a private firm, but the engineer should recuse himself or herself even if the client or the employer with an interest in the decision is another governmental (or quasigovernmental) agency. The rule makes no exception in the case of "full disclosure." The idea seems to be that engineers serving in government (in whatever capacity) or in a quasigovernmental agency (such as AMTRAK or the U.S. Postal Service) are supposed to put their independent judgment at the public's service. Disclosure of a conflict of interest to the relevant agency does not, as such, protect the public. Even the agency's informed consent does nothing to ensure protection of the public interest. The disclosure would have to be made to the public directly in a way that allows the public to take appropriate action. This can seldom happen when the engineer is advising a public agency (as it can when an engineer is speaking to the public directly). Disclosure to the relevant agency does not necessarily reach the public, and even when it does, the agency and not the public would ordinarily make the decision. So, the only way to protect the public from an engineer's conflict of interest when the engineer's judgment, though exercised in behalf of the public, works through a public agency, is to have the engineer avoid participation in the decision.

Rule II.4e adopts the same strategy with respect to soliciting or accepting "a contract from a governmental body on which a principal or officer of their organization serves as a member." (For some reason, this rule is silent concerning quasigovernmental bodies.) Again, neither mere disclosure of the conflict nor disclosure with consent is enough. The engineer must never solicit or accept such a contract. Although Rule II.4e concerns conflict of interest, it is not designed to protect the engineer's judgment (as the others are) but is designed to protect the judgment of the principal or the officer of the organization that the engineer serves. Indeed, it seems to be designed to protect the principal or the officer in question from the appearance of conflict as well as from actual conflict. There is no requirement that the principal or officer know of the contract or have anything to do with obtaining it. Protecting the principal or officer in question from the appearance of conflict of interest is part of being a faithful agent or trustee.

Rule II.5b consists of three long sentences mostly concerned with bribery, but a part of the first sentence seems designed to avoid both certain conflicts of interest and the mere appearance of them (as well as actual bribes): "Engineers shall not . . . receive, either directly or indirectly, any contribution to influence the award of a contract by public authority, or which may be reasonably construed by the public as having the effect or intent of influencing the awarding of a contract." The expression "reasonably construed" is, of course, a somewhat lower standard than "perceived," as used in Rule II.4a. "Perceived" may be interpreted to include unreasonable as well as reasonable construal. The reason for the change in terms is not obvious (or known). One explanation is that what the public might reasonably construe as taking a bribe or as being a threat to judgment is too close to dishonesty (the concern of Rule II.5) to be good for engineering's reputation. However, what might unreasonably be so construed is not. There are other ways to deal with unreasonable construal; for example, pointing out how unreasonable it is. In this context, an engineer should be above "reasonable suspicion" but cannot avoid all suspicion.

One problem with the use of "the appearance [or perception] of conflict of interest" is its subjectivity. What appears to be is in part a matter of the psychology of the person doing the perceiving. The mad, the overly suspicious, or the profoundly cynical might see a conflict of interest where no one else would. In contrast, what might reasonably be construed as a conflict of interest, given the evidence available to the person doing the construing, is an objective matter. Even if we know that there is no conflict of interest (for example, because we know that the investments in question are in a blind trust), we can see that the public would be right to draw the opposite conclusion if all it knew was, say, that the engineer in question held the compromising investment. The public's construal of the situation is, on the basis of the evidence, reasonable.

Although the distinction between reasonable construal and unreasonable construal is important, it may not be as important to interpreting the NSPE code as it seems. All codes of ethics must be applied by using reasonable interpretive principles. One principle of reasonable interpretation is that, unless it is unavoidable, an interpretation should not lead to logical impossibility or practical absurdity. Because the avoidance of all perception or appearance of conflict of interest is probably impossible or at least unreasonable, it seems likely that even the code provisions that do not specify the "reasonableness" of the perception or appearance in fact assume it—or, at least, should be interpreted as so doing.

Professional Obligations

So far we have been examining the part of the NSPE Code of Ethics called Part II. Rules of Practice. That part explicitly provides interpretations of Fundamental Canons 1 to 5, rules designed to protect the public, client, and employer. We now turn to the next part, Part III. Professional Obligations, rules that seem to offer interpretations of the remaining Fundamental Canon, which requires engineers to "Conduct themselves honorably, responsibly, ethically, and lawfully so as to enhance the honor, reputation, and usefulness of the profession." This section has nine main rules, numbered like the Rules of Practice, but not obviously derived from the wording of either the preamble or the Fundamental Canons. Except for not overlapping much with the Rules of Practice, there is no obvious unity in the subject matter of Part III. It is, in effect, a code within a code concerned (primarily) with enhancing the honor, reputation, and usefulness of the profession rather than with protecting the public, the client, or the employer (though following its rules would often have that effect too). Part III has three rules concerning conflict of interest: Rules III.4, III.5, and III.6.

Rule III.4 protects the confidentiality of business and technical information that engineers learn while they are acting in a professional capacity. Rule III.4a is concerned with the unreliability in judgment that arises from trying to judge as one would if one did not know what one in fact knows. That rule forbids engineers "without the consent of all interested parties, [to] promote or arrange for new employment or practice in connection with a specific project for which the engineer has gained particular and specialized knowledge." The engineer must have the consent of "all interested parties," generally, the old employer and the new one (as well as clients, if any), because she or he would be in an ethically untenable position otherwise. The engineer has an obligation to maintain the confidentiality of all specific business and technical information learned at the present employer (apart from what has become the engineer's skill, experience, or general knowledge). At the new job, the engineer will have an obligation to act as a faithful agent, using her or his best engineering judgment on behalf of the new employer (or client), just as she or he did at the old employer. The engineer cannot use her or his best engineering judgment while trying to ignore some of what she or he knows (say, the specifics of a new product under development). If the engineer "bends over backward" to be fair to the previous employer, she or he will not treat her or his new employer as she or he should. The engineer will give the new employer less than her or his best. If, however, the engineer does not bend over backward to be fair, she or he cannot know that she or he has treated the old employer as she or he should. (To avoid revealing too much, the engineer needs a margin of safety, which means revealing too little.) Without guidance from the fully informed "interested parties," the engineer is likely to fail the past employer, the new employer, or both. Because much technical and business information consists of trade secrets, the engineer may even provoke a lawsuit between the past and the present employer.

The only way to avoid all of these troubles, apart from never changing jobs or never seeking new employment closely related to projects that one has worked on before, is to have the parties work out an arrangement in advance of the move from one company to another. The arrangement may be as simple as the new employer agreeing to buy a right to use the technology in question or as complicated as an agreement stating what kinds of projects the engineer can work on for a specified period (say, 2 years).

Why does Rule III.4a not simply forbid engineers to seek employment too closely related to previous work? Why does it allow the consent of interested parties to resolve the conflict of interest problem (even if it does not resolve the underlying threat to judgment)? The (primary) moral wrong that conflict of interest threatens is a betrayal of justified reliance (rather than actual biased judgment). Engineers undertake to provide a certain level of service, that is, to be a reliable source of independent professional judgment concerning engineering. Conflict of interest means that an engineer can no longer safely be relied on for such judgment within a certain range of activities. If an interested party, that is, someone justified in relying on that judgment, is alerted to the problem by its disclosure and, by its (informed) consent, accepts the risk, the possibility of betrayal (in that respect) is eliminated. The profession's honor and reputation for honor are preserved. What remains is only a practical problem of protecting the various interests at stake from biased judgment (that is, protecting engineering's usefulness and its reputation for usefulness). One of those interests is the public's interest in the productive use of what the engineer knows. Forbidding engineers to move from one job to a closely related one would waste some of what the engineer has learned (a social resource as well as a personal one) and make it harder for employers to find the engineers that they need.

The rationale for Rule III.4b is similar. The rule forbids engineers, "without the consent of all interested parties, [to] participate in or represent an adversary interest in connection with a specific project or proceeding in which the engineer has gained particular specialized knowledge on behalf of a former client or employer." Engineers frequently testify in court, arbitration hearings, and similar proceedings on behalf of one side or the other. The United States does not have a system of official experts for tribunals to rely on. Representation or even participating in an adversary representation (for example, by testifying as an expert witness for one side or the other) may seem like a betrayal of trust or reliance (whether or not it is), if the engineer's expertise derives even in part from specialized knowledge gained in the course of working for the adverse party ("biting the hand that once fed him or her," so to speak). The engineer should appear as an expert in such a proceeding (or otherwise participate in it) only if all the interested parties welcome the engineer as an independent expert or at least as someone who is not going to betray their justified trust or reliance. Again, the honor and the reputation of engineering are preserved. (The number of engineers makes it unlikely that the adverse party will fail to find a qualified witness even if one party rejects the first engineer for conflict of interest.)

Rule III.5 forbids engineers to "be influenced in their professional duties by conflicting interests." The rule should not be interpreted as forbidding engineers to be influenced by conflicts of interest because, so interpreted, it would be inconsistent with all of the rules discussed so far, which permit conflicts of interest when there are full disclosure and consent (however, the interests, in fact, influence the decision). The only way to avoid being influenced by a conflict of interest is to avoid the conflict of interest or, having failed to avoid it, to recuse oneself. There is no other way to ensure that the decision in question is not influenced. (Disclosure and consent protect against betrayal of trust, not the loss of independent judgment itself.) So, Rule III.5 must instead be understood as forbidding certain kinds of interests, those that always (or at least too often) conflict with an engineer's professional duties.

The two rules under Rule III.5 confirm this inference. Rule III.5a bars the acceptance of "financial or other considerations, including free engineering designs, from material or equipment suppliers for specifying their product." (Free engineering designs, sometimes including free software, are the engineering equivalent both of the free samples of drugs that physicians receive and of drug company-sponsored courses.) Rule III.5b also bars the acceptance of "commissions or allowances, directly or indirectly, from contractors or other parties dealing with clients or employers of the engineer in connection with work for which the engineer is responsible." There is no exception for disclosure and consent. The engineer can easily avoid such interests without failing to do anything that an engineer should do for the public, a client, or an employer. The engineer should not put his or her interests in financial gain ahead of the interests of the public, a client, or an employer in having the engineer's independent judgment.

Finally, Rule III.6 is concerned with obtaining employment. Although most of the rules under it have nothing to do with conflict of interest, one does. Rule III.6a forbids engineers to "request, propose, or accept a commission on a contingent basis under circumstances in which their judgment may be compromised." At one time, most engineering codes simply forbade engineers from working on a "contingent basis" (that is, where payment, all or just part, depends on success). One consequence of a series of antitrust cases brought against professions in the 1970s was that the rule against contingent fees was declared an unreasonable restraint of trade. The NSPE then sought to restate the rule to make clear its intent, which was not to raise the fees that engineers could charge for failure but to protect engineering judgment. Engineers might, it was thought, take chances that they should not take if their income depended even in part on "success"—success not in the sense in which engineers understand it (which takes into account the public's long-term interests) but in the sense in which a client or employer might understand it (for example, getting a product out the door by a certain date). Hence, Rule III.6a is another absolute rule. The consent neither of the client nor of the employer would permit an engineer to enter a fee contingent arrangement that might compromise her or his judgment.

That completes the survey of how the NSPE code of ethics regulates conflict of interest. That does not, however, complete the survey of NSPE's regulation of conflict of interest. In addition to the code, the NSPE maintains the Board of Ethical Review (BER), which receives inquiries from NSPE members concerning questions of ethics and issues opinions in response.[64] BER publishes between 6 and 13 opinions each year. About

[64] Many of these, including most since 1990, are available at www.niee.org/cases/.

a quarter of these are indexed under "conflict of interest" (among other categories). Space does not allow for an examination of these, but such an examination would only confirm the guiding principles sketched so far: avoid all conflicts of interest that can reasonably be avoided, whether they are actual, potential, or merely apparent. Tolerate the remainder only if full disclosure to interested parties and their informed consent give them the tools that they need to protect against less reliable judgment. Neither consent nor disclosure is enough when an affected party cannot protect itself once it is fully informed.

ABET Code

The ABET code consists of two major parts: the Code of Ethics proper, which is a short document (210 words), and the much longer Suggested Guidelines for Use with the Fundamental Canons of Ethics (2,667 words). The Code of Ethics is divided into Fundamental Principles (which have much the same content as the NSPE preamble) and Fundamental Canons (which have much the same content as NSPE's Fundamental Canons). The ABET guidelines correspond to the rest of the NSPE code (Parts II and III).

For the purposes of this paper, the only significant difference between the two codes (apart from the guidelines) is that ABET's Fundamental Canon 4 has been amended to append to the language of the NSPE code a comma and the words "and shall avoid conflicts of interest." Most engineering codes of ethics now include that amendment, the result of a scandal in the middle 1970s that ended in a $7.5 million judgment against ASME.[65] Some volunteers in one of ASME's standard-setting bodies, although faithful agents and trustees of their employer (as Fundamental Canon 4 then required), had a conflict of interest when acting as members of the committee. Because the engineers involved were members of ASME, as well as volunteers, ASME had not been their client or employer (in the ordinary sense of these terms). They had not (it seemed) violated Fundamental Canon 4 (or any other rule in effect at the time). Yet, most engineers thought that they had clearly done something that an engineer should not do. Since Fundamental Canon 4 did not seem to cover the case, although it should have, ABET revised Fundamental Canon 4 (adding the reference to conflict of interest), and most other engineering societies followed (with the notable exception of NSPE—which dealt with the problem by adding or amending rules *under* its equivalent of Fundamental Canon 4).

---

[65] See *ASME v. Hydrolevel Corp.*, 456 U.S. 556 (1982).

ABET Guidelines

Although the ABET Guidelines were explicitly designed for use with the Fundamental Canons, they are an independent code in structure (and they were in fact the body of the code itself until 1977). The guidelines consist of seven main divisions, each of which is identical to one of the code's Fundamental Canons (and carries the same number). Under each of these are lettered sections and sometimes numbered subsections interpreting or applying the canon. Many of the sections are identical in language to provisions of the NSPE code. Some differ in ways not important here. For example, ABET Rule 3d differs from NSPE Rule III.3c in using "engineering matter" rather than "technical matter," by requiring engineers to identify themselves (as well as the party for whom they are speaking), and requiring them to describe any "pecuniary interest" that they may have in what they are about to say (rather than just any interest). In what follows, we ignore such small differences, focusing on rules that add something important to what we found in the NSPE code. There are only two such rules. They are, not surprisingly, both under Canon 4 (the canon explicitly concerned with avoiding conflict of interest).

Rule 4a of ABET's code differs from its NSPE counterpart (Rule II.4a) in requiring engineers to "avoid all known conflicts of interest" (rather than simply to disclose them) and to disclose promptly to their clients or employers the rest, what the NSPE code identified as "potential" conflicts of interest: "any business association, interests, or circumstances which *could* influence their judgment or the quality of their services" (emphasis added). This guideline makes explicit what we had found implicit in NSPE's Rule II.4a. The ABET rule may, nonetheless, be less demanding than its NSPE counterpart. If the adjective "business" applies to "interest" and "circumstance" as well as to "association" (a natural reading), then Rule 4a does not require disclosure of all conflicts of interest but only those arising from business associations, business interests, or business circumstances.

The theme of avoidance is carried through the rest of the conflict of interest provisions under Rules 4b to 4g—all of which, except for Rule 4b, are (more or less) identical to the rules in the NSPE code (and, in fact, date from some of the earliest codes of engineering ethics). The exception, Rule 4b, forbids engineers to "knowingly undertake any assignments which would knowingly create a potential conflict of interest between themselves and their clients or their employers." The two uses of "knowingly" suggests not only sloppy editing but also a great concern that engineers not be blamed for undertaking such assignments inadvertently. The requirement of knowledge is a break with the ABET code's general policy, which is to require avoidance or disclosure without providing for the excuse "I did not know." (In other words, engineering codes generally treat ethical conduct as a question of competence for which "I did not know" is an admission of wrongdoing and not an excuse.) There is only one other use of "knowingly" in the entire code, one of which is unrelated to conflict of interest (Rule 6a, avoiding association with a disreputable business). Rule 4a's knowledge requirement (like the use of "conflict of interest") is new to the 1977 code. However, it is an innovation that some other codes have followed. For example, Rule 4b in ASME's current code (2002) is simply a cleaner version of ABET's: "Engineers shall not undertake any assignments which would knowingly create a potential conflict of interest between themselves and their clients or their employers."

Conclusions from Survey of Engineering Codes

For engineering, then, conflict of interest is a threat to the profession's usefulness (the reliability of its judgment) as well as to its honor and reputation. For most purposes, the best response to an actual or potential conflict of interest is to avoid it as soon as one learns of it. In a few cases, recusal is allowed (or required); in others, those cases in which (1) disclosure allows the public, client, and employer an adequate response and (2) the engineer cannot be replaced or cannot be replaced at reasonable cost, tolerance of a conflict of interest is allowable. However, it is only allowable. Even then, there is a risk to all who rely on the engineer's judgment that the engineer's judgment will not be as good as it should be (and would be but for the conflict of interest). Disclosure is not a cure-all.

COMPARATIVE OVERVIEW

This survey has discussed both similarities and differences in the treatment of conflicts of interest by four important professions. What can be learned from this survey of lawyers, certified public accountants, architects, and engineers? The obvious point is that all four professions take conflict of interest in professional practice very seriously. The recent history of public accountancy shows that failure to take conflicts of interest seriously enough can result in federal regulation. Engineering had a similar experience three decades ago with civil liability.[66]

With the exception of engineering, these professions do not undertake the kind of scientific research carried out by some in the medical

[66] *American Society of Mechanical Engineering, Inc. v. Hydrolevel Corp.*, 456 U.S. 556 (1982), in which the U.S. Supreme Court held that ASME was strictly liable for the acts of its agent (the chairman of ASME's Boiler and Pressure Vessel Codes Committee) if those acts are in breach of antitrust laws (the chairman, an officer in the competitor of Hydrolevel, had a financial interest in his committee, finding that Hydrolevel's product did not meet ASME's code).

profession.[67] They have therefore not had to deal with controversies over conflicts of interest in research. Although each profession sets standards for providers of continuing professional education, they have, it seems, not faced any significant conflict of interest in education either.[68]

One reason for the relatively low level of attention given to conflicts of interest in research and education may be that lawyers and accountants do not act as gatekeepers for significant numbers of products and services as physicians do when they prescribe medications, use medical devices, order diagnostic tests, and the like. To the extent that architects and engineers are gatekeepers for supplies, their codes of ethics carefully regulate relationships with suppliers, gifts from suppliers, and other entanglements with suppliers that might threaten their professional judgment.

All four professions treat conflict of interest situations as risk situations; bias, breach of confidentiality, fraud, and malpractice are dealt with separately. Conflicts of interest are understood to threaten the quality of the individual professional's judgment and, as a consequence, the well-being of the client or employer in question, the profession's usefulness to the public (depending on the specific circumstance), and the reputation of the profession as a whole. The four professions express concern about conflict of interest in somewhat different ways and justify their management measures by appealing to different core values. The three most prominent values are loyalty to the client (or the employer), professional judgment, and public service. Beyond the fact that the four professions share these three most prominent values, we can draw at least 13 other conclusions:

1. Each profession has, over time, developed at least one detailed national code of professional ethics. Each of these codes is generally adopted (sometimes with amendments) by state-level professional organizations, licensing boards, or both. All these codes include general principles as well as more specific rules. A substantial part of each of these codes addresses conflicts of interest, describing what the profession understands conflict of interest to mean and how members of the profession should deal with

[67] Publishable engineering research generally goes on in (1) universities, (2) government laboratories, or (3) private laboratories (such as IBM's Watson Research Center). Most of this engineering research is scientific and is therefore subject to federal conflict of interest rules much as most medical research is. Relatively little engineering research is the equivalent of testing by the FDA. Some is, however, for example, the testing done by Underwriters Laboratories. So far, it seems, engineering's strict rules concerning conflict of interest seem to have protected it from the sorts of scandals medical research has suffered.

[68] Nevertheless, some guidance on conflict of interest in scholarship is available from the Association of American Law Schools, which requires that professors disclose any economic interest that they have in the subject matter of their scholarship. Insofar as professors are themselves members of their respective professions, they will be subject to the same conflict of interest rules and codes of conduct as their nonscholarly colleagues.

specific conflicts of interest (usually describing which conflicts will be prohibited, consentable, or allowable even without consent).

2. Compliance with each profession's codes of ethics depends—as the AICPA code of ethics says—"primarily on members' understanding and voluntary actions, secondarily on reinforcement by peers and public opinion, and ultimately on disciplinary proceedings, when necessary, against members who fail to comply with the Rules." In other words, the codes of ethics of all four professions are enforced in much the same way that the AMA enforces its code of ethics. They are not designed for use by state licensing boards.

3. Protecting against conflict of interest occurs not only at the level of the professional society and state licensing board. Some conflicts of interest constitute malpractice or breach of criminal law or civil regulation (e.g., the Sarbanes-Oxley Act and its regulations). Some failures to deal properly with conflicts of interest can have serious consequences for the professionals involved. Statutes and case law, however, generally sets a standard for conduct lower than that set by codes of ethics: law is designed to set minimum standards below which no member of the profession should fall, whereas codes of ethics are designed at least in part to set a higher standard (something closer to the best that can reasonably be expected of members of the profession). For many professions, the minimum standard with respect to conflict of interest has risen substantially over the last four decades. There is no reason to expect that trend to change anytime soon.

4. There is general agreement that professionals will find themselves in some conflict of interest situations even when all reasonable precautions have been taken to avoid them. When avoidance cannot reasonably be expected or has failed, censure attaches not so much to having a conflict of interest (except for prohibited relationships) as to a professional's failure to take proper steps to deal with it.

5. The conflicts of interest discussed in this paper can arise in at least three ways:

- The interests of two or more of a professional's current or former clients (or employers) can conflict and the professional can therefore be in a situation in which serving one client competently (for example, preserving confidential information) would mean not serving another client competently (that is, the professional is not able to use all of the information that he or she knows). This is a major concern for lawyers as well as for engineers.
- The financial, familial, or other interests or relationships of a professional can conflict with the interests of one or more clients (or employers) and thereby compromise judgment (a major concern for all four professions).

- The interests of a client (or employer) can conflict with the public interest and thereby risk compromising the quality of the professional's judgment (a major concern for CPAs, particularly when they conduct audits, but also a concern for architects working as adjudicators or making public statements and for engineers making public statements or working for or with government).

6. Each of the professions, as a general matter, understands that conflicts of interest can be created not only by financial considerations but also by other considerations, such as nonmonetary gifts, friendships, family relationships, and previous employment. The crucial question is always the known or suspected tendency of the fact in question to affect professional judgment adversely.

7. Each profession understands that conflict of interest is in part a threat to the trustworthiness (or reliability) of the profession as well as to judgments in specific cases. This is clear from the way in which the professions, each in a somewhat different way, address appearances. In general, members of these professions are supposed to avoid giving clients, employers, and the public even a plausible reason to suppose that they have an interest, relationship, or the like that might impair their objectivity (the reliability of their judgment).

8. Not all conflicts of interest are treated in the same way. We may distinguish three ways of treating them. The codes of ethics for each of the four professions begin with the instruction to avoid conflicts of interest. This general instruction is then modified or further refined by distinguishing between (1) conflicts of interest that must be avoided regardless of the specific circumstances (i.e., conflict of interest situations that are prohibited), (2) those that are permitted under certain circumstances following disclosure and, generally, that are accompanied by the informed consent of the client or other parties directly affected or some other management strategy, and (3) those conflicts of interest that are permitted because of their relative insignificance. Because clients or employers are often sophisticated individuals or businesses, they are capable of refusing consent or setting conditions for consent (once a conflict is disclosed). Modifiers such as "substantial" or "significant" as well as "direct" (in contrast to "indirect") indicate that not all conflicts of interest are of equal concern. The professions understandably attempt to focus their rules on interests that seem likely to have more than a minor impact on professional judgment or on trust in the profession.

9. Because so many conflicts of interest are either prohibited outright, require disclosure and consent, or are hard to manage, avoidance is, all else being equal, the preferred technique for dealing with conflict of interest. Avoidance is facilitated by certain practices; for example, a lawyer runs a "conflicts check" inside the firm before a new file is accepted. In all four

professions, the avoidance of a conflict of interest sometimes means forgoing personal gain or gain for a client or an employer, a fact that all four professions acknowledge. Avoiding conflict of interest certainly has costs (as well as benefits).

10. When the conflict of interest has not been avoided (for whatever reason and whether intentionally or unintentionally), various options to escape from or manage the conflict exist. Recusal is one option. For example, engineers who are members, advisors, or employees of a governmental department must withdraw from decisions in which they, their employers, or their clients have an interest. The engineer must comply with this ethical rule even if governmental regulation allows for disclosure and consent as an alternative way of managing the conflict. Despite the general requirement to avoid conflicts of interest, professionals can proceed despite a conflict of interest under specified circumstances. Generally, certain precautions must then be taken: (1) disclosure of the interest to the parties concerned (who can include current and former clients, current and former employers, and third parties), (2) the informed consent of these parties (although, occasionally, disclosure alone is sufficient), and (3) the implementation of additional management measures (for instance, the use of screens in law firms). The codes try to make clear when disclosure followed by consent (or disclosure alone) will be considered sufficient to preserve both the fact and the appearance of proper judgment (independence, loyalty to client, reliability, or the like). When proper judgment cannot be ensured, the conflict must be avoided, despite the advantages (to the professional, the professional's employer or client, or any other party) of accepting it.

11. Patterns of difference between (what lawyers call) "consentable" and "nonconsentable" conflicts of interest are sometimes difficult to discern (and, indeed, may be evolving). Overall, it seems that the more dependent that the client, employer, or public is on the professional and the less ability that the client, employer, or public has to manage the conflict, the more likely that consent, even after full disclosure, will not override the general prohibition of conflict of interest. In legal practice, for example, a typical nonconsentable conflict of interest arises if a lawyer undertakes the drafting of a will granting him or her a substantial gift from a client. A typical consentable conflict of interest arises if, for example, a lawyer bought a share in a hotel owned by a client (what lawyers call an "arm's-length" business transaction).

12. Instruction in understanding, identifying, and managing conflicts of interest is included in graduate education, licensing examinations, and (often) in mandated CPE for all of the professions evaluated here.

13. CPE in law, accounting, architecture, and engineering is provided by companies that are authorized by the relevant state-designated licensing boards or a national accreditation body to provide CPE. Individual pro-

fessionals must regularly complete a set amount of CPE, often including training in conflict of interest, to maintain their professional licenses. They or their employers pay the cost of the CPE, although some CPE courses are offered for free by local or national professional organizations.

Table C-1 summarizes the responses of the four professions discussed here to conflicts of interest.

TABLE C-1 Summary of the Responses of Four Professions to Conflicts of Interest

Conflict of Interest	Lawyers	Certified Public Accountants	Architects	Engineers
Gifts or rebates	Lawyers cannot solicit or prepare instruments to receive substantial gifts.	Gifts are prohibited unless the value is "clearly insignificant to the recipient."	Gifts cannot be accepted. Rebates are permitted only with the informed consent of all relevant parties.	Engineers cannot solicit or receive gifts or other valuable consideration.
Public speaking, speaking about professional issues	Not addressed.	Public speaking is not addressed, except to the extent that audits and attestations are public statements (conflict of interest management is very strict in such cases).	Architects must disclose any personal financial interests in public statements.	Engineers are forbidden from making statements on technical matters "that are inspired or paid for by interested parties," unless the engineer prefaces the statement with disclosure of the interest.
Financial or other relationships with client	Some fair financial relationships (business transactions, real estate, etc.) with a client are possible following disclosure and informed consent. Many personal relationships are nonconsentable.	Neither a CPA nor members of a firm can have direct or many indirect financial interests or familial interests in the client being audited. Restrictions on nonaudit services are offered during the time of audit.	Disclosure and consent are required if the client is not aware.	No contingent fee under conditions that could affect professional judgment is allowed. Disclosure and consent are required if the client is not aware.

Financial or other relationships with relevant (opposing) nonclients	No representation of opposing parties in litigation is allowed. Representation following disclosure and consent of both parties at other times is allowed.	Few restrictions.	Disclosure and consent of all interested parties are required.	Such relationships are generally prohibited. Exceptions (such as testifying in court as an expert witness) are allowed with full disclosure and consent.
Sponsorship of CPE	CPE is usually paid for by the lawyer or his or her firm.	CPE is paid for by the accountant or his or her firm. CPE is not approved if it is "devoted to the promotion of particular products or services."	AIA or NCARB provides CPE. CPE is paid for by the architect or the firm when it is not provided for free.	CPE is primarily required for a PE license, generally state certified. Most engineers are not required to take CPE, but whether it is required or not, it is generally paid for by the engineer or the employer.

D

How Psychological Research Can Inform Policies for Dealing with Conflicts of Interest in Medicine

*Jason Dana**

Physicians take an altruistic pledge to consider their patient's interests ahead of their own in clinical practice. Likewise, medical researchers have a professional obligation to conduct their research ethically in their search of truth. A conflict of interest is a set of circumstances that creates a substantial risk that professional judgment or actions regarding a primary interest will be unduly influenced by a secondary interest. Although the information in this report can be applicable to many types of conflict of interest, it focuses on financial conflicts of interest, which can occur when medical professionals interact with the pharmaceutical industry. For example, when physicians accept support for clinical research or continuing education programs, accept consultantships and appointments to industry-sponsored speakers bureaus, or have informal meetings with pharmaceutical sales representatives who buy lunch and bring drug samples, there is concern about the impact of these relationships on prescribing behaviors and professional responsibilities (Marco et al., 2006).

The purpose of this paper is to bring basic psychological research to bear on understanding financial conflicts of interest in medicine and effectively dealing with these conflicts. A particular focus will be research on self-serving biases in judgments of what is fair. This research shows that when individuals stand to gain by reaching a particular conclusion, they tend to unconsciously and unintentionally weigh evidence in a biased fashion that favors that conclusion. Furthermore, the process of weighing

* Jason Dana, Ph.D., is professor of psychology in the Department of Psychology, University of Pennsylvania, Philadelphia.

evidence can happen beneath the individual's level of awareness, such that a biased individual will sincerely claim objectivity. Application of this research to medical conflicts of interest suggests that physicians who strive to maintain objectivity and policy makers who seek to limit the negative effects of physician-industry interaction face a number of challenges. This research explains how even well-intentioned individuals can succumb to conflicts of interest and why the effects of conflicts of interest are so insidious and difficult to combat.

The section Unconscious and Unintentional Bias describes the psychological research on bias in more detail, and its relevance to financial conflicts of interest will be made clearer. The section Parallel Evidence in the Medical Literature then provides a brief review that demonstrates the correspondence between the findings from studies of conflicts of interest in the medical field and the findings from basic studies of bias in the field of psychology. The section Implications for Policies Dealing with Medical Conflict of Interest details for policy makers how approaches including educational initiatives, mandatory disclosure, penalties, and limiting the size or type of gifts can be informed by the psychological bias literature. The Methods and Limitations of the Data briefly addresses the propriety of applying psychological experiments to professionalism in medicine. Finally, a conclusions section summarizes what can be learned from the psychological literature.

UNCONSCIOUS AND UNINTENTIONAL BIAS

One intuitive view of financial conflicts of interest is that the physicians who are swayed by them are corrupt. Physicians have taken an oath to put their professional obligations first, so that if they are indeed influenced by private financial incentives, they have chosen not to uphold that oath. Although there may indeed be a minority of individuals who are fundamentally corrupt, most physicians certainly try to uphold ethical standards. This intuition is implicit in the guidelines set forth by the American Medical Association, the American College of Physicians, and the self-imposed guidelines of the Pharmaceutical Manufacturers Association, all of which stress that gifts accepted by physicians should primarily entail a benefit to patients and should not be of substantial value, suggesting that the temptation to provide or accept large or personal gifts is a concern. This view perhaps suggests that physician relationships with the pharmaceutical industry are problematic and can elicit hostility from some physicians. Understandably, most physicians see themselves as ethical people who would not place their objectivity for sale, and so they believe that they can be trusted to navigate these conflicts when dealing with industry. Compounding matters, many enticements from industry are of relatively small financial value. This prompts responses that physicians are "above sacrificing their self-esteem for penlights" (Hume, 1990) or that if panelists on a scientific committee are influenced by receiving reimbursement for travel and expenses, someone "bought their opinions" and "they obviously come cheap" (Coyne, 2005).

This view is also compatible with an orthodox economic approach, which casts succumbing to conflicts of interest as the rational output of a cost-benefit calculation. In that case, solutions to problems of conflicts of interest would involve better monitoring and punishment, hopefully to the point at which ethical lapses would be too costly to indulge.

Evidence from psychology offers us a different view, one in which our judgments may be distorted or biased in ways of which we are unaware. Some of the most compelling evidence of bias comes in the domain of optimism about the self. There is, for example, much evidence that people engage in self-deception that enhances their views of their own abilities (Gilovich, 1991). One of the most oft cited and humorous examples of self-enhancement is found in a study that reported that 90 percent of people thought they were better drivers than the average driver (Svenson, 1981). Such biases have been dubbed "self-serving" (Miller and Ross, 1975) when they lead one to take credit for good outcomes and blame bad outcomes on external sources. Although an unrealistic optimism about the self is sometimes adaptive and healthy (Taylor and Brown, 1988), these biases can lead to judgments that are unwise or unjust in situations in which we are epistemically responsible for being correct.

Perhaps most relevant to the issue of financial conflicts of interest are well-known self-serving biases in the interpretation of what allocations are fair or just. A classic demonstration of self-serving bias in fairness comes from a study by van Avermaet (reported by Messick, 1985). Subjects were instructed to fill out questionnaires until they were told to stop. When the subjects finished, the experimenter left them with money that they could use to pay themselves and send in an envelope as pay for another subject who had already left. In four different conditions, the subject was told one of the following four different conditions: (1) the other subject had put in half as much time and had completed half as many surveys, (2) the other subject had put in half as much time but had completed twice as many surveys, (3) the other subject had put in twice as much time but had completed half as many surveys, or (4) the other subject had put in twice as much time and had completed twice as many surveys.

It is first interesting to note that almost everyone took the trouble to send the other person a share of the money, even though they were free to keep it all. It was not clear to the author that the rare cases of nonreturn were not due to a mistake or a lost envelope. Clearly, the subjects' sense of ethics served as a powerful constraint on their behavior: keeping all of the money would be unjustifiably selfish and unfair because the other subject at least did similar work, so most subjects shared it. How they shared the money, however, provides an interesting insight into human nature. The subjects who worked twice as long and completed twice as much kept twice as much money, on average, a simple application of a merit principle to pay. The subjects kept more than half of the money, however, both under the condition in which they worked longer and completed less and under the condition in which they completed more work and did not work as long. Again, their behavior was consistent with a merit principle, but the principle chosen, on average, systematically favored the subject making the allocation. Finally, when the subjects completed only half as much work and worked only half as long, they did not, on average, give the other subject twice as much money. Instead, the subjects kept about half of the money, on average, consistent with a rule of equal division rather than merit.

What we can take away from the van Avermaet study is that most people are not unabashedly selfish; they have a sense of what is fair and tend to abide by it. Yet, that does not mean that judgments of fairness are not systematically biased to favor the self. When people are free to choose among competing principles of fair behavior, they tend to gravitate toward those principles that most favor their own interests. Other early experiments have similarly found that interpretations of fair allocations of pay are self-servingly biased (Messick and Sentis, 1979). One potential shortcoming of these experiments, however, is that they used a survey methodology. Thus, the subjects' self-interest was imagined, and they had no motivation to honestly report what they thought was fair. Thus, although it is apparent that the subjects had malleable interpretations of what was fair, it is not always clear whether these interpretations reflected a bias or, for example, a strategic effort on the part of the subjects. In that case, one wonders if the use of sufficient compensation would erase the effect.

A series of experiments by behavioral economists (Loewenstein et al., 1992; Babcock et al., 1995) addresses this problem through the use of real money incentives without deception and establishes that self-serving interpretations can arise as unwitting and unintentional biases. Simulating pretrial bargaining, Loewenstein et al. (1992) conducted bargaining experiments in which subjects were presented with case materials (depositions, police reports, etc.) from an actual law suit. The subjects were randomly assigned to the role of either the plaintiff or the defendant and were asked to negotiate a settlement in the form of a payment from the defendant to the plaintiff. At the outset, the experimenters gave the defendants a monetary endowment to finance the settlement, and the division of the endowment that the subjects agreed upon through bargaining was what they took home as pay. The longer that it took the parties to agree to a settlement, the more that both were penalized by having the endowment of money that they were dividing shrink. If they failed to settle, the defendant's payment to the plaintiff, based on the smaller endowment size, was determined by a neutral judge who had reviewed all of the case materials. Before they negotiated, both the plaintiffs and the defendants were asked to predict how the neutral judge would rule in the case and were also paid for the accuracy of this prediction.

The subjects in this experiment had every incentive to be objective in seeking a settlement; if their demands were unreasonable, the pot of money would only shrink and ultimately the award would be determined by a neutral and informed party. If the subjects' estimates of a fair settlement were biased in a self-serving manner, however, they might be inclined to view the other party's offer as unjust and unacceptable. Indeed, the subjects were often unable to settle, to their own detriment. Direct evidence that the self-serving bias played a role in this failure to settle came in the form of the predictions of the judge's ruling. The plaintiffs' predictions of the judge's award to them were, on average, substantially higher than those of the defendants, even though the estimates were secret and had no bearing on the settlement and both parties were paid to be accurate in their estimates. Furthermore, the larger that the discrepancy between a particular plaintiff's and defendant's estimates was, the lower was their likelihood of settlement, and hence, they both left the experiment worse off in terms of payment. This evidence suggests that self-serving biases are unintentional because people are often unable to avoid being biased, even when it is in their best interest to do so.

In subsequent experiments that used the same paradigm (Babcock et al., 1995), the settlement rates were markedly improved by assigning subjects their roles only after they had read the transcripts. In this way, any motivation to interpret evidence as favorable to one side over another while the subjects were reading and evaluating the materials was removed. Without the subjects having a self-interested conclusion to reach, interpretations of fairness, as measured by predictions of the judge's ruling, looked more like those of a neutral third party than an interested party. In principle, of course, these judgments were exactly like a third party's judgment. The finding is important, however, because these subjects still had the same bargaining task as in the earlier experiments. Thus, one cannot conclude that the majority of failures to settle were due to the subjects being overly competitive or having a poor strategy. Rather, manipulations targeting the objectivity of the fair ruling judgment increased the settlement rates. This finding suggests that self-serving biases work by way of distorting the way that people seek out and weigh information when they perceive that they have a stake in the conclusion.

The motivated reasoning displayed by the subjects in the study of Loewenstein et al. (1992) confirms the general findings from social psychology research. Gilovich (1991) describes the different evidential standards that people typically use to evaluate propositions that they wish to be true versus propositions that they wish to be false. When they evaluate an agreeable proposition, people ask, "Can I believe this?" When they evaluate a disagreeable position, people ask, "Must I believe this?" The former question implies a more permissive evidential standard because it requires the decision maker only to seek out confirmatory evidence, whereas the latter question implies that the proposition must survive a search for disconfirming evidence.

These different evidential standards are exemplified by studies that use a variant of the classic Wason card selection task (Wason, 1966). The Wason task asks subjects to test an abstract logical rule by choosing which pieces of information that they want to be revealed to them. An overwhelming majority of subjects, even those with high levels of formal education, fail to reason through this task properly. The most common mistake that they make is selecting information that could confirm the rule but that is useless for testing it while failing to select information necessary for testing the rule because it could disconfirm it.

Dawson and colleagues (2002) modified the Wason card selection task by having subjects sometimes test hypotheses that they did not want to believe, such as those that implied their own early death. Providing motivation not to believe in this manner improved the subjects' performance over that in situations in which the subjects were testing nonthreatening or agreeable hypotheses. This finding is interesting because it shows not only that people approach the problem differently when the hypothesis is agreeable or disagreeable but also that the proper motivations can lead them to solve problems that they are otherwise incapable of solving. Thus, motivated reasoning appears to operate at a preconscious level.

The "can I?" versus "must I?" distinction in the motivated evaluation of evidence could be applied to thinking in many financial conflict of interest situations. For example, a physician may evaluate evidence that a particular treatment is effective. If that physician stands to make money by prescribing that treatment, the motivation of financial gain may make his or her evaluation of the drug's effectiveness hold to a weaker evidential standard.

In further studies on the self-serving bias, Babcock et al. (1995) attempted to reduce bias by educating subjects, describing to them the behavioral regularities of bias that lead to disagreement, and testing the subjects to make sure that they understood. This intervention, on average, had little success in improving settlement rates. It did help the subjects recognize bias, but mostly in their negotiating opponents rather than in themselves. Moreover, those subjects who did concede that they might be somewhat biased tended to drastically underestimate how strong their bias was. This finding suggests not only that bias is unconscious but also that conscious attention alone cannot be expected to remove bias.

This finding—that teaching people about bias makes them recognize it in others but not themselves—has since been confirmed and extended. Several studies of the "bias blind spot" (Pronin et al., 2002) have found that for any number of cognitive and motivational biases that the researchers can describe, subjects will, on average, see themselves as less subject to the bias than the "average American," classmates in a seminar, and fellow airport travelers. That is, the average subject repeatedly sees himself or herself as less biased than average, a logical impossibility in the aggregate that suggests that self-evaluations of bias are systematically biased. Furthermore, experiments have shown that when people rate themselves as being less biased than they rate the average person, they subsequently tend to insist that their ratings are objective (Pronin et al., 2002; Ehrlinger et al., 2005). Much like in the study of Loewenstein et al. (1992), this insistence persists even after the subjects read a description of how they could have been affected by the relevant bias. Why do people recognize less bias in themselves than in others, and why does education not make this bias go away?

Further studies of the bias blind spot (Ehrlinger et al., 2005; Pronin and Kugler, 2007) have identified a mechanism behind this behavior that they term an "introspective illusion." Being privileged to their own thoughts, people use introspection to assess bias in themselves. Because biases like the self-serving bias operate below the level of conscious awareness, they can "see" that they are not biased; at least, they have no experience of bias and so conclude that they are not biased. When they assess bias in others, however, people do not have the privilege of knowing what a person thought and must rely on inferences based on the situation. If another's behavior is consistent with a bias, people will often conclude that the other is biased. Learning about various cognitive and motivational biases can exacerbate these "I'm better-than-average" effects. People will often still hold that they are not biased because they "know" their own thoughts, but they will now know what to look for in a situation that could bias others. The bias blind spot gives us one way of understanding why such strong disagreements can take place over whether conflicts of interest are problematic.

In summary, psychological research suggests that people are prone to having optimistic biases about themselves. Judgments about what is fair or ethical are often biased in a self-serving fashion, leading even ethical people to behave poorly by objective standards. Self-serving bias is unconscious and unintentional, and people often fall prey to it even when they do not want to do so and they do not know they are doing it. The bias works by influencing the way in which information is sought and evaluated when the decision maker has a stake in the conclusion (financial or otherwise). The bias thus leads to the use of more lax evidentiary standards when the decision maker wants to believe something than when the decision maker does not. Teaching about egocentric biases like the self-serving bias does little to mitigate them because when people examine their own thinking, they do not experience themselves as being biased. People do learn to look for bias in others, however, which can lead them to conclude that others are biased while they themselves are not.

PARALLEL EVIDENCE IN THE MEDICAL LITERATURE

Medical research on conflicts of interest—such as research on attitudes about or the influences of gifts to physicians from industry—has not set out to research whether unintentional bias exists. The findings in the medical literature, however, correspond nicely with the findings from basic psychological studies of bias. This correspondence serves as support for the idea that the model of unconscious and unintentional bias can help us understand conflicts of interest in medicine.

Most prominently, although some physicians may admit to the possibility of being influenced, physicians typically deny that they are influenced by interactions with and gifts from industry, even though research suggests otherwise (Avorn et al., 1982; Lurie et al., 1990; Wateska, 1992; Caudill et al., 1996; Orlowski and Gibbons et al., 1998; Adair and Holmgren, 2005). The question is whether these denials by and large reflect a sincere belief in one's objectivity. Accumulating evidence suggests that physicians believe that other physicians are more likely to be influenced by gifts than they themselves are (McKinney et al., 1990).

A study of medical residents (Steinman et al., 2001) found that 61 percent reported that "promotions don't influence my practice," while only 16 percent believed the same about other physicians. Findings that residents in general believe that others are more likely to be influenced by interactions with industry than they are have been confirmed in a more recent review (Zipkin and Steinman, 2005). Morgan et al. (2006) found that for all of four different gifts, ranging in size from a drug sample to an offer of a well-paid consultancy based only on prescribing volume, physicians rated themselves as less likely, on average, to be influenced by their acceptance of a gift than their colleagues. Even medical students see gifts of equal value as being more problematic for other professions than their own (Palmisano and Edelstein, 1980).

There is even some direct evidence that physicians do not appreciate industry's influence on them. Orlowski and Wateska (1992) tracked the pharmacy inventory usage reports for two drugs after the companies producing the drugs sponsored 20 physicians at their institution to attend continuing medical education seminars. The rates of use of the drugs described at these seminars increased, both in time series analysis of the rate of use of the drugs at the institution and in comparison with the national average rate of use during the same period. However, before they attended the seminars, all but one of the physicians denied that the seminars would influence their behavior. Being asked about bias should make physicians more aware of the potential of bias entering into the seminar, yet this did not prevent the seminar from apparently having an impact on the physicians' decisions.

A retrospective study (Springarn et al., 1996) tracked house staff who attended a grand rounds sponsored by a pharmaceutical company and found that they were more likely to indicate that the company's drug was the treatment of choice than were their colleagues who had not attended the session. Interestingly, these same physicians were often not even able to recall the sponsored grand rounds, so they were not consciously aware that it had any influence on their decisions.

If conflicts of interest in medicine can indeed be understood as unconscious and unintentional, how might that affect how policy makers approach dealing with them?

IMPLICATIONS FOR POLICIES DEALING WITH MEDICAL CONFLICTS OF INTEREST

Short of eliminating conflicts of interest altogether, there are several interventions that universities, professional societies, and other policy makers frequently employ to guard against the inappropriate influence of industry on medical practice and research. These interventions may be implicitly predicated on the view that succumbing to conflicts of interest is a conscious choice, however, and thus they may have limited or surprising effects if physicians are subject to unconscious bias. The psychological research reviewed here suggests that policy makers may wish to be cautious in their expectations of success for these policies, as they are not tailored to deal with unconscious bias. Policy makers may also wish to consider some possible perverse consequences that can result from using these interventions.

Education

Educational initiatives can be thought of as taking two forms: substantive education in ethics and education aimed specifically at describing and explaining institutional policies and enforcement and individual responsibilities.

Perhaps the biggest barrier to the effectiveness of teaching about bias specifically is the bias blind spot. Certainly, some value exists in teaching physicians about potential conflicts of interest when they are dealing with industry. Simply knowing about the potential for bias, however, does not prevent one from being biased. The bias blind spot (Pronin et al., 2002) research described earlier suggests that simply teaching about biases is more likely to help physicians recognize bias in other physicians than in themselves. The blind spot suggests one reason why many physicians deny that they are personally influenced by gifts from industry, despite evidence that gifts and interactions do influence decision making (e.g., Orlowski and Wateska, 1992; Caudill et al., 1996; Wazana, 2000).

Even if people are taught about bias, they are still prone to it. Navigating relationships with industry and accepting gifts while remaining completely objective, then, is not a simple imperative that physicians can be easily trained to follow. Indeed, the research of Loewenstein et al. (1992) suggests that knowing about bias is not sufficient to prevent it even if one is determined to be objective. Thus, recommendations for physicians, such as "If nominal gifts are accepted, make certain that they do not influence your prescribing or ordering of drugs" (Marco et al., 2006), are not practical. Perhaps an effective use of education is to help physicians recognize which relationships lead to bias so that those relationships may be preemptively avoided.

There is, however, some indication that teaching specifically about the unconscious aspect of bias could help in one respect (Pronin and Kugler, 2007). That is, limited evidence suggests that such teaching reduces the gap between perceptions of bias in self and others, and thus, education could reduce the sharpness of disagreement about whether bias exists.

Education aimed at conveying institutional guidelines about the receipt of gifts has produced mixed results. On the one hand (Brett et al., 2003; Agrawal et al., 2004; Schneider et al., 2006), after successfully completing such educational initiatives, residents can identify practices that are appropriate and inappropriate consistent with institutional guidelines. On the other hand, these behaviors, which are mostly of a self-report nature on a survey, do not suggest much about how residents will behave, and several authors have raised questions about how long lasting these effects are (Agrawal et al., 2004; Schneider et al., 2006; Carroll et al., 2007). Furthermore, it seems that there are also some perverse effects from familiarizing students with how to interact with industry. Although theirs was not a study about education as such, Fitz et al. (2007) found that even though clinical and preclinical students had the same knowledge about industry, their attitudes about the appropriateness of gifts could still differ, with clinical students far more likely to believe that accepting gifts is appropriate. Hyman et al. (2007) found that although students generally believed that they were not educated enough to deal with industry, students who reported feeling better educated about the pharmaceutical industry were less skeptical about the industry and were more likely to view interactions with the pharmaceutical industry as appropriate. We cannot tell from this sort of self-reporting what the exact nature of this education was.

When guidelines are voluntary, many physicians interact with industry without familiarizing themselves with the guidelines. Morgan et al. (2006) found that although most physicians had contact with the pharmaceutical industry—as evidenced by the fact that more than 93 percent of them had received drug samples—less than two-thirds were aware of the guidelines for interaction with the industry set forth by the college to which the physician belonged, and only one-third were familiar with the guidelines of the American Medical Association. Therefore, requiring education on the content of the guidelines might be a useful point of intervention if many physicians are unaware of them.

Penalties

Deterring bias through punishment is more likely to be effective if people are knowingly influenced by financial considerations. The psychological research reviewed above, however, suggests that bias due to conflicts of interest can often arise unconsciously and unintentionally, such that people cannot overcome bias even when it is in their best interest to do so. One concern, then, is that aligning self-interest with guidelines through punishment may not be as effective as we would wish.

Perhaps even more difficult, though, is establishing whether a case of bias exists. Research identifies statistical evidence of bias by analyzing aggregated sample information, ideally against some control sample. That is much different from establishing that an individual is biased. Law typically requires that each case be considered individually, but without adequate comparisons, it cannot be established that a physician's beliefs and practices were unduly influenced by nonproscribed relationships with industry, as opposed to being genuine and objective. The prospect of penalties can, of course, help deter cases of blatant corruption and may encourage conformance to policies requiring disclosure of financial interests. The vast majority of industry's influence on physicians, however, is likely of a more nuanced nature, the result of basically ethical individuals being subtly biased. There are thus serious barriers to effective penalties.

Disclosure

One common policy response is to require physicians with potential conflicts of interest to disclose them to those whom they advise. In this way, patients or those hearing a presentation can consider the potential for bias, and the physician may perhaps be mindful of this when he or she enters into relationships with industry. For several reasons, this policy is problematic, and disclosure may be largely ineffective by itself and in some instances could have perverse effects.

As an example, consider a physician who advises a patient to pursue some treatment and discloses a possible financial conflict of interest. How should the patient rationally discount the physician's advice in light of the disclosure? Even if the physician has private incentives, it does not follow that the advice is not genuine. Furthermore, even if the physician is likely to be biased, that does not mean that the advice is incorrect. Often it will be the case that the patient can either take or ignore the physician's advice, and the disclosure does little to alleviate uncertainty. In addition, patients are in often a vulnerable situation with a need to trust their physicians.

Forcing the physician to disclose a possible conflict of interest may also have perverse effects. For example, now that the disclosure has taken place, the physician may expect that the patient will be skeptical and respond by making the message more forceful, a sort of strategic exaggeration (Cain et al., 2005). If patients metaphorically cover their ears, physicians who believe that they must get their message across will yell louder. Although the exaggerated advice may perhaps be discounted, it may still be followed.

Decades of psychological research on anchoring and insufficient adjustment has shown that when judgment begins from even a random anchor that people know is incorrect, judgment will not be adjusted sufficiently far from the anchor. For example, experimenters ostensibly spun a wheel of fortune that actually always landed on 65 or 10 and then asked two questions (Tversky and Kahneman, 1974): "Is the proportion of African nations in the United Nations less than or greater than (10/65)?" and "What is the proportion of African nations in the United Nations?" The median response when the wheel was spun to 10 was much lower (25) than the median response when the wheel was spun to 65 (45). Although the subjects did adjust away from the implausible anchors that they were given, they were still affected by those anchors, even though they knew that the values of the anchors were irrelevant. This effect is one of the strongest in the judgment and decision-making literature. One implication, then, is that even if advisees know that the advice is exaggerated, they will still be influenced by it.

An experimental study of the effects of disclosure has found just that (Cain et al., 2005). Experimental "advisers" were asked to give advice on the worth of a jar of coins that they could get close to and hold. Their advisees earned money by accurately guessing the value in the jar, whereas the advisers earned money by inducing higher guesses from the advisee. Perversely, when advisers had to disclose these incentives, advisees were made significantly worse off. This effect was in part due to the fact that the advisers exaggerated their advice in light of disclosure, whereas the advisees were unable to sufficiently adjust down from the inflated advice.

Limiting Gifts by Size or Use

Policies on gifts often suggest that any gifts accepted by physicians individually should primarily entail a benefit to patients and should not be of substantial value. Certainly, small gifts are preferable to large gifts. Because bias is unintentional and not a matter of corruption, however, small gifts may still produce results and therefore should not be assumed to be benign. Katz and colleagues (2003) reviewed and synthesized a sizeable body of social science literature that suggests that small gifts induce feelings of reciprocity, get a message across by mere exposure (pens, notepads, etc.), and can be effective in changing behavior. Even the sheer ubiquity of trinkets like pens and notepads suggests that this is true. Why else would profit-minded entities who conduct market research on their practices continue to supply them if their efforts did not fetch a return?

The ethical distinction of a gift having versus not having a primary patient benefit, though intuitively appealing, may also be meaningless. The distinction may reveal a lack of appreciation of the fungibility of money, as first pointed out in Thaler's treatise on mental accounting (1980). For example, if a physician receives a $100 anatomical model, then he or she does not have to buy it, and that frees up $100 to buy something else for themselves, such as a golf bag or a nice dinner. This situation is consequentially equivalent to the company giving the physician an inappropriate monetary gift, even though our intuitions may tell us that the latter is much worse because we place it in the "extravagance" account rather than the "patient care" account. The research evidence cannot tell us what is ethical, but the policy maker should keep in mind that any gift is still a gift, because the economic value is exchangeable whether it is received in the "extravagance" account or the "patient care" account.

Even gifts with clear patient benefit—like the ubiquitous drug sample—have been associated with problems. Physicians and their staff frequently end up using the samples that are intended for patients (Westfall et al., 1997), which can also provide a covert means for pharmaceutical representatives to supply physicians with free medications for personal or family use. Furthermore, there is evidence that physicians with access to drug samples will end up prescribing more advertised, expensive drugs in the future (Adair and Holmgren, 2005), so that these gifts can also drive up health care costs.

Limitations on the size and use of gifts may not be a bad policy in terms of limiting corruption, but there may still be influence associated with gifts that are permitted under many current policies.

METHODS AND LIMITATIONS OF THE DATA

A common problem with data from psychology experiments is that they overly rely on college undergraduates as a sample of convenience. This problem is perhaps serious in that it raises questions about the generality of the results. Whereas care should be used in extrapolating the findings of experiments conducted with populations composed entirely of college students, there are reasons to take the findings on unconscious bias seriously. First, the phenomenon in question is less likely to suffer from a lack of generality because it is proposed to be a function of the human brain and is not dependent much on context or experience. Because the brain development of college students has mostly been completed, these findings should hypothetically generalize to older adults. Second, absent a theory of how physicians differ from other college students, there is no reason to suspect that they will not be subject to unconscious bias. As support for this idea, the applicability of the psychological research to other professionals (auditors) was also drawn into question when findings of unconscious bias were suggested as a cause for financial malfeasance. Yet, when a study was done with a sample of actual auditors (Moore et al., 2006), the findings of bias were much as what would be expected in the laboratory with college students.

Perhaps more importantly, the types of decisions and incentives studied in psychological experiments are considerably different in quality from the treatment decisions made by physicians who have relationships with industry. The intention of this paper is not to overstate the similarity between the two. That does not mean, however, that the concept of unconscious bias does not raise valid concerns over how to deal with conflicts of interest. Indeed, the fact that the findings from research on bias in medicine (and other professions) mirror the findings from the psychological research on bias suggests that the concept of unconscious bias is a good tool to be used to obtain an understanding of conflicts of interest in medicine.

CONCLUSIONS

Psychological research tells us that people are prone to having optimistic biases regarding themselves, including judgments about whether their own behavior is objective. A large body of literature has shown that these biases are unconscious and unintentional: people fall prey to them even when they do not want to or think that they do. Although it may seem to be intuitively and easily recognized that people are biased in assessing themselves, the fact that these biases are often unconscious and unintentional is not intuitive and is largely underappreciated. The findings of research on the influence of industry on medical practice corresponds closely to the findings of psychological research, suggesting that we might view the biasing effect of conflicts of interest in medicine to result from an unconscious and unintended bias.

Although this view is kind to physicians, in that it allows the biased individual to be understood as basically being well intended, it is also a cause for concern, in that research suggests that such unconscious biases are quite difficult to combat on the large scale. For example, teaching about egocentric biases does not mitigate them because when we examine ourselves, we do not experience ourselves as being biased. This distinction is not merely an academic argument about human nature; several policies that we expect to combat the effects of conflict of interest may not be effective if unconscious bias is an important factor, and the effects of these policies could even be perversely counterproductive. Policy makers may benefit from recognizing and accommodating a more psychologically nuanced view of conflicts of interest in their interventions.

REFERENCES

Adair, R., Holmgren, L. (2005). Do drug samples influence resident prescribing behavior? A randomized trial. *The American Journal of Medicine*, 118, 881–884.

Agrawal, S., Saluja, I., Kaczorowski, J. (2004). A prospective before-and-after trial of an educational intervention about pharmaceutical marketing. *Academic Medicine*, 79, 1046–1050.

Avorn, J., Chen, M., Hartley, R. (1982). Scientific versus commercial sources of influence on the prescribing behavior of physicians. *American Journal of Medicine*, 73, 4–8.

Babcock, L., Loewenstein, G., Issacharoff, S., Camerer, C. (1995). Biased judgments of fairness in bargaining. *American Economic Review*, 85, 1337–1342.

Brett, A., Burr, W., Moloo, J. (2003). Are gifts from pharmaceutical companies ethically problematic? *Archives of Internal Medicine*, 163, 2213–2218.

Cain, D., Loewenstein, G., Moore, D. (2005). The dirt on coming clean: The perverse effects of disclosing conflicts of interest. *Journal of Legal Studies*, 34, 1–25.

Carroll, A., Vreeman, R., Buddenbaum, J., Inui, T. (2007). To what extent do educational interventions impact medical trainees' attitudes and behaviors regarding industry-trainee and industry-physician relationships? *Pediatrics*, 120, e1528–e1535.

Caudill, T., Johnson, M., Rich, E., McKinney, P. (1996). Physicians, pharmaceutical sales representatives, and the cost of prescribing. *Archives of Family Medicine*, 5, 201–206.

Coyne, J. (2005). Industry funded bioethics articles (letter). *The Lancet*, 366, 1077–1078.

Dana, J., Weber, R., J. X. Kuang. (2007). Exploiting moral wriggle room: Experiments demonstrating an illusory preference for fairness. *Economic Theory*, 33, 67–80.

Dawson, E., Gilovich, T., Regan, D. T. (2002). Motivated reasoning and performance on the Wason selection task. *Personality and Social Psychology Bulletin*, 28, 1379–1387.

Ehrlinger, J., Gilovich, T., Ross, L. (2005). Peering into the bias blindspot: People's assessments of bias in themselves and others. *Personality and Social Psychology Bulletin*, 31, 680–692.

Fitz, M., Homan, D., Reddy, S., Griffith, C., III, Baker, E., Simpson, K. (2007). The hidden curriculum: Medical students' changing opinions toward the pharmaceutical industry. *Academic Medicine*, 82(10 Suppl), S1–S3.

Gibbons, R., Landry, F., Blouch, D., Jones, D., Williams, F., Lucey, C. (1998). A comparison of physicians' and patients' attitudes toward pharmaceutical industry gifts. *Journal of General Internal Medicine*, 13, 151–154.

Gilovich, T. (1991). *How We Know What Isn't So: The Fallibility of Human Reason in Everyday Life*. New York: The Free Press.

Hume, A. (1990). Doctors, drug companies, and gifts. *Journal of the American Medical Association*, 263, 2177–2178.

Hyman, P., Hochman, M., Shaw, J., Steinman, M. (2007). Attitudes of preclinical and clinical medical students toward interactions with the pharmaceutical industry. *Academic Medicine*, 82, 94–99.

Katz, D., Caplan, A. L., Merz, J. F. (2003). All gifts large and small: Toward an understanding of the ethics of pharmaceutical industry gift giving. *The American Journal of Bioethics*, 3, 39–46.

Loewenstein, G., Issacharoff, S., Camerer, C., Babcock, L. (1992). Self-serving assessments of fairness and pretrial bargaining. *Journal of Legal Studies*, 12, 135–159.

Lurie, N., Rich, E., Simpson, D., et al. (1990). Pharmaceutical representatives in academic medical centers: interaction with faculty and housestaff. *Journal of General Internal Medicine*, 5, 240–243.

Marco, C., Moskop, J., Solomon, R., Geiderman, J., Larkin, G. (2006). Gifts to physicians from the pharmaceutical industry: An ethical analysis. *Annals of Emergency Medicine*, 48, 513–521.

McKinney, W., Schiedermayer, D., Lurie, N., Simpson, D., Goodman, J., Rich, E. (1990). Attitudes of internal medicine faculty and residents toward professional interaction with pharmaceutical sales representatives. *Journal of the American Medical Association*, 264, 1693–1697.

Messick, D. (1985). Social interdependence and decisionmaking. In G. Wright (ed.), *Behavioral Decision Making* (pp. 87–109). New York: Plenum.

Messick, D., Sentis, K. (1979). Fairness and preference. *Journal of Experimental Social Psychology*, 15, 418–434.

Miller, D. T., Ross, M. (1975). Self-serving biases in the attribution of causality: Fact or fiction? *Psychological Bulletin*, 82, 213–225.

Moore, D., Tetlock, P., Tanlu, L., Bazerman, M. (2006). Conflicts of interest and the case of auditor independence: Moral seduction and strategic issue cycling. *Academy of Management Review*, 31, 10–29.

Morgan, M. A., Dana, J., Loewenstein, G., Zinberg, S., Schulkin, J. (2006). Physician interactions with the pharmaceutical industry. *Journal of Medical Ethics*, 32, 559–563.

Orlowski, J., Wateska, L. (1992). The effects of pharmaceutical firm enticements on physician prescribing patterns. *Chest*, 102, 270–273.

Palmisano, P., Edelstein, J. (1980). Teaching drug promotion abuses to health profession students. *Journal of Medical Education*, 55, 453–455.

Pronin, E., Kugler, M. B. (2007). Valuing thoughts, ignoring behavior: The introspection illusion as a source of the bias blind spot. *Journal of Experimental Social Psychology*, 43, 565–578.

Pronin, E., Lin, D. Y., Ross, L. (2002). The bias blind spot: Perception of bias in self versus others. *Personality and Social Psychology Bulletin*, 12, 83–87.

Pronin, E., Gilovich, T., Ross, L. (2004). Objectivity in the eye of the beholder: Divergent perceptions of bias in self versus others. *Psychological Review*, 111, 781–799.

Schneider, J., Arora, V., Kasza, K., Van Harrison, R., Humphrey, H. (2006). Residents' perceptions over time of pharmaceutical industry interactions and gifts and the effect of an educational intervention. *Academic Medicine*, 81, 595–602.

Springarn, R., Berlin, J., Strom, B. (1996). When pharmaceutical manufacturers' employees present grand rounds, what do residents remember? *Academic Medicine*, 71, 86–88.

Steinman, M., Shlipak, M., McPhee, S. (2001). Of principles and pens: attitudes of medicine housestaff toward pharmaceutical industry promotions. *American Journal of Medicine*, 110, 551–557.

Svenson, O. (1981). Are we all less risky and more skillful than our fellow drivers? *Acta Psychologica*, 47, 143–148.

Taylor, S., Brown, J. (1988). Illusion and well-being: A social psychological perspective on mental health. *Psychological Bulletin*, 103, 193–210.

Thaler, R. (1980). Towards a positive theory of consumer choice. *Journal of Economic Behavior and Organization*, 1, 39–60.

Tversky, A., Kahneman, D. (1974). Judgment under uncertainty: Heuristics and biases. *Science*, 185, 1124–1131.

Wason, P. (1966). Reasoning. In B. M. Foss (ed.), *New Horizons in Psychology*. Harmondsworth, United Kingdom: Penguin.

Wazana, A. (2000). Physicians and the pharmaceutical industry: Is a gift ever just a gift? *Journal of the American Medical Association*, 283, 373–380.

Westfall, J., McCabe, J., Nicholas, R. (1997). Personal use of drug samples by physicians and office staff. *Journal of the American Medical Association*, 278, 141–143.

Zipkin, D., Steinman, M. (2005). Interactions between pharmaceutical representatives and doctors in training: A thematic review. *Journal of General Internal Medicine*, 20, 777–786.

E

The Pathway from Idea to Regulatory Approval: Examples for Drug Development

*Peter Corr and David Williams**

IN BRIEF: FROM IDEA TO MARKET AND CLINICAL PRACTICE

For small-molecule drugs, the path to a marketed drug involves a long and exhaustive journey through basic research, discovery of the medicine, preclinical development tests, increasingly complicated clinical trials with humans, and regulatory approval by the Food and Drug Administration (FDA). Several years—usually 10 to 15—and hundreds of millions of dollars later, under the best of circumstances, a new drug will be approved for marketing. Because of its complexity, drug discovery and development is widely recognized as one of the most financially risky endeavors in all of science and a major challenge for the biomedical industry. Much of this cost comes from failures, which account for 75 percent of the total research and development costs. Although these failures are disappointing and costly, they still contribute to the body of knowledge on disease processes. Academic health centers and research institutions play major roles in defining the targets applicable for small molecules and carrying out the clinical trials that are needed. The discovery and development process for therapeutic proteins or biologics is similarly long and difficult, and success is far from certain. Biologics are derived from living sources, including humans, other animals, bacteria, and viruses. From these sources come products such as vaccines and monoclonal antibodies, which also are regulated by the FDA. Academic health centers and research institutions have led the development of many biological agents, many of which have been successfully codeveloped with pharmaceutical and biotechnology companies.

---

* Peter B. Corr, Ph.D., and David A. Williams, M.D., are members of the Committee on Conflict of Interest in Medical Research, Education, and Practice.

Medical devices include a range of technologies, from surgical gloves, syringes, and thermometers to sophisticated prosthetics, imaging equipment, artificial heart valves, and electronic neurostimulators. Reflecting this diversity, the path from idea to product development for medical devices can be quite variable and quite different from that for drugs and biologics. The same is true for the extent of collaboration among academic, industry, and government researchers. Before they can market complex devices, device manufacturers must seek either premarket clearance (which is most common and which generally does not require clinical data) or premarket approval (which is required for only a small number of devices—often implanted devices—and which does require clinical data) from the FDA. As is the case for drugs, obtaining premarket approval is a complicated process that can take many years. For complex medical devices, the research team may include physicists, materials scientists, engineers, and mathematicians, as well as biologists and physiologists. Physicians often play a critical role in defining the needs for devices and the initial testing of prototypes in human clinical trials. In some cases, the basic idea for important medical devices can come from individuals who are not involved in basic or clinical research. For example, the idea (and crude first model) for a device to drain the buildup of cerebrospinal fluid in individuals with hydrocephalus came from a self-described mechanic who was the parent of an affected infant (Baru et al., 2001).

The following sections briefly describe the sequence of events for small-molecule drugs from concept to a marketed product. Figure E-1 (developed by the authors) depicts the process in graphic form for each of the following seven sections. (A more thorough review of the research and development process for small molecules, therapeutic proteins, vaccines, medical devices, and diagnostics can be found at www.rdguide.org.)

BASIC RESEARCH: THE IDEA

Long before a new drug can even be imagined, scientists are working to gain a basic understanding of a disease or of specific normal chemical pathways that are subverted in an abnormal cell. This research might be conducted in academic laboratories and research institutes around the world, and some of it is paid for by industry. Industry also plays a large role in the development of novel technologies, such as new approaches to sequencing of the human genome.

Along the road toward developing new medications, researchers have to acquire a basic understanding of bacterial, animal, and human genomes. They study which genes are involved in specific diseases. They also look at how gene products—or proteins—contribute to the derailments in cellular processes that result in the initiation or maintenance of a disease.

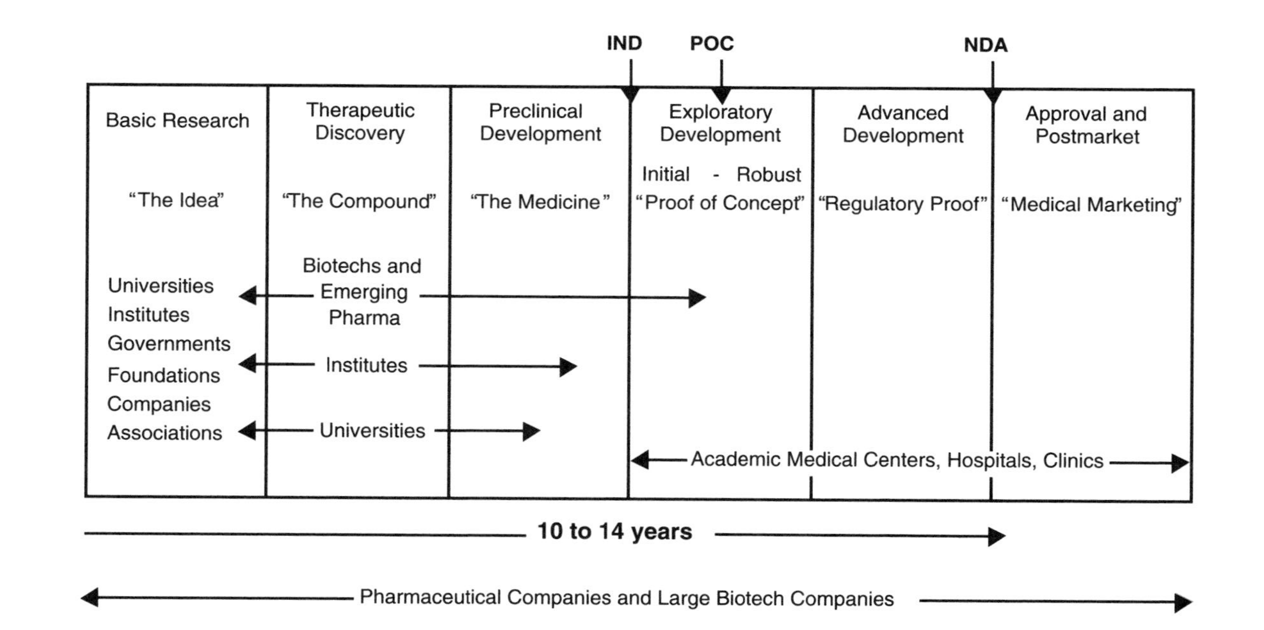

FIGURE E-1 Defining biomedical research from idea to market. IND = Investigational New Drug application; POC = proof of concept; NDA = New Drug Application; Pharma = pharmaceutical companies. SOURCE: Adapted from Corr, 2008.

In a kind of medical reconnaissance mission, biologists seek out and identify targets that might be attacked with a new drug. These targets are proteins, as well as the genes that define how those proteins are structured. Either may play a role in the onset or progression of a particular disease.

Until recently, researchers were limited to studying the biology (the function or the structure of molecules and cells) of only about 500 target proteins or genes. Now, with scientific advances, such as knowledge of the sequence of the human genome, the number of available biological targets has soared. Despite these gains, however, researchers still know very little about the role that many of these new targets play in causing or maintaining diseases.

Once researchers have identified a target, they then validate them by determining whether the target is relevant to the disease that they are studying. They must then determine if a drug could affect the target enough to alter the course of the disease. To do this, they use biochemical, cellular, or animal models to validate the biological mechanism of the target gene or protein.

Box E-1 summarizes an example of successful, extended, and complex collaboration that involved scientists from the National Institutes of Health as well as academic and industry scientists. Chapter 4 of the committee report cites additional examples.

Searching for Compounds

When a potentially relevant target for an identified disease is validated, chemists then mount a massive search for chemicals that might modify the target or targets. They screen vast compound libraries to develop a list of potential chemicals that might some day become a new medicine. This sophisticated process can be divided into three distinct steps: (1) development and maintenance of large compound libraries, (2) specific assay development, and (3) high-throughput screening.

Assays are analyses that quantify the interaction of the biological target and the compound that the researchers are investigating. They also might measure how the presence of the compound changes the way in which the biological target behaves.

The chemical compounds tested in these assays are maintained in large compound libraries, some of which contain more than 5 million chemicals. Products from natural sources like plants, fungi, bacteria, and sea organisms can be integrated within compound libraries. Most compounds, though, are derived through the use of chemical synthesis techniques, in which researchers create chemical compounds by manipulating chemicals. They might also use combinatorial chemistry, in which researchers create

BOX E-1
Case Example of Successful Collaboration in Drug Discovery and Development

In 2002, the biotechnology company Sugen and the Salk Institute published the human kinome, a subset of the human genome (Manning et al., 2002). Kinases regulate proteins and, in turn, have multiple functions in cells in both the normal and the disease states. On the basis of that work, scientists now know that there are 518 kinases in humans. These findings have revolutionized the approach to the inhibition of these kinases by drugs used to treat cancer and other diseases and that are currently on the market.

Elsewhere, researchers knowledgeable about patients with severe combined immunodeficiency disease (popularly referred to as the "bubble boy syndrome") had identified these patients as having mutations within the JAK-3 kinase, which suggested that a possible mechanism for affecting the deficiency of the immune system could be achieved through a JAK-3 inhibitor (Russell et al., 1995). This research was done at the National Institutes of Health.

Industry scientists at Pfizer spent several years discovering a compound that is active against JAK-3. The goal was to find a compound that would not block JAK-1 or JAK-2 kinase but that would be effective as an immunosuppressant by specifically and partially blocking JAK-3 without causing severe side effects.

Pfizer focused first on the drug's role as a potential antirejection drug for patients who have received an organ transplant. It collaborated with the transplant center at Stanford University to conduct studies with primates, with promising results (see, e.g., Borie et al. [2004]). The drug is being tested with human transplant recipients. It is also being investigated as a treatment for rheumatoid arthritis (see, e.g., Changelian et al. [2008] and Stanczyk et al. [2008]).

new chemical compounds in large masses and test them rapidly for desirable properties.

Testing of the expanding number of available biological targets against millions of chemical entities requires some highly sophisticated screening methods. Researchers use robotics, for example, to simultaneously test thousands of distinct chemical compounds in functional and binding assays. Many times, academic researchers with expert knowledge of specific pathways may guide the development of assays in collaboration with industry.

The chemical compounds identified through this kind of screening can provide powerful research tools that help provide a better understanding of biological processes. This, in turn, may lead to new targets for potential drug discoveries.

The purpose of this chemistry stage is to refine the compound. Hundreds and possibly thousands of related compounds may be tested to determine if they have greater effectiveness, less toxicity, or improved pharmacological behavior, such as better absorption after a patient takes the drug orally.

To optimize the molecules being investigated, scientists use computers to model the structure of the lead compounds and how they link to the target protein. This approach to structure-based design is known as in silico modeling (the word "silico" refers to the silicon technology that powers computers). This kind of structural information gives chemists a chance to modify the molecules or compounds selected in a more rational way. Lead optimization produces a drug candidate that has promising biological and chemical properties for the treatment of a disease.

The drug candidate is then tested for its pharmacokinetic behavior in animals, including its gastrointestinal absorption, body distribution, metabolism, and excretion. It is also tested for its pharmacodynamics, which refers to the relative effectiveness of the molecule.

Preclinical Studies: The Medicine

Once a single compound is selected, preclinical studies are performed to evaluate a drug's safety, efficacy, and potential toxicity in animal models. These studies are also designed to prove that a drug is not carcinogenic (i.e., it does not cause cancer when it is used at therapeutic doses, even over long treatment intervals), mutagenic (i.e., it does not cause genetic alterations), or teratogenic (i.e., it does not cause fetal malformations). Because a patient's ability to excrete a drug can be just as important as the patient's ability to absorb the drug, both of these factors are studied in detail at this stage of preclinical development.

Preclinical studies also help researchers design proposed Phase I studies to be conducted with human. For example, preclinical studies with animals help determine the initial dose to be evaluated in the clinical trial and help identify safety evaluation criteria. The latter include factors such as patient signs and symptoms that should be monitored closely during clinical trials.

The result of work at this stage is a pharmacological profile of the drug that will be beneficial long into the drug's future. Researchers can use the profile to develop the initial manufacturing process and pharmaceutical formulation to be used for testing with humans. Industry has particular strengths in these areas, and most development efforts at this stage are based in biotechnology or pharmaceutical companies. They can also use specifications assigned in this stage to evaluate the chemical quality and purity of the drug, its stability, and the reproducibility of the quality and purity during repeat manufacturing procedures. At this stage, and before testing with humans begins, an Investigational New Drug (IND) application is filed with the FDA. If the IND application is approved, then clinical trials can begin.

Phase I Clinical Trials: Safety

Phase I trials are the first time that a drug is tested in humans. These trials may involve small numbers (20 to 100) of healthy volunteers, or they may include patients with specific conditions for which targeted pathways have been identified as potentially relevant to the disease under study. A Phase I study may last for several months. The focus of a Phase I study is the evaluation of a new drug's safety, the determination of a safe dosage range, the identification of side effects, and the detection of early evidence of effectiveness if the drug is studied in patients with disease, for example in patients with cancer. From Phase I clinical trials, researchers gain important information about

- the drug's effect when it is administered with another drug (the effect is often unpredictable and sometimes results in an increase in the action of either substance or creates an entirely new adverse effect not usually associated with either drug when it is used alone);
- the drug's pharmacokinetics (absorption, distribution, metabolism, and excretion) to better understand a drug's actions in the body;
- the acceptability of the drug's balance of potency, pharmacokinetic properties, and toxicity or the ability of the drug to zero in on its target and not another biological process; and
- the tolerated dose range of the drug to minimize its possible side effects.

Phase II Clinical Trials: Proof of Concept

In Phase II clinical trials, the study drug is tested for the first time for its efficacy in patients with the disease or the condition targeted by the medication. These studies may have up to several hundred patients and may last from several months to a few years. They help determine the correct dosage, common short-term side effects and the best regimen to be used in larger clinical trials. This usually begins with Phase IIa clinical trials, in which the goal is to obtain an initial proof of concept (POC). The POC demonstrates that the drug did what it was intended to do, that is, interacted correctly with its molecular target and, in turn, altered the disease. Phases I and IIa are sometimes referred to as "exploratory development." The Phase IIb trials are larger and may use comparator agents and broader dosages to obtain a much more robust POC.

Phase III Clinical Trials: Regulatory Proof

Phase III clinical trials are designed to prove the candidate drug's benefit in a large targeted patient population with the disease. These trials confirm efficacy, monitor side effects, and sometimes compare the drug candidate to commonly used treatments. Researchers also use these clinical trials to collect additional information on the overall risk-benefit relationship of the drug and to provide an adequate basis for labeling after successful approval of the drug.

Phase III studies are conducted with large populations consisting of several hundred to several thousand patients with the disease or the condition of interest. They typically take place over several years and at multiple clinical centers around the world. These studies provide the proof needed to satisfy regulators that the medicine meets the legal requirements needed to be approved for marketing. The study drug may be compared with existing treatments or a placebo. Phase III trials are, ideally, double blinded; that is, neither the patient nor the researcher knows which patients are receiving the drug and which patients are receiving placebos during the course of the trial. Phase III trials are usually required for FDA approval of the drug. If the trials are successful, then a New Drug Application is submitted to the FDA. The process of review usually takes 10 to 12 months and may include an advisory committee review, but such a review is at the discretion of the FDA.

Phase IV Clinical Trials: Marketing and Safety Monitoring

Phase IV trials are studies conducted after a drug receives regulatory approval from the FDA. They may be used primarily for medical marketing. In some cases, the FDA may require or companies may voluntarily undertake postapproval studies to generate additional information about a drug's long-term safety and efficacy, including its risks, benefits, and optimal use. These studies may take a variety of forms, including studies that use data from the administrative databases of health plans as well as observational studies and additional clinical trials.

Postapproval trials may also be designed to test the drug with additional patient populations (e.g., with children), in new delivery modes (e.g., as a timed-release capsule), or for new uses or indications (i.e., for the treatment of a different medical condition). Because these postapproval trials are intended to provide the basis for FDA approval of further uses or delivery modes, they must meet the same standards as the Phase III trials conducted for initial approval.

REFERENCES

Baru, J. S., D. A. Bloom, K. Muraszko, and C. E. Koop. 2001. John Holter's shunt. *Journal of the American College of Surgeons* 192(1):79-85.

Borie, D. C., J. J. O'Shea, and P. S. Changelian. 2004. JAK3 inhibition, a viable new modality of immunosuppression for solid organ transplants. *Trends in Molecular Medicine* 10(11):532-541.

Changelian, P. S., D. Moshinsky, C. F. Kuhn, M. E. Flanagan, M. J. Munchhof, T. M. Harris, J. L. Doty, et al. 2008. The specificity of JAK3 kinase inhibitors. *Blood* 111(4):2155-2157.

IOM (Institute of Medicine). 2009. *Breakthrough Business Models: Drug Development for Rare and Neglected Diseases and Individualized Therapies*. Washington, DC: The National Academies Press.

Manning, G., D. B. Whyte, R. Martinez, T. Hunter, and S. Sudarsanam. 2002. The protein kinase complement of the human genome. *Science* 298(5600):1912-1934.

Russell, S. M., N. Tayebi, H. Nakajima, M. C. Riedy, J. L. Roberts, M. J. Aman, T. S. Migone, et al. 1995. Mutation of Jak3 in a patient with SCID: Essential role of Jak3 in lymphoid development. *Science* 270(5237):797-800.

Stanczyk, J., C. Ospelt, and S. Gay. 2008. Is there a future for small molecule drugs in the treatment of rheumatic diseases? *Current Opinion in Rheumatology* 20(3):257-262.

F

Model for Broader Disclosure

This appendix has two parts. The first is a proposal by three committee members for a model for broader disclosure of financial relationships and conflicts of interest than is presented in the committee report. The second is a response by the other committee members.

I. A PROPOSED MODEL FOR BROADER DISCLOSURE

Lisa A. Bero, Robert M. Krughoff, and George Loewenstein

We believe that the recommendations in Chapter 3 regarding disclosure of financial relationships or conflicts of interest would be greatly improved if they explicitly called for more extensive and standardized public disclosure by researchers, physicians, and senior officials of institutions. We believe that—with the help of interpretation by the press, public-interest groups, researchers, health care consultants, patient representatives, and other information intermediaries—expanded disclosure would provide important information for physicians, patients, researchers, health plans, regulators, policy makers, financial donors, and others who rely on research, practice guidelines, educational programs, and the quality and efficiency of medical care.

We believe that the recommendations should be extended to a "broader-disclosure model" in which

- The consensus-development process described in Recommendation 3.3 would not only set out the standardized content, formats, and procedures for disclosure to institutions but also design a secure national online database system that could be used to report the same information to appropriate institutions and to the public.

- The consensus-development process would set out minimum standards as to the data elements that must be reported by people in specific roles (such as physician researchers and hospital administrators) to their institutions and would allow institutions to have higher standards if they so choose.
- Each institution would require that any information on financial relationships or conflicts of interest that must be reported to it—or at least all information included in the consensus-defined minimum standards—also be made available to the public through the online system.

We envision the broader-disclosure model working as follows:

- The first time that a person was required to report information on financial relationships or conflicts of interest to an institution, he or she would register on the secure national online database system; create a profile with name, location, and other nonconfidential information; select a permanent ID; and get a confidential password. The system would have procedures for verifying the person's identity. The person's profile associated with the ID would be sufficient to identify the person to public users of the database. (In the case of physicians, the profile might include a field for the National Provider Identifier number.)
- The person would enter, in a standardized format dictated by the database system, at least the minimum standard information on all financial relationships or conflicts of interest that he or she was required to report to an institution. Depending on the person's role in each institution with which he or she had a relationship, more or less information might be required.
- When the person instructed the database to make any information available to any institution, the same information would automatically become available to the public. (Provisions might be made to protect some details of intellectual property, for example, of a drug formula until patent registration.)
- The person-reported information in the database designed by the consensus-development process would ideally be linked to industry-reported information called for in Recommendation 3.4. One objective of the consensus-development process would be to make it convenient to find—in one place, in one format, for any person—any information reported by the person (to an institution) or by industry. Each database could be used to check the completeness of reporting in the other.

We stress the following elements of the model:

- The model would require public reporting only by persons already required to report to institutions and would not add any reporting burden—just "one more press of the button." In fact, the model would probably reduce the overall burden on people by eliminating the need to re-enter information for reporting to multiple institutions.
- The model would make it easier to report correctly by providing explicit standards and instructions.
- The vast majority of practicing physicians do not have to report relationships or conflicts to institutions, so they would not be required to report to the public.
- The information that people would have to report would be limited to financial relationships and conflicts of interests related to drug, medical-device, or biotechnology companies, not other financial or personal information.
- The person-reported information available to the public would add to what would be reported by industry according to Recommendation 3.4 in that it would include information on equity ownership in companies and testing facilities, patent rights, and other types of interests (see list in Table 3-3), not just payments from industry.
- The system of person-reported information would allow people to incorporate more explanatory material about payments received (for example, reasons for payments for consulting) than would probably be reported by industry.
- The centralized nature of the system would make it easier to update reporting requirements for everyone involved if future consensus-development processes deemed it important to include different types of information in standard reports.
- The model would allow persons who might rely on information on financial relationships or conflicts of interest to obtain it when they want it—for example, before enrolling in a continuing medical education program or long after participating in one, or when meeting with family and friends before or after meeting with a surgeon rather than in the brief time with the surgeon.

We believe this model would be a strong and flexible tool for managing conflicts of interest. In key areas of health care, including those in the conflict of interest charge as the committee has defined it for purposes of this report, we are troubled by the possible harms that might arise from conflicts between commercial interests and patient and public interests. This is true in research, in education, and in the development of practice guidelines. But we believe that in each of these areas, totally eliminating all conflicts—for instance, removing all industry roles in translational research or barring all educational organizations from having any direct or indirect support from industry (even for research or for an endowed chair)—might involve more change than could be justified in light of how research, education, and medical-care systems have evolved. We conclude that greatly expanded requirements for public disclosure would create incentives and monitoring tools that would reduce the risk posed by some of the conflicts that it might not be practical to eliminate.

As documented throughout this report, there are serious limitations in the accuracy, completeness, comparability, and timeliness of conflict of interest information reported to institutions and to the public—for example, as conflicts are shown in National Guideline Clearinghouse documentation of practice guidelines or as conflicts are reported by speakers in continuing medical education programs. These limitations make it difficult for patients, students, clinicians, and others who might be affected by conflicts to make timely assessments of their presence or severity. These limitations also make it difficult for researchers, the press, policy makers, and others to assess the extent of conflicts and the effectiveness of efforts to manage them. We believe that the broader-disclosure model would help to overcome the limitations of currently available information and that the information made available by the model would encourage and facilitate expanded efforts by researchers, the press, public-interest groups, and other information intermediaries to assess and compare conflict of interest policies and practices of all relevant parties.

Even if information on financial relationships or conflicts of interest were rarely used by patients, physicians, or others to make decisions, the fact of public reporting would probably motivate some researchers, physicians, and senior officials to eliminate unproductive conflicts. The model would also create incentives for people to report to institutions completely and accurately to avoid the risk of being identified as having failed to do so.

We recognize the challenges of reaching broad agreement on standard content, formats, and procedures for reporting in an online system—even if the information would be reported only to institutions and not the public. But we believe, on the basis of academic research and experiences in our own organizations, that the cost of maintaining such a system would be minor. Knowing that the information would be public would encourage organizations to participate in planning and designing the system.

We are aware that proposals for public disclosure often elicit concerns about compromising personal privacy. But most people would not have information on financial relationships or conflicts of interest to report and so would have nothing to report publicly. Most mutual-fund shares, stocks, bonds, bank accounts, salaries from institutions, income from medical practice, and other forms of assets and income would ordinarily not be reported. We assume that even among people who would have relevant financial interests or conflicts of interest to report, the financial interests involved would usually constitute a relatively minor part of their financial affairs and not be a meaningful indicator of individual or family income or wealth; if this assumption is not accurate, public reporting of the information would be all the more important.

There are numerous examples of public reporting of financial information currently in effect that have not been shown to have substantial adverse consequences or to discourage people from participating in the institutions or programs that require reporting—for example, the required public disclosure of salaries of government employees, the public disclosure of individual contributions to political candidates, the public disclosure (on Internal Revenue Service Form 990) of salaries of higher-paid employees of most tax-exempt nonprofit organizations, and, most pertinent, the currently required public accessibility, under state freedom of information laws, of financial relationships or conflicts of interest reported to state universities and health care systems.

We are not persuaded by arguments that the model would create an unfair imbalance in reporting requirements between physicians who work for institutions and physicians who work only in private practice. We note that physicians who have relationships with universities and other institutions already have reporting requirements (to the institutions and subject to public release in the case of public institutions) that other physicians do not have. And we believe that the distinction between institution-affiliated physicians and other physicians is logical: physicians affiliated with institutions are more likely than other physicians to have equity interests, intellectual-property interests, and other interests that may represent conflicts, whereas reporting by every practicing physician would create a large and burdensome system that would not contribute much public information beyond that expected to be included in the industry disclosures under Recommendation 3.4.

We are aware that there might be concerns about misinterpretation of the disclosed information. In a society with freedom of speech and press, any type of information can be misinterpreted or overemphasized. But we believe that the very discipline of free speech, armed with widely available information, would lead generally to better decisions than would result from less complete information.

II. THE RESPONSE OF THE COMMITTEE MAJORITY TO THE PROPOSED MODEL FOR BROADER DISCLOSURE

Wendy Baldwin, Lisa Bellini, Eric G. Campbell, James F. Childress, Peter B. Corr, Todd Dorman, Deborah Grady, Timothy S. Jost, Robert P. Kelch, Bernard Lo, Joel Perlmutter, Neil R. Powe, Dennis F. Thompson, and David A. Williams

As described in Chapter 3 of the report, the full committee supports the development of a public database for company reporting of payments and generally favors making more information on financial relationships and conflicts of interest public. We do not, however, endorse the proposed broader-disclosure model, which calls for institutions that require disclosure from physicians and researchers to require that those individuals also make their disclosures public each time that they report a financial relationship or conflict of interest to those or any other institutions. (That is, the institution would impose the requirement, but the individual would transmit the information.)

We do not endorse the proposed broader-disclosure model for several reasons. First, most members were not convinced of the value that would be added by the suggested expansion of institutional requirements if the other recommendations made in this report were adopted. According to Recommendation 3.4, pharmaceutical, medical-device, and biotechnology companies would be required to report their payments to various individuals and institutions, and that information would be available in a public searchable database. Depending on how many institutions adopted the additional public-disclosure requirements, the proposed expansion might yield some additional information about relationships or interests, such as holdings in publicly traded stock and possibly some expert-witness fees. Such relationships might already be public in specific contexts, for example, in connection with a journal article or educational presentation. In contrast, congressional action on the Medicare Payment Advisory Commission (MedPAC) proposal for the disclosure of physician-ownership interests in health care facilities would provide information about conflicts of interest that are more likely to influence physician decisions about patient care.

A second concern of the committee majority involved intrusions on privacy if physicians and researchers were required to make public the additional information that they disclose to academic medical centers and other institutions. It is likely that many people will not want further exposure to the risks of identify theft, mischaracterization by the mass media, or other kinds of harm, particularly if the database of expanded disclosures is privately managed. The privacy of family members is also at stake because some institutions require the disclosure of the financial relationships of spouses or domestic partners and children for some purposes. Managing a secure and up-to-date website with personal information requires resources and expertise to protect against errors in disclosure, to offer ways to correct errors, and to clarify disclosures with supplementary information. If the information becomes public without such safeguards, there could be allegations of intentional deception when honest mistakes occur or when a person discloses information to other institutions that have different requirements or formats for disclosure. A system would also need to protect against the malicious entry of erroneous information. We believe the committee did not have the expertise to investigate many matters like these.

A third concern was the additional cost of expanded public disclosure. For example, the proposed unified database would require that the additional disclosures be approved for integration into a federally mandated and overseen database of company-reported payments, or, alternatively, some party would have to create and manage an integrated, secure private database. Either would involve additional costs for creating, maintaining, updating, and correcting the integrated database and maintaining security. In an era of increasing cost pressures on medical institutions and governments, the committee is not convinced that spending for additional, marginal public disclosures can be justified over such alternatives as spending for electronic medical records. In addition, in the committee's experience, estimates of costs for information systems, even seemingly straightforward ones, often fall short of actual costs.

Fourth, we were concerned about setting up a disparity, in particular, between university faculty and private practitioners and between medical institutions that require additional disclosure and ones that do not. Although it is not clear how many institutions would choose to require physicians and researchers to make public their disclosures to all institutions, the institutions that did so would place an extra burden on people who, for the most part, are faculty members whose relationships and conflicts of interest are already overseen by their academic institutions. In contrast, many physicians in private practice have no reporting requirements and no oversight. Thus, the expansion of disclosure is not targeted to higher-risk situations. Furthermore, unless the additional public reporting of institutional disclosure was mandated by the U.S. Congress, there could be perverse consequences for academic or other institutions that required people to make public the information that they disclose both to those institutions and to other institutions. Some physicians and researchers might be attracted by such transparency; but we believe that others would prefer to work at institutions that kept their disclosures confidential, except when disclosure is required for specific purposes, such as publication of a journal article or participation in the development of a clinical-practice guideline.

Finally, we are concerned about other risks and unintended adverse consequences of requiring additional public disclosure beyond company-reported payments. For example, the requirement would add to the risk that information from different sources might fail to match exactly because of technical errors or differences in reporting requirements, procedures, or periods.[1] Some might seize on the lack of an exact match as evidence of misbehavior—that is, a deliberately incomplete or inaccurate disclosure—on the part of institutions or individuals, who then might have to respond to public accusations; this would distract from their primary responsibilities for research, education, or clinical care. Misinterpretation already may occur with the reporting of payments by companies to physicians; for example, reporters may treat scientific and promotional consulting as equivalent and deserving of the same criticism.

Overall, the majority of committee members thought that making public the information that physicians and researchers report to institutions was not supported by the principle of proportionality and that responses to conflicts of interest should be based on assessment of their severity. The likely burdens on individuals and institutions of an expanded public-disclosure system beyond that proposed in Recommendation 3.4 or already in place in accordance with other public or private policies are disproportionate to any benefits from the marginal amount of additional information that would be provided.

---

[1]According to Recommendation 3.3, consistency in institutional disclosure requirements and formats would increase and reporting burdens would decrease for people who must make disclosures to multiple institutions.

G

Committee Biographies

Bernard Lo, M.D. (*Chair*) is professor of medicine and director of the Program in Medical Ethics at the University of California, San Francisco (UCSF). At UCSF, he directs the Research Ethics Component of the Clinical and Translational Sciences Institute, which is funded by the National Institutes of Health (NIH), and he codirects the Policy and Ethics Core, Center for AIDS Prevention Studies. He is national program director of the Greenwall Faculty Scholars Program in Bioethics. He is a member of the Institute of Medicine (IOM), serves on the IOM Council, and has served as chair of the Board on Health Sciences Policy and as chair or member of several IOM committees. He cochairs the Scientific and Medical Accountability Standards Working Group of the California Institute for Regenerative Medicine and serves on the Medicare Evidence Development and Coverage Advisory Committee at the Centers for Medicare and Medicaid Services, the Medical Advisory Panel for the Blue Cross Blue Shield Association Technology Evaluation Center, the Ethics Advisory Committee (uncompensated) for Affymetrix (which develops and supplies genetic research products), and two Data and Safety Monitoring Committees at NIH. In the past he served on the National Bioethics Advisory Committee, the Ethics Working Group of the NIH-sponsored HIV Prevention Trials Network, and the Ethics Committee of the American College of Physicians. Dr. Lo is the author of numerous publications, including *Resolving Ethical Dilemmas: A Guide for Clinicians*. He is board certified in internal medicine and currently teaches courses on clinical ethics and the responsible conduct of research.

Wendy Baldwin, Ph.D., is director of the Population Council's Poverty, Gender, and Youth program. Before coming to the council, she served as executive vice president for research (EVPR) at the University of Kentucky,

Lexington. The EVPR is responsible for grant and contract oversight, including technology transfer and evaluation of conflicts of interest. She also spent three decades at the National Institutes of Health (NIH), completing her service as the deputy director for extramural research, a program that represents more than 80 percent of the NIH budget and that applies conflict of interest policies for researchers who receive NIH funds. Dr. Baldwin, who is a social demographer, has served on the National Research Council Committees on Assessing Behavioral and Social Science Research on Aging and Assessing Interactions Among Social, Behavioral, and Genetic Factors in Health.

Lisa Bellini, M.D., is associate dean for graduate medical education and is also vice chair for education in the Department of Medicine, University of Pennsylvania. Her primary responsibilities revolve around directing educational programs for residents and fellows. She is the program director of the Internal Medicine Residency program, which has 150 residents. In her role as vice chair, she is also responsible for overseeing all of the subspecialty fellowship programs. She spends a large portion of her time teaching trainees at all levels. Given the concentration of her teaching experiences on inpatient services, Dr. Bellini is responsible for the organization and maintenance of inpatient medicine services for over 220 beds and 15,000 admissions per year. In 2005, she assumed responsibility for all of the graduate medical education for the health system. As associate dean, she oversees the education and training of over 850 residents across 61 different programs. Her primary research interests involve the design, implementation, and evaluation of new educational initiatives. Current interests involve issues related to quality of life for the house staff, including sleep deprivation, depression, burnout, and empathy. Her clinical interests include general pulmonary medicine, particularly advanced lung disease.

Lisa A. Bero, Ph.D., is a professor in the Department of Clinical Pharmacy, School of Pharmacy and Institute for Health Policy Studies, School of Medicine, University of California, San Francisco (UCSF). She is vice chair in the Department of Clinical Pharmacy and chair of the UCSF Conflict of Interest Committee. She is also a member of the UCSF Academic Senate Vendor Relations Task Force and has served on numerous institutional and international committees related to conflicts of interest. In addition, Dr. Bero is a member of the World Health Organization (WHO) Essential Medicines Committee and has participated in advising on guidelines related to conflict of interest disclosure for the WHO guidelines development process. She is codirector of the San Francisco Branch of the U.S. Cochrane Center; a member of the Steering Group of the Cochrane Collaboration; and editor for the Cochrane Effective Practice and Organization of Care Group, which is conducting a meta-analysis of the literature on interventions that are used to change the behavior of health care professionals. She was involved in drafting and incorporating international commentary on the Cochrane Collaboration's Commercial Sponsorship Policy and is currently the funding arbiter for the Cochrane Collaboration. Dr. Bero is a consultant to the *British Medical Journal*. She is a pharmacologist with primary interests in how clinical and basic sciences are translated into clinical practice and health care policy. Her program of research includes examination of the influences on the design and conduct of clinical research and publication of research findings. She also conducts research on university-industry relationships and university conflict of interest policies.

Eric G. Campbell, Ph.D., is an associate professor at the Institute for Health Policy and the Department of Medicine at Massachusetts General Hospital and Harvard Medical School. His main research interests lie in understanding the effects of academic-industry relationships on the processes and outcomes of biomedical research, investigating the effects of local health care market competition on the activities and attitudes of medical school faculty, and understanding the impact of data sharing and withholding on academic science. In addition, he is researching the role of organizational culture in promoting patient safety, and he is participating in a national evaluation of the use of health information technology for the Office of the National Coordinator of Health Information Technology. Dr. Campbell has published numerous articles in professional journals and has delivered numerous presentations at local, national, and international conferences on health care policy, medical education, and science policy. He served on the Institute of Medicine Committee on Alternative Funding Strategies for the U.S. Department of Defense's Biomedical Research Program.

James F. Childress, Ph.D., is the John Allen Hollingsworth Professor of Ethics at the University of Virginia, where he teaches in the Department of Religious Studies and directs the Institute for Practical Ethics and Public Life. He has served as chair of the University's Department of Religious Studies and as codirector of the Virginia Health Policy Center. He is the coauthor of the widely used and cited textbook *Principles of Biomedical Ethics*. Dr. Childress was vice chair of the national Task Force on Organ Transplantation and was a member of the presidentially appointed National Bioethics Advisory Commission (1996 to 2001). He has also served on the board of directors of the nonprofit United Network for Organ Sharing (UNOS), the UNOS Ethics Committee, the Recombinant DNA Advisory Committee of the National Institutes of Health (NIH), the Human Gene Therapy Subcommittee of that committee, and several Data and Safety Monitoring Boards for NIH clinical trials. He is a member of ethics advisory panels for

Roche (on tissue banking and clinical research) and Johnson & Johnson (on stem cell research). He chaired the Institute of Medicine (IOM) Committee on Increasing Rates of Organ Donation, cochaired the National Research Council Subcommittee on Use of Third Party Toxicity Research with Human Test Subjects, and served as a member of IOM committees on assessing genetic risks and establishing a national cord blood stem cell bank program. Dr. Childress is a member of the IOM.

Peter B. Corr, Ph.D., is founder and general partner of Celtic Therapeutics L.L.L.P., a private equity firm focused on the development of innovative therapeutics, the development of alliances that advance solutions for diseases of the developing world, and global advocacy for biomedical innovation. Dr. Corr retired from Pfizer Inc. at the end of 2006, where he served as senior vice president for science and technology. Before that, he served as executive vice president of Pfizer Global Research and Development and president of Worldwide Development. Before joining Pfizer in 2000, Dr. Corr was president of pharmaceutical research and development at Warner Lambert/Parke Davis (until the merger with Pfizer), and he previously served as senior vice president of discovery research at Monsanto/Searle. Dr. Corr also spent 18 years as a researcher in molecular biology and pharmacology at Washington University in St. Louis, Missouri, where he was a professor of medicine (cardiology) and a professor of pharmacology and molecular biology. Dr. Corr owns stock and retains stock options in Pfizer Inc. from his employment at the company, and he sits on the Boards of Directors of CBio, an Australian biotechnology company, and Cibus, an agricultural biotechnology firm headquartered in San Diego, California. His research has been published in more than 160 scientific manuscripts. Dr. Corr serves on the Board of Governors of the New York Academy of Sciences, the Board of Regents of Georgetown University, and several other nonprofit and for-profit boards. He is also a member of the Institute of Medicine's Forum on Drug Discovery, Development, and Translation.

Todd Dorman, M.D., is associate dean and director of continuing medical education as well as a professor of anesthesiology and critical care medicine at the Johns Hopkins Medical Center (JHMC). Among other posts, he is the vice chair for critical care services. Dr. Dorman's research interests include informatics applications in the intensive care unit (ICU), such as remote monitoring of critically ill patients; leadership strategies in the ICU; the creation of a culture of safety; and the application of pharmacokinetic models to drug administration in critically ill patients. He has participated in the development and application of conflict of interest policies in a number of areas within and outside JHMC, including continuing medical education, medical center relationships with commercial entities, guidelines development, and scientific journal publication. He served as a co-principal investigator on the project on the effectiveness of continuing medical education funded by the Agency for Healthcare Research and Quality. Dr. Dorman is president of the American Society of Anesthesiologists and vice president of the Society for Academic CME.

Deborah Grady, M.D., M.P.H., is a professor of medicine, associate dean for clinical and translational research, and director of the Women's Health Clinical Research Center at the University of California, San Francisco (UCSF). She is a general internist who provides clinical care for adult women and is an expert on the risks and benefits of postmenopausal hormone therapy. Dr. Grady has received funding for independent research from the National Institutes of Health (NIH) and nonprofit and commercial sources and has led several large, long-term clinical studies. In addition to six current NIH-funded activities, she is currently investigator for one study of the treatment for metastatic breast cancer and two studies of treatments for menopause symptoms that are supported by Bionovo through awards to UCSF under university policies that provide for university ownership of the research data, information, and reports resulting from the research and for independence in the publication of research findings. University policies also state that faculty conducting research that is privately sponsored shall not receive honoraria, consulting fees, or other compensation from the sponsor or serve on any board or in other decision-making capacity for the sponsor during the course of the research. She is one of the directors of the UCSF Clinical and Translational Science Institute and coedited *Designing Clinical Research*, a textbook on clinical research methods. Dr. Grady is also a member of the Executive Committee of the San Francisco Coordinating Center, which provides coordination services for multicenter studies in women's health, aging, and related areas. She has participated in the development of practice guidelines and evidence reviews in a number of areas of women's health and served on the Institute of Medicine committee that assessed the need for clinical trials of testosterone replacement therapy.

Timothy S. Jost, J.D., is the Robert L. Willett Family Professor of Law at the Washington and Lee University School of Law. He is a coauthor of the widely used teaching book, *Health Law*, now in its sixth edition, and is the author of *Readings in Comparative Health Law and Bioethics*, *Health Care at Risk: A Critique of the Consumer-Driven Movement, and Disentitlement*, and the editor of *Health Care Coverage Determinations: An International Comparative Study and Regulation of the Healthcare Professions*. He has written numerous articles and book chapters on health care regulation and comparative health law and policy. Professor Jost was a member of the Institute of Medicine (IOM) committee that assessed and recommended improvements in the U.S. system for protecting human research participants and was a scholar in residence at the IOM in 2005.

Robert P. Kelch, M.D., is executive vice president for medical affairs at the University of Michigan, Ann Arbor, and chief executive officer of the University of Michigan Health System. He oversees the University of Michigan Hospitals and Health Centers and the University of Michigan Medical School, including their policies governing conflicts of interest in research, education, patient care, and other areas. Earlier, Dr. Kelch served as vice president of the University of Iowa Health System and was previously chair of the Department of Pediatrics at the University of Michigan and physician-in-chief of C. S. Mott Children's Hospital. He has been president of the Society for Pediatric Research and chairman of the American Board of Pediatrics. Dr. Kelch has also served on the American Association of Medical Colleges task force on conflicts of interest as well as numerous other association committees. He is a member of the U.S. Department of Veterans Affairs National Research Advisory Council. His research has focused on pediatric endocrinology. Dr. Kelch is a member of the Institute of Medicine.

Robert M. Krughoff, J.D., is founder and president of Consumers' CHECKBOOK/Center for the Study of Services, an independent, nonprofit consumer organization founded in 1974. The organization publishes local versions of *Consumers' CHECKBOOK* magazine in seven major metropolitan areas (Boston, Massachusetts; Chicago, Illinois; Minneapolis/St. Paul, Minnesota; Philadelphia, Pennsylvania; San Francisco/Oakland/San Jose, California; Seattle/Tacoma, Washington; and Washington, D.C.). The magazine evaluates local service firms such as hospitals, auto repair shops, and banks. The center also has developed the *Consumers' Guide to Hospitals*, *Guide to Health Plans for Federal Employees*, and other materials and services for consumers. Before founding the Center for the Study of Services, Mr. Krughoff served in the U.S. Department of Health, Education, and Welfare (now the U.S. Department of Health and Human Services) as director of the Office of Research and Evaluation Planning and as special assistant to the Assistant Secretary for Planning and Evaluation. He currently serves on the board of directors of the Consumer Federation of America (1984 to the present) and has served on the board of directors of Consumers Union, publisher of *Consumer Reports* magazine. He chairs the Technology Assessment Advisory Committee for the ECRI Institute. Mr. Krughoff is a member of the New York Bar and District of Columbia Bar.

George Loewenstein, Ph.D., is the Herbert A. Simon Professor of Economics and Psychology in the Department of Social and Decision Sciences at

Carnegie Mellon University. Previously, he was on the faculty of the University of Chicago's Graduate School of Business. His research focuses on behavioral economics and neuroeconomics. He is a fellow of the American Psychological Association and was a member of the National Research Council Committee on a Research Agenda for the Social Psychology of Aging. Dr. Loewenstein is coeditor of *Conflicts of Interest: Challenges and Solutions in Business, Law, Medicine, and Public Policy* as well as the author of numerous articles, book chapters, and other publications on topics in economics, psychology, and public policy.

Joel Perlmutter, M.D., is Elliot Stein Family Professor of Neurology and Professor of Radiology, Physical Therapy and Occupational Therapy at Washington University in St. Louis, Missouri, where he is head of movement disorders. He is director of the American Parkinson Disease Association Advanced Research Center for Parkinson Disease, the Huntington Disease Center of Excellence, and the NeuroClinical Research Unit and the Brain, Behavior, and Performance Unit at Washington University. Dr. Perlmutter is a member of the American Academy of Neurology, the Parkinson's Study Group, the Huntington's Study Group, and the Dystonia Study Group and is a fellow of the American Neurological Association. One of Dr. Perlmutter's main research interests is brain imaging investigation of the pathophysiology of Parkinson's disease and related movement disorders. He has participated in the development of conflict of interest policies for clinical research, patient care, and education.

Neil R. Powe, M.D., M.P.H., M.B.A., is University Distinguished Service Professor of Medicine and Epidemiology at the Johns Hopkins School of Medicine and Bloomberg School of Public Health and director of the Welch Center for Prevention, Epidemiology, and Clinical Research, a multidisciplinary clinical research and training center at Johns Hopkins. Dr. Powe also directs the Clinical Research Scholars Program and the Predoctoral Clinical Research Training Program. He is a member of the Institute of Medicine. He is also a member of the Agency for Healthcare Research and Quality National Advisory Committee, the Board of Trustees of the Foundation for Anaemia Research (an independent medical research charity), and the Secretary's Advisory Committee on Human Research Protections (U.S. Department of Health and Human Services). Dr. Powe's research bridges medicine and public health and includes prevention and screening, clinical epidemiology, patient outcomes research, quality of care, technology assessment, and cost-effectiveness analysis. He has participated in the development of clinical practice guidelines and studied their implementation.

Dennis F. Thompson, Ph.D., is Alfred North Whitehead Professor of Political Philosophy in the Government Department and a professor of public policy at the Kennedy School, Harvard University. He was founding director of the universitywide Edmond J. Safra Foundation Center for Ethics from 1986 to 2007 and served as associate provost and later as the senior adviser to the president of the university until 2004. His books include *Restoring Responsibility: Ethics in Government, Business and Healthcare*; *Political Ethics and Public Office*; and *Ethics in Congress: From Individual to Institutional Corruption*. He is also the author (jointly with Amy Gutmann) of *Why Deliberative Democracy?* and *Democracy & Disagreement*. Dr. Thompson, a political scientist, has served as a consultant to the Joint Ethics Committee of the South African Parliament, the American Medical Association, the U.S. Senate Select Committee on Ethics, the U.S. Office of Personnel Management, and the U.S. Department of Health and Human Services.

David A. Williams, M.D., is chief of hematology/oncology and director of translational research at Children's Hospital Boston. He is also Leland Fikes Professor of Pediatrics, Harvard Medical School. He was previously director of the Division of Experimental Hematology and associate chair for translational research at Cincinnati Children's Hospital Medical Center. He served as the inaugural director of the Herman B. Wells Center for Pediatric Research at the Indiana University School of Medicine and was an investigator of the Howard Hughes Medical Institute for 16 years. Dr. William's research focuses on the study of blood stem cell biology, blood formation, leukemia, and the treatment of genetic blood disorders using gene therapy. He has received several patents, including, among others, three on methods to increase the efficiency of gene transfer for genetic therapies. Dr. Williams is actively involved in gene therapy trials for congenital immunodeficiencies and pediatric cancer. His policy interests include physician-scientist training and the development of more effective approaches to translational research. He is a member of the Institute of Medicine.

Study Staff

Marilyn J. Field, Ph.D., study director, is a senior program officer at the Institute of Medicine (IOM). Her recent projects at the IOM have examined the safety of pediatric medical devices and clinical research involving children. Among earlier projects, she has directed three studies of the development and use of clinical practice guidelines, two studies of palliative and end-of-life care, and congressionally requested studies of employment-based health insurance and Medicare coverage of preventive services. Past positions include associate director of the Physician Payment Review

Commission, executive director for Health Benefits Management at the Blue Cross and Blue Shield Association, and assistant professor of public administration at the Maxwell School of Citizenship and Public Affairs, Syracuse University. Her doctorate in political science is from the University of Michigan, Ann Arbor.

Franklin Branch is a research associate for the Board on Health Sciences Policy. Before joining the Institute of Medicine, he worked for the Adolescent Health Research Group at Johns Hopkins University and at the American Association of People with Disabilities. Mr. Branch graduated with a B.A. in psychology from the University of Michigan, Ann Arbor.

Robin E. Parsell is a senior program assistant for the Board on Health Sciences Policy. Before joining the Institute of Medicine, she gained 3 years of community-based preparatory research experience with special populations at the Johns Hopkins University Center on Aging and Health and other applied research experience at the Pennsylvania State University. Ms. Parsell graduated with a B.S. in biology (focus in molecular genetics and biochemistry) and a Certificate in Gerontology from the University of Alabama at Birmingham.

Index

A

D

E

G

H

I

J

K

L

M

Q

R

S

T

U

W